D0765689

AUTISM IN
ADOLESCENTS
AND ADULTS

CURRENT ISSUES IN AUTISM
Series Editors: Eric Schopler and Gary B. Mesibov

University of North Carolina School of Medicine
Chapel Hill, North Carolina

AUTISM IN ADOLESCENTS AND ADULTS
Edited by Eric Schopler and Gary B. Mesibov

AUTISM IN ADOLESCENTS AND ADULTS

Edited by

Eric Schopler
and
Gary B. Mesibov

University of North Carolina School of Medicine
Chapel Hill, North Carolina

PLENUM PRESS • NEW YORK AND LONDON

Library of Congress Cataloging in Publication Data

Main entry under title:

Autism in adolescents and adults.

  (Current issues in autism)
  Includes bibliographical references and index.
  1. Autism. 2. Adolescent psychopathology. 3. Autism — Patients — United States —
Services for. I. Schopler, Eric. II. Mesibov, Gary B., 1945-   . III. Series. [DNLM: 1.
Autism — In adolescence. 2. Autism — In adulthood. WM 203.5.A9375]
RJ506.A9A9224 1982   616.89′82   82-22314
ISBN 0-306-41057-5

First Printing — February 1983
Second Printing — October 1985

© 1983 Plenum Press, New York
A Division of Plenum Publishing Corporation
233 Spring Street, New York, N.Y. 10013

Printed in the United States of America

Contributors

WAYNE V. ADAMS • Alfred I. duPont Institute, Child Diagnostic and Development Clinic, P.O. Box 269, Wilmington, Delaware 19899

VICTOR L. BALDWIN • Teaching Research Infant and Child Center, Monmouth, Oregon 97361

MARIE M. BRISTOL • Carolina Institute for Research on Early Education of the Handicapped, Frank Porter Graham Child Development Center, University of North Carolina, Chapel Hill, North Carolina 27514

JAY BUCKLEY • Teaching Research Infant and Child Center, Monmouth, Oregon 97361

JOANNA S. DALLDORF • Biological Sciences Research Center, University of North Carolina School of Medicine, Chapel Hill, North Carolina 27514

MARIAN K. DeMYER • Institute of Psychiatric Research, Department of Psychiatry, School of Medicine, Indiana University, Indianapolis, Indiana 46223

MARGARET AVERY DEWEY • 2301 Woodside Road, Ann Arbor, Michigan 48104

JUDITH E. FAVELL • Western Carolina Center, Morganton, North Carolina 28655

H. D. BUD FREDERICKS • Teaching Research Infant and Child Center, Monmouth, Oregon 97361

LAWRENCE A. FROLIK • School of Law, University of Pittsburgh, Pittsburgh, Pennsylvania   15260

PEG GOLDBERG • Institute for Psychiatric Research, Department of Psychiatry, Indiana University School of Medicine, Indianapolis, Indiana   46233

GARY W. LaVIGNA • 1596 E. Cipres Street, Camarillo, California   93010; formerly of Jay Nolan Center, Newhall, California   91321

AMY L. LETTICK • Benhaven, New Haven, Connecticut   06511

SIDNEY M. LEVY • Department of Special Education, George Peabody College, Vanderbilt University, Nashville, Tennessee   37203

CATHERINE LORD • Department of Psychology, Glenrose Hospital, Edmonton, Alberta, Canada   T56 OB7

MARY B. MELONE • Benhaven, New Haven, Connecticut   06511

GARY B. MESIBOV • Division TEACCH, University of North Carolina School of Medicine, Chapel Hill, North Carolina   27514

WILLIAM MOORE • Teaching Research Infant and Child Center, Monmouth, Oregon   97361

PATRICIA J. O'NEILL • St. Paul Program for Autistic Children and Social Development, St. Paul, Minnesota   55119

CLARA CLAIBORNE PARK • 29 Hoxsey Street, Williamstown, Massachusetts   02167

ERIC SCHOPLER • Division TEACCH, Department of Psychiatry, University of North Carolina School of Medicine, Chapel Hill, North Carolina   27514

DAVID V. SHESLOW • Child Diagnostic and Development Clinic, Alfred I. duPont Institute, Wilmington, Delaware   19899

JERRY L. SLOAN • Southeastern TEACCH Center, Wilmington, North Carolina   28401

KATHLEEN STREMEL-CAMPBELL • Teaching Research Infant and Child Center, Monmouth, Oregon   97361

PAUL WEHMAN • Division of Educational Services, Virginia Commonwealth University, Richmond, Virginia   23284

LORNA WING • MRC Social Psychiatry Unit, Institute of Psychiatry, De Crespigny Park, Camberwell, London   SE5 8AF, England

Preface

The state of North Carolina has had a longstanding concern and commitment to the understanding and treatment of autistic, communications-handicapped children and their families. This commitment found expression in the only comprehensive statewide program for families confronted with this disability, Division for the Treatment and Education of Autistic and related Communication handicapped CHildren (Division TEACCH). Our program staff has been privileged to respond to this commitment by developing and providing the needed services, and to engage in research informed by our clinical experience. Although many of the problems concerning these developmentally disabled children remain to be solved, substantial progress has been made during this past decade of collaboration among professionals, parents, and their government representatives.

The TEACCH staff has resolved to mark the effectiveness of this collaboration by holding a series of annual conferences focused on the several major issues confronting these children and their families. The conferences are held in order to bring together the best research knowledge available to us from throughout the country, and to encourage participation by the different professional disciplines and concerned parents. In addition these annual meetings form the basis for a series of books based on the conference theme. These books are, however, not merely the published proceedings of the presented papers: some chapters are expanded from conference presentations and many others were solicited from experts in the related areas of research and their service application. Each volume is intended to provide the most current knowledge and professional practice available.

Our first conference was held in Greensboro, North Carolina, in 1979. Most of the chapters have been prepared since that time. Our theme, "Autism in Adolescents and Adults" is especially timely, as the chronic nature of autism had been either ignored or misunderstood in the past. This volume provides an overview of the historical context of the autistic disorder, a series of chapters on the handicaps and needs presented by the children, their families, and their community programs.

We were fortunate in obtaining contributions from many outstanding experts whose work is generated from different regions and interests. However, they all share what we believe to be valuable information useful to all of us concerned with the emerging adulthood of people with autism.

Most of all, we dedicate this series to the many families and young adults whose heroic struggles have informed our work, and to their representatives in the North Carolina General Assembly and the state agencies who have responded to their needs.

Eric Schopler
Gary B. Mesibov

Acknowledgments

It is our pleasure to acknowledge the many sources of help we have had during various phases of this project. First, our thanks to Peter Coogan, who helped with the arrangements for the conference that was the starting point for this book. We would also like to acknowledge the secretarial and typing assistance from Cindy Fesmire and Raymina Y. Mays. The editorial assistance of Judy Davis has been invaluable in strengthening many of the individual chapters. We would also like to thank our many thoughtful and creative colleagues in the TEACCH program for their stimulating work and thoughts about the older age group.

Finally, and most important, the book would not have materialized without the families of the autistic adolescents and adults in North Carolina. They both sensitized us to the importance of this topic and provided us with many valuable insights.

E.S.
G.B.M.

Contents

Part II: Individual Needs

Chapter 4

LANGUAGE AND COMMUNICATION NEEDS OF
ADOLESCENTS WITH AUTISM   57

Catherine Lord and Patricia J. O'Neill

Chapter 5

THE EDUCATION NEEDS OF THE AUTISTIC ADOLESCENT   79

H. D. Bud Fredericks, Jay Buckley, Victor L. Baldwin,
William Moore, and Kathleen Stremel-Campbell

Chapter 6

RECREATION AND LEISURE NEEDS: A COMMUNITY
INTEGRATION APPROACH   111

Paul Wehman

Chapter 7

SCHOOL DOESN'T LAST FOREVER; THEN WHAT?
SOME VOCATIONAL ALTERNATIVES   133

Sidney M. Levy

Chapter 8

MEDICAL NEEDS OF THE AUTISTIC ADOLESCENT   149

Joanna S. Dalldorf

Chapter 9

SEX EDUCATION AT BENHAVEN   169

Mary B. Melone and Amy L. Lettick

Chapter 10

THE MANAGEMENT OF AGGRESSIVE BEHAVIOR   187

Judith E. Favell

Part III: Family Perspectives

Chapter 11

FAMILY NEEDS OF THE AUTISTIC ADOLESCENT   225

Marian K. DeMyer and Peg Goldberg

Chapter 12

STRESS AND COPING IN FAMILIES OF AUTISTIC ADOLESCENTS   251

Marie M. Bristol and Eric Schopler

Chapter 13

GROWING OUT OF AUTISM   279

Clara Claiborne Park

Chapter 14

PARENTAL PERSPECTIVE OF NEEDS   297

Margaret Avery Dewey

Chapter 15

LEGAL NEEDS   319

Lawrence A. Frolik

Part IV: Social and Community Programs

Chapter 16

SOCIAL AND INTERPERSONAL NEEDS   337

Lorna Wing

Chapter 17

BENHAVEN   355

Amy L. Lettick

Chapter 18

THE JAY NOLAN CENTER: A COMMUNITY-BASED PROGRAM   381

Gary W. LaVigna

Chapter 19

SERVICE DEVELOPMENT FOR ADOLESCENTS AND ADULTS IN
NORTH CAROLINA'S TEACCH PROGRAM   411

Gary B. Mesibov, Eric Schopler, and Jerry L. Sloan

INDEX   433

Overview

Introduction
Can an Adolescent or Adult Have Autism?

ERIC SCHOPLER

When that question was asked one or two decades ago, most people familiar with the term "autism" would have said "Certainly not." They had heard of Leo Kanner's work (Kanner, 1943). He had used the term "infantile autism." It meant a psychiatric disorder of early childhood involving severe disturbances of human relationships, speech, communication, and cognitive functions. It also involved all kinds of behavior problems, including repetitive behaviors and resistance to their change.

According to that definition the only way the diagnosis could be made for an adult was retroactively, from a person's early history. But if you met an adult whose early history you did not know, most people had no idea what characteristics and current behaviors might be expected to make up the diagnosis of autism.

The reason for this state of ignorance is not very mysterious. Kanner's descriptive reports on young children had only been on the books for four decades. Empirical research initiated by behaviorists had only begun in the 1960s, and those of us, including parents, who were concerned with these problems then directed most of our attention to the younger children. Autism was defined by Kanner's criteria. We literally had not met and were not familiar with autistic children who had grown up. We did not know what to expect, what kind of behavior to look for, let alone what needs and what kinds of help they might need, and where to find such adolescents. Would we look in mental institutions or psychiatric wards? In those days autism was considered the earliest form of

ERIC SCHOPLER ● Division TEACCH, School of Medicine, Department of Psychiatry, University of North Carolina Chapel Hill, North Carolina 27514.

childhood schizophrenia. Such children were usually regarded as "untestable" and could easily be mistaken for the mentally retarded. Or should we look in the so-called normal population, since autistic children were often confused with "artistic" children with high intellectual potential? These questions were largely ignored during the 1960s. Clinicians and researchers had their hands full just trying to understand autism in young children, replacing misconceptions with research data and developing appropriate services.

The first group to demand attention for understanding and help for autistic adolescents were their parents. Some of their children were growing up and at adolescence facing a world oblivious to their existence, unfamiliar with their needs. But even the National Society for Autistic Children (NSAC), which had given much clearer direction to professional thinking and social policy for the younger children, was caught up in the attention lag for autistic adolescents. As late as 1977 a motion was introduced to the executive board of NSAC recommending that the name of the organization be changed from National Society for Autistic Children to the National Society for Autistic Citizens—to include adolescents and adults. The motion was defeated at that time. However, the growing interest in adolescents and adults was not.

By publishing this volume we have affirmed our view that autistic adolescents and adults indeed exist. Moreover they have attracted an increasing cadre of talented workers concerned with improving our understanding and treatment of this long-neglected older group. Many of these contributions are represented in the following chapters. Although this is the first book published on autism past adolescence, we disclaim any implication of having discovered the diagnostic group. Instead it is our view that the growing body of empirical research developed during the past 20 years has both classified and broadened the definition of autism. Below is a brief historical review of how this development led to the recognition of these handicapped adults.

Kanner's first description of infantile autism continues to be the milestone contribution among the severe disorders of childhood. The post–World War II period brought with it a proliferation of diagnostic labels referring to severely disturbed children. Laufer and Gair (1969) identified more than 20 such labels, with no substantial agreement among professionals as to how they distinguished different groups of children. The best known of these included symbiotic psychosis, atypical child, borderline psychosis, and childhood schizophrenia. Most of these diagnostic terms have faded into obscurity. Kanner's autism category, however, has withstood the changes in professional interest and increased research information. If anything, the term "autism" will continue to stimulate wider use and research efforts in the future. The primary reason for this some-what unique development in the mental health field is that many of the other psychiatric labels were dependent on theoretical explanations based on psychodynamic concepts, unverified or disproved by empirical data. For example, the infant's experience with sexuality, excessively close mother–infant ties, and other forms of psychodynamic theory were the bases of many labels. On the other hand, Kanner's directly behavioral, clinical observations facilitated the development of empirical research which confirmed, modified, and built on his original formulations in ways not possible for the theory-based diagnostic labels. However, even some of Kanner's early hypotheses and interpretations were modified by sub-sequent research. In several respects this led to a broadening of the autism definition and also to the trend of identifying adolescents and adults with autism. The following five changes will illustrate this trend.

1. *The Social-Withdrawal Hypothesis.* Autism was first regarded as an affective disorder. Although Kanner considered the possibility of con-stitutional origins, his major causal emphasis was on parental personality, specifically that parents were emotionally cold, intellectual, and compul-sive, all personality traits which encouraged their autistic child to with-draw from social contacts with them. A number of subsequent studies summarized by Cantwell, Baker, and Rutter (1978) presented compelling evidence that parents of autistic children were not significantly different from parents of so-called normal children, with the exception that they had perplexingly handicapped children with needs for special under-standing and care. While autism was first thought to be an affective or emotional disorder, it is now widely recognized as a developmental dis-ability (Schopler, Rutter, & Chess, 1979) with a range of handicapping conditions along a continuum of severity (Wing & Gould, 1978).

2. *Parental Social Class Status.* Not only were parental personality characteristics believed to be the primary cause for their child's autistic development, these same characteristics were also thought to be part and parcel of their higher socioeconomic status (SES). However, as larger samples of families with autistic children were studied, it became evident that these parents also came from middle- and lower-class origins (Ritvo, Cantwell, Johnson, Clements, Benbrook, Slagle, Kelley, & Ritz, 1971; Wing, 1980). Moreover, Schopler, Andrews, and Strupp (1979) showed that a number of selection factors were responsible for the predominance of upper SES families reported in many small sample studies. In their large North Carolina study the parental SES measured by the Hollings-head–Redlich Index (Hollingshead & Redlich, 1958) showed a predomi-nance of lower-middle-class families.

3. *The Single-Disease Hypothesis.* Initially Kanner believed that the

autism syndrome indicated a unitary, underlying disease process. This was later widely interpreted to mean that the symptoms were primarily caused by parental pathology. During the last decade research data from diverse sources have shown beyond reasonable doubt that the autistic disorder can be the result of multiple biological causes and nonspecific forms of brain abnormality. For example, Rutter and Lockyer (1967) reported that 18% of their follow-up cases had developed seizures at adolescence, when no hard signs of brain malfunction were identified in neurological examinations during the early years. Genetic factors have been demonstrated in a twin study (Folstein & Rutter, 1977). Chess (1977) has shown the rubella virus associated with autism. Darby (1976) found neuropathology, as in cerebral lipidosis and tuberous sclerosis. In short, increasing evidence shows that a variety of biological factors may produce the syndrome of autism.

4. *Autism and Childhood Schizophrenia.* Initially autism was regarded as the earliest form of childhood schizophrenia. More recent follow-up studies (Rutter & Lockyer, 1967, DeMyer et al., 1973) have shown that most autistic children grow into adulthood without resembling schizophrenia, but more often appearing mentally retarded. Moreover, Kolvin (1971) found a biomodal distribution in his sample, according to age of onset. Most of his autistic subjects had early onset of their disorder before 3 years of age, while the schizophrenic group was found more frequently with onset during late childhood and adolescence. While the distinction between autism and childhood schizophrenia tended to restrict the number of severely disturbed children who would be defined as autistic, the opposite direction occurred regarding autism and mental retardation.

5. *Mental Retardation and Peak Skills.* Kanner had first been impressed by the unusual skills, musical abilities, rote memory feats, and number manipulations skills he observed in autistic children. These unusual peak skills were believed to indicate that autistic children had normal or better intellectual potential. This hypothesis was further supported by reports that autistic children were generally "untestable" on standard psychological tests. Alpern (1967) and Gittelman and Birch (1967) have shown that autistic children are indeed testable when test items to which they do not respond are replaced by lower level, easier items, and when appropriate, non-language-dependent tests are used (Schopler & Reichler, 1971). Since that time most studies with access to larger samples of autistic children have shown that the majority of cases suffer from severe to mild degrees of retardation (DeMyer et al., 1974; Schopler, Andrews, and Strupp, 1979) and that the early-onset autistic group had lower IQs than the late-onset schizophrenic group (Kolvin, 1971). By now it is widely

accepted that autism and mental retardation coexist and are not necessarily different diagnostic categories (Rutter, 1978).

In summary, empirical research illustrated in the five points above,
and stimulated by Kanner's (1943) first series of 11 case studies, has had
the effect of broadening his original definition of autism. Research distin-
guishing autism from childhood schizophrenia by age of onset is an exception to this trend as it provided a basis for separating autism from
schizophrenia. However, the other four points show how the increase of
knowledge broadened the definition of autism and thus contributed to the
recognition of adolescents and adults with autism.

As autism became established as a developmental disability rather
than an emotional disorder resulting from parental psychopathology, parents were less consumed by guilt. Instead of trying to cope on an individual
basis, they formed parent groups who lobbied for services even after their
autistic children grew up. During the early Kanner era only the well-to-
do upper-class parents had the resources for private help. As it became
established that autism was not confined to the upper social classes, a
larger number of families expressed their right to public services. As
services developed and the social stigma against autism was reduced,
increasing numbers of families with grown autistic children expressed
their needs by seeking these public services. In a similar vein, as the
autism syndrome was associated with other developmental handicaps like
tuberous sclerosis, rubella, and genetic factors, families with such medical
histories joined forces with those whose children suffered from the classic
Kanner syndrome. The latter were characterized by peak skills, suggestive
of normal or better intellectual potential. However, in most cases such
peak skills did not result in the realization of the anticipated normal potential, and as they became adults many of these individuals were also
mentally retarded. As the association between mental retardation and
autism was more extensively demonstrated, parents of such adolescents
and adults increasingly sought appropriate diagnosis and treatment. These
trends lead to the work represented in this volume.

This book brings together the experience and studies of contributors
from a variety of sources. Because the recognition of adolescents and
adults with autism is of recent origin, some chapters represent the current
state of knowledge rather than established research. We anticipate that
future research will confirm some of the conclusions and practices presented by our authors, while others will be modified.

The book is organized in four parts, with the first offering an overview
for the scope of the older age group. From their extensive work with
normal adolescents, Adams and Sheslow identify the range of issues and

problems presented by the adolescent transition to adulthood for any child. These are shared by the developmentally handicapped and complicated by their disorders, as elaborated in Mesibov's chapter "Current Perspectives and Issues in Autism and Adolescence," discussing the special issues presented by the autistic handicaps.

The second, and largest, section of the book includes the range of needs to be met if optimum personal adaptation between the growing adults and their environment is to be achieved. Language and communication problems cut across the entire range of autistic clients. Lord and O'Neill review how the relationship between language assessment and intervention leads to improved communication skills. These cut across all other needs, including the special adjustments required in educational activities and curriculum. From their experience, Fredericks and his collaborators link the special needs posed by mental retardation with those of autistic persons in Chapter 5. The frequently ignored relationship between special education and training for use of leisure time in recreation is brought into focus by Wehman in Chapter 6. The special needs presented in these three chapters have immediate bearing on the vocational expectations confronted by the emerging adult. In Chapter 7 Levy discusses vocational needs and placements which can often be realized with the assistance of a vocational advocate.

The combination of adolescence and developmental disability also manifests itself in special medical issues. In Chapter 8 Dalldorf reviews such issues as medical management, special diagnostic procedures, and interventions currently available. The adolescent's emerging sexuality is an ever-present source of concern compounded in perplexity by the autistic syndrome. Melone and Lettick provide forthright and sensible guidelines for sex education from their experience with youngsters at Benhaven. Second only to the cultural preoccupations and worry about the management of sexuality is the concern about the threat of aggression. In Chapter 10 Favell gives a clear account of the humane management of aggression when viewed in the context of behavior theory.

The personal adjustment needs covered in Part II are familiar concerns to families of autistic adolescents. The chapters providing a family perspective are grouped in Part III. How the problems of autistic adolescents influence their families is reported by DeMyer and Goldberg in Chapter 11. Their report is based on questionnaires and interviews of over 40 parents. Bristol and Schopler in Chapter 12 deal with the special stress generated in families of developmentally handicapped children and how it may be mediated by formal and informal support groups. Data are included from a larger family stress research project. The next two chapters were prepared by two parents of autistic adults. These are not presented as formal research, but rather as intensive case studies forged from the crucible of their direct experience with their own children's life span. Chapter 13 is an extension of Park's (1982) influential monograph covering her daughter's childhood years. Dewey, in Chapter 14, on the other hand offers an account of her adult son, a higher level young man with autism, who struggles for independent living. These two chapters present an interesting contrast to the more objective research approaches of DeMyer and Bristol. The parents' accounts are animated by personal resourcefulness motivated by the effort to overcome a family handicap. These important qualities are not readily accessible through research methodology. Increasing recognition of autistic adults brought with it awareness of their legal rights for social services and family needs for estate planning and limited guardianship, issues which Frolik discusses in Chapter 15.

Social needs and community programs are included in Part IV. From her longstanding interest in and studies of childhood autism, Wing presents her well-informed study of social and interpersonal needs in Chapter 16. This is followed by three chapters describing well-established programs for autistic adolescents and adults. Lettick describes the philosophy and program of her residential facility, Benhaven, in Chapter 17. LaVigna covers the Jay Nolan Center in Los Angeles, California, in Chapter 18. Mesibov, Schopler, and Sloan discuss the extension of the North Carolina TEACCH program to services for adolescents and adults.

Although this volume could not include all the productive activity and experience with the older age group, it was our intent to represent the major trends in this area for the 1980s.

REFERENCES

Alpern, G. D. Measurement of "untestable" autistic children. *Journal of Abnormal Psychology,* 1967, *72,* 478–486.

Cantwell, D. P., Baker, L., & Rutter, M. Family Factors. In *Autism: Reappraisal of Concepts and Treatment* (M. Rutter & E. Schopler, eds.), New York: Plenum Press, 1978.

Chess, S. Follow-up report on autism in cogenital rubella. *Journal of Autism and Childhood Schizophrenia,* 1977, *7,* 68–81.

Darby, J. K. Neuropathologic aspects of psychosis in children. *Journal of Autism and Childhood Schizophrenia,* 1976, *6,* 339–352.

DeMyer, M. K., Barton, S., DeMyer, W. E., Norton, J. A., Allen, J., & Steele, R. Prognosis in autism: A follow-up study. *Journal of Autism and Childhood Schizophrenia,* 1973, *3,* 199–246.

DeMyer, M. K., Barton, S., Alpern, G. D., Kimberlin, C., Allen, J., Yang, E., & Steele, R. The measured intelligence of autistic children. *Journal of Autism and Childhood Schizophrenia,* 1974, *4,* 42–60.

Folstein, S., & Rutter, M. Genetic influences and infantile autism. *Nature,* 1977, *265,* 726–728.

Gittelman, M., & Birch, H. G. Childhood schizophrenia: Intellect, neurological status, prenatal risks, prognosis, and family pathology. *Archives of General Psychiatry*, 1967, *17*, 16–25.

Hollingshead, A., & Redlich, F. *Social class and mental illness*. New York: Wiley, 1958.

Kanner, L. Autistic disturbances of affective contact. *Nervous Child*, 1943, *2*, 217–250.

Kolvin, I. Studies in the childhood psychoses: Diagnostic criteria and classification. *British Journal of Psychiatry*, 1971, *118*, 38–384.

Laufer, M. W., & Gair, D. S. Childhood schizophrenia. In *The Schizophrenic Syndrome* (L. Bellak and L. Loeb, eds.) New York: Grune & Stratton, 1969.

Park, C. C. *The Seige*, 2nd ed. Boston: Little, Brown, 1982.

Ritvo, E., Cantwell, D., Johnson, E., Clements, M., Benbrook, F., Slagle, S., Kelley, P., & Ritz, M. Social class factors in autism. *Journal of Autism and Childhood Schizophrenia*, 1971, *1*, 297–310.

Rutter, M. Diagnosis and definition of childhood autism. *Journal of Autism and Childhood Schizophrenia*, 1978, *8*, 139–161.

Rutter, M., & Lockyer, L. A five to fifteen year follow-up study of childhood psychosis. *British Journal of Psychiatry*, 1967, *113*, 1169–1182.

Schopler, E., & Reichler, R. J. Problems in the developmental assessment of psychotic children. *Excerpta Medica International Conference Series*, 1971, *274*, 1307–1311.

Schopler, E., Andrews, C. E., & Strupp, K. Do autistic childrem come from upper middle class parents? *Journal of Autism and Developmental Disorders*, 1979, *9*, 139–159.

Schopler, E., Rutter, M., & Chess, S. Editorial: Change of journal scope and title. *Journal of Autism and Developmental Disorders*, 1979, *9*, 1–10.

Wing, L. Childhood autism and social class: A question of selection? *British Journal of Psychology*, 1980, *137*, 410–417.

Wing, L., & Gould, J. Systematic recording of behaviors and skills of retarded and psychotic children. *Journal of Autism and Childhood Schizophrenia*, 1978, *8*, 79–97.

2

A Developmental Perspective of Adolescence

WAYNE V. ADAMS and DAVID V. SHESLOW

Our understanding of "normal adolescence" is full of unknowns and speculation; the study of the exceptional adolescent is just beginning. It is the aim of this chapter to give an overview of what is known of normal adolescence so we might better understand the issues faced by the autistic teenager and his family in terms of developmental changes and behavioral expectations. After a brief historical perspective we will focus on three major aspects which define adolescence: physical development, cognitive development, and social-emotional development. At the end of each of these sections some comments will be made concerning what is known about the autistic adolescent within each of these three major areas of development. At the end of the chapter additional comments will be made as to the challenge which awaits parents, researchers, and the autistic adolescent himself.

A HISTORICAL GLANCE

The study of adolescence as a formal discipline originated almost 100 years ago with the work of G. Stanley Hall, one of America's early and influential American psychologists. From those early beginnings the field decreased in popularity and has evolved at a much slower rate than other areas of developmental psychology and is often isolated from much of the rest of general psychology. Clinical advances have been even more limited than empirical or theoretical progress.

WAYNE V. ADAMS and DAVID V. SHESLOW ● Child Diagnostic and Development Clinic, Alfred I. duPont Institute, Wilmington, Delaware 19899.

From its early beginnings the field of adolescent study was strongly influenced by the ideas of Darwin and Freud. However, with the emergence of anthropological investigation in the 1920s and 1930s it became apparent that adolescence was not a *necessary* biological or evolutionary stage as inferred from Darwin and Freud. Further, those who felt adolescence *had* to have "storm and stress" associated with it relented when Mead (1928) reported societies in which tranquility was the hallmark of adolescence. Today it is recognized that normal adolescence is a period whose psychological impact is more dependent on cultural than biological influences.

Accordingly, in America today the majority of adolescents do not find this period to be filled with conflict or turmoil (Offer, Marcus, & Offer, 1970). Almost 80% of today's 45 million U.S. adolescents registered general satisfaction with major aspects of their lives (Conger, 1977). Conversely, adolescents who indicate they are having difficulty adjusting during this developmental stage should be given heed and not be ignored.

The study of early infantile autism has a much shorter history, beginning in 1943 with Kanner's "Autistic Disturbances of Affective Contact." Although almost three decades have passed since Dr. Kanner's early observations, the sum of what we know formally about the nature of autism in adolescence is gleaned from subjective reports from parents (Everard, Note 1), detailed case studies (Kanner, Rodriguez, & Ashenden, 1972), and a few well-reported follow-up studies (DeMyer, Barton, DeMyer, Norton, Allen, & Steele, 1973; Lotter, 1974; Rutter, Greenfield, & Lockyer, 1967). As indicated from these outcome studies, the general prognosis associated with early infantile autism is poor. Some 50% fail to develop useful language by adolescence. And 50%–80% are either maintained at home or in long-term residential facilities. A near-normal social life and satisfactory functioning at work *or* school is reported in only 10%–15% of cases. It is typically reported that not more than 5% of autistic adolescents and young adults are gainfully employed. While adolescence may not emerge as a particularly distinct period in the development of the autistic person in terms of radical behavioral changes, there are changes in expectation within both the family and society that may make adolescence a particularly stressful developmental stage.

PHYSICAL ASPECTS OF ADOLESCENCE

For many, adolescence is defined by the various physical changes associated with this developmental stage. The physiological changes occurring are largely attributable to a complex hormonal interaction system involving areas of the brain and various glands. We are yet unsure as to what triggers the onset of these physical changes and what brings this biologically unique period to an end. Chapter 8 in this book nicely describes in detail the biological aspects associated with adolescence. However, let us here mention key aspects.

Body Changes

Marked height and weight increases are among the most dramatic physical changes apparent during adolescence, and begin around 12 years of age for females and about 2 years later for males. Other changes occurring during early adolescence include marked increases in bone width and length, and for males, increases in muscle strength, number of red blood cells, and heart size (Tanner, 1978). The skin becomes coarser and the sebaceous glands with their increased production fill the enlarged pores, which may lead to complexion problems.

Changes in the Reproduction System

The word "puberty" (literally translated, "age of manhood") usually connotes reproductive capacity. The onset of puberty is experienced earlier by today's adolescents than it was by those of earlier times. It seems likely that improved nutrition and eradication of many childhood diseases are mainly responsible (Tanner, 1978).

The answer to the question "When does puberty begin?" is somewhat dependent on the criterion of puberty selected. For example, in girls the onset of breast development often occurs before pubic hair growth, which itself preceeds the menarche (the first menstruation). Therefore the age at which puberty begins for girls could range between 10 and 13, depending on the measure selected. Puberty for boys is 1½–2 years later. Wide variation exists between onset and sequence of physical changes within normal adolescence for both sexes. In Figures 1 and 2 the normal range of ages for various physical events is given by the figures placed directly at the start and finish of each event. Note that considerable variability exists, and "normal" adolescents of the same age can manifest very different degrees of physical development.

Cortical Changes

While these more obvious external physical changes are occurring, more subtle internal changes are also being influenced by the biochemical

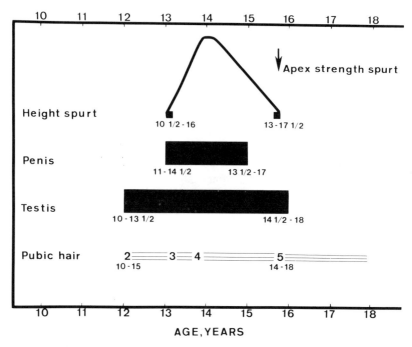

Figure 1. Sequence of events at adolescence in boys. An average boy is represented; the range of ages within which each event may normally occur is given by the figures placed directly below the event. (Reprinted with permission from J. M. Tanner, *Growth at Adolescence* [2nd ed.]. London: Blackwell, 1962, p. 30.)

alterations as puberty. It is commonly accepted that those experiencing head injuries prior to puberty have a much better prognosis for recovery than those injured thereafter (Reitan, 1972). It also appears that the qualitative complexity of our thinking continues to develop until about puberty, after which point we seem to plateau (Piaget, 1966). Although we continue to acquire new information and capitalize upon our experience, the basic "programming plan" we use to solve problems and interpret the world around us becomes fixed. Consequently a retarded or normal child continues to develop cognitively until about puberty, but at this age the rate of intellectual development levels off (Inhelder, 1968).

At early adolescence there is an increased probability that a seizure disorder will occur, reversing the trend of a gradually decreasing incidence from infancy (Livingston, 1972). Other support that central nervous system changes are occurring around puberty comes from Salamy (1978), who reported that neurotransmission time between cerebral hemispheres peaks at adolescence and remains relatively constant into adulthood.

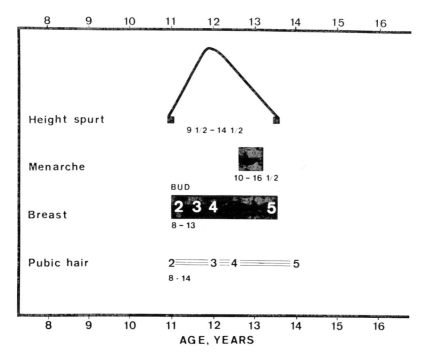

Figure 2. Sequence of events at adolescence in girls. An average girl is represented; the range of ages within which each event may normally occur is given by the figures placed directly below the event. (Reprinted with permission from J. M. Tanner, *Growth at Adolescence* [2nd ed.]. London: Blackwell, 1962, p. 36.)

Psychological Effects of Physiological Change

The physical changes which characterize puberty are universal and yet they evoke considerable psychological meaning for both the adolescent and those around him. As a child begins to look more and more like an adult his culture begins to give him more responsibility and to have higher expectations from him—all without formal announcement. The adolescent finds himself with a modified or inconsistent set of rules for interacting, and his attitudes toward himself and others often need adjustment to fit these new expectations.

Certain physical changes frequently seem to dominate this psychological reevaluation. Breast development may play a large part in a girl's perception of her own femininity, sometimes feeling troubled because of "less than adequate" development after a year of breast enlargement, not knowing that breast development often takes 3 years (Reynolds &

Wines, 1951). Boys too develop anxiety over physical characteristics such as some degree of breast development (which is common temporarily in males too) or delay in penis growth. If an adolescent has a small penis he may begin to question his manliness and ability to give sexual satisfaction to a future mate, although research has shown no relationship either between overall male stature and penis size or between penis size and the ability to give sexual satisfaction (Masters & Johnson, 1966). Obesity, voice changes, hair growth or lack of it, and acne are other common characteristics which cause major adolescent worries.

It seems likely that physical attributes do contribute to the development of a person's social and emotional makeup. Children rated as physically handsome or pretty are more popular among their peers (Cavior & Dokecki, 1973). The major determinant of how much a person is liked on a first date is how attractive he or she is; no relationship was found for such things as overall personality ratings, intelligence, or academic achievement (Walster, Aronson, Abrahams, & Rottman, 1966).

Research on the effect of maturing earlier as opposed to later than one's peers suggests that earlier maturation is perceived as a disadvantage by females whereas for males it is perceived as an advantage. Accordingly, later maturing males perceive themselves more negatively than their earlier maturing counterparts. Later maturing females perceive themselves in a manner similar to the so-called normal maturing female (Weatherley, 1964).

The sex difference found with regard to early and later maturers' self-perceptions may exist because for the early-maturing girl few of the boys and a small number of female peers are experiencing puberty. The female's physical changes are conspicuous and probably produce some anxiety and embarrassment. The early-maturing girl is interested in boys but only older boys are receptive, and older, more emotionally mature girls offer difficult competition. The later maturing boy is not as likely to be as strong or as fast as the early-maturing boy at a time when physical feats (as in athletic competitions) take on particular importance for the developing self-concept.

For girls there does not seem to be any long-term consequence to perceptions of early or late maturing. However, Ames (1957) found that the negative self-perceptions of the later maturing male may result in lower occupational levels and less formal as well as informal social participation during young adulthood.

Adolescent Sexuality

With the onset of puberty a number of sexual impulses are felt with greater intensity. How adolescents deal with these is for the most part a learned phenomenon although the learning tends to be relatively informal and inconsistent. Research in sexual practices among U.S. adolescents has been gathered over the past few decades. The following generalizations seem justified. While still the most common sexual outlet, the incidence of masturbation among male adolescents has decreased somewhat while a slight increase by younger females has also occurred. By the end of adolescence a substantial majority of males and about half of females have masturbated (Sorensen, 1972). Almost half of all adolescents report some feelings of anxiety or guilt because they feared masturbation might have undesirable consequences (Shipman, 1968). Most males have not been given information by their parents concerning ejaculation prior to its first occurrence, which is usually either during masturbation or during sleep (a nocturnal emission).

Despite what appeared to be a more relaxed attitude concerning homosexuality, the incidence of homosexual behaviors among older adolescents seems to be less now than during the 1940s for both sexes. It is commonly held (although the generalization does not seem to be well grounded in empirical support) that homosexual behavior peaks during adolescence. To date there is no agreed-upon cause for homosexuality, although parenting as well as biological explanations have been advanced. More than 80% of all males and over 90% of females report having had no homosexual experiences by the end of adolescence (Sorensen, 1972); figures which correspond closely to these were reported by Kinsey and his colleagues (Kinsey, Pomeroy, & Martin, 1948; Kinsey, Pomeroy, Martin, & Gebhardt, 1953) 20 years earlier.

Petting now occurs earlier, with greater frequency, and tends to be associated with greater expressions of intimacy. By age 19 some form of petting is nearly a universal experience for both sexes.

With respect to premarital sexual behavior, teenage males appear to engage in greater frequency of intercourse (and all other forms of sexual behavior) than females. By 15 years of age almost half the males and almost a third of the females have experienced intercourse. This is an almost tenfold increase for females when comparing the more current findings (Sorensen, 1972) with those obtained in the Kinsey studies during the 1940s. Comparing the older findings with those more recently obtained, little difference appears in the percent of males having engaged in intercourse by age 19 (72%), although again among females the incidence has almost tripled (57%). Therefore the so-called sexual revolution seems to be more a phenomenon among female teens and younger adolescents of both sexes. Among the U.S. college population forms of physical intimacy including intercourse seem to be reserved for a relatively small number of partners and at frequencies much lower than foreign college student counterparts (Luckey & Nass, 1969).

Despite considerable efforts by public schools to include sex education courses in their curriculum, there is a disturbing ignorance or carelessness about contraceptive use and knowledge of veneral disease. For example, when asked whether any birth control method was utilized during their first sexual encounter over two-thirds of the teenagers said "no" or "do not know." As disturbing are the 13- to 15-year-old subjects' responses to the truthfulness of the statement "if the girl does not want to have a baby she won't get pregnant even though she may have sex without taking any birth control method"; over one-third of the adolescents in this age group indicated that they agreed with the statement's accuracy (Sorensen, 1972).

There has been and continues to be an increase in reported cases of syphilis, gonorrhea, and other types of venereal disease among teens. Gordon (1973) estimates that there are at least a half-million people in the U.S. with undetected and therefore untreated syphilis. Adolescents tend to have less information about VD than about other areas of sexuality.

As Zelnik and Kantner (1974) have said, "to marry and then to conceive is the exception among teenagers." Three out of four live births among adolescents were conceived prior to marriage. Most teenage mothers do not choose to abort their children or surrender the child for adoption. Consequently almost a million teenage girls become mothers each year, with two-thirds of these pregnancies unintentional.

Among the million or so teenagers who do marry in the U.S. there is a 2–4 times greater chance that the relationship will end in divorce compared to those who wait until their early 20s (Lowrie, 1965). When asked about the wisdom of their early marriages, most teenagers indicate that if they had to do it over again they would wait longer. Some of the difficulties during early marriage include lack of true financial independence (and therefore forced dependency on parents), relatively insufficient education for job aspirations, unrealistic ideas of what marriage would be like, and general emotional immaturity which makes the great demands of the new role as parent and spouse particularly difficult.

Autism and Puberty

There is little information available which would suggest that the manifestation of physical changes in autistic adolescents differs from that typically found. A few studies examining physical growth of autistic children have suggested delays in height and skeletal maturation (Campbell, Petti, Greene, Cohen, Genieser, & David, 1980; Simon & Gillies, 1976), which may lead to the expectation that the onset of puberty may be slightly delayed for some autistic persons. This, however, remains to be documented more precisely.

With the onset of the physical changes associated with puberty the moderately impaired autistic adolescent is often in need of more formal training to ensure a developmentally appropriate understanding of these changes, to develop those new behaviors to ensure appropriate personal hygiene, and to provide social skills training to promote greater social awareness of the expectations that others hold for the physically mature (Liberman & Malone, 1979). DeMyer (1979) notes that most of the parents of autistic persons interviewed reported that, for males, there is little drive toward sexual intercourse. Concern, however, is present for the autistic female who may "passively" accept a convincing invitation as a result of inadequate judgment. While parents of the normal adolescent naturally have concerns about extramarital pregnancy, the concerns of parents of autistic adolescents are further heightened by their awareness of the youngsters' social immaturity and poverty of adaptational skills. Overall, few overt sexual problems are reported for the autistic teenager (Dewey & Everard, 1974), although DeMyer (1979) found that parents report that more autistic youngsters masturbated (63%) than normal controls (45%), and in contrast to the normal children a small minority of autistic children (6%) were reported to masturbate "very frequently" or "most of the time." For some mildly autistic teenagers there may be interest in heterosexual contact. Approaches, though, may be rebuffed as a result of the poor social and verbal skills of the autistic youth. The scant literature on autistic adolescent development is notable for the lack of reference to autistic heterosexual or homosexual relationships with normal or other autistic youth.

Along with the external bodily changes that mark adolescence may be changes within the central nervous system of the autistic adolescent. In the Maudsley Hospital series 28% of youngsters who were seizure free during childhood developed epilepsy in adolescence (Rutter, 1970). Deykin and MacMahon (1980) found the highest risk of developing seizures occurred at the time of puberty (11–14 years) for their autistic group. The rate of seizuring among autistic adolescents appears to be many times greater than for normal adolescents (Deykin & MacMahon, 1980). The hyperactivity common to the autistic child was in some replaced by "inert underactivity" so that the lack of drive became a problem. Further, approximately 10% of the youngsters followed by Rutter (1970) demonstrated progressive mental deterioration in adolescence.

COGNITIVE ASPECTS OF ADOLESCENCE

"Cognition" is a term which refers to those mental processes used to perceive, organize, remember, and otherwise "think" about the world outside and within us. The term "intelligence" is closely related to cognition, and in the U.S. was originally defined in terms of what intelligence tests measured. The most common and reputable intelligence tests used with adolescents include the Wechsler Intelligence Scale for Children—Revised (for youngsters up through 16 years of age) (Wechsler, 1974) and the Wechsler Adult Intelligence Scale (for those 16 years of age and older). Each of these tests samples a broad range of behavior and has a similar format with assessments of verbal forms of intelligence (common sense and abstract verbal reasoning, memory for facts, numerical reasoning) and nonverbal forms (such as those skills necessary to construct puzzles, logically arrange in sequence pictures of stories, and extract essential visual relationships in abstract designs). The Wechsler tests yield a Verbal Scale IQ score, a Performance Scale IQ score and a Full Scale IQ score. Each scale IQ score may be thought of as a summary of a person's problem-solving abilities averaged over the samples of behaviors examined. The Full Scale scores may be thought of as the average of verbal and nonverbal problem-solving skills. Each scale score and the Full Scale score compares the adolescent's performance with that obtained by age peers. The IQ score per se is used for comparisons across ages. Therefore an IQ score can be achieved by a number of "routes." For example, good verbal skills and low nonverbal skills could result in an IQ numerically equivalent to that of another individual whose strengths are in nonverbal areas but having verbal deficits. Obviously, then, the rate of development in one intellectual skill can be faster than for another, despite what might be suggested in a single summary score like an IQ.

IQ scores obtained in middle to late childhood are quite predictive of scores obtained in adolescence and young adulthood (Bayley, 1970). IQ scores are affected by a number of environmental factors such as socioeconomic class and emotional well-being, as well as biological characteristics making up the central nervous system (Bayley, 1970). While IQs are relatively stable through adolescence, variations of up to 15 points between testings are common. Currently it seems that intelligence, while a more global trait during infancy and childhood, becomes increasingly more specific to the subskills necessary to perform a variety of tasks in the adult world (Bayley, 1970). While IQ and high school academic achievement are predictors of each other and related to the level of job attainment, intelligence test performance is not a good predictor of job success (McClelland, 1973).

Ever since the early 1920s, when intelligence testing was becoming a major area of investigation, it was observed that the older the child or adolescent became, the more efficiently would information be stored, the faster would problems be solved, and the more complex could the problems be that allowed solution (Cole & Hall, 1970). Most American researchers interpreted this as indicating that older children and adolescents simply had more of the basic "stuff" of intelligence than did younger children.

A very different view was emerging in Europe, and one of its principal proponents was Jean Piaget. While Piaget recognized that adolescents knew more and thought in more complex ways than did younger children, he did not feel it was justified to conclude that this was because they simply had more of the same kind of "intelligence" that an infant or young child had. Rather, Piaget (1966) postulated, and through a series of very clever observations demonstrated, that there are four relatively discrete qualitative stages through which a child's logical thinking progresses. For most children these sequential stages have approximate transition times of 2 years, 6 years, and 12 years of age. At each of these points a new level of *logical operations* would emerge, incorporating all the previous ones, and by adding additional logical operations result in a reasoning ability which was more than the sum of the previous stages. That is, Piaget argued that the adolescent was capable of thinking at levels beyond his 9- or 10-year-old counterpart not because of more experience but because of the qualitatively different ways which could be used to interpret the same information. Piaget felt that the adolescent during the cognitive stage called *formal operations* was, for the first time in his life, capable of thinking about conditions he had not experienced or even conditions contrary to fact. For example, he could generate and analyze possible solutions to the question "What would happen if people never died?" Moreover the adolescent now was capable of the systematic and logical thinking known as scientific inquiry.

This degree of cognitive complexity frees the adolescent thinker from having to use concrete events to solve problems, a characteristic of the preadolescent, and allows him or her to consider the hypothetical. Now the adolescent is capable of examining himself, his parents, his moral training, and the political system under which he lives. The preadolsecent shows little interest in these abstract entities, Piaget says, because he is incapable of processing at this degree of complexity since he lacks the necessary logical operations to do so.

Therefore a Piagetian views adolescence as a time when a revolution in conceptualization occurs. Using this conceptual position one could understand why adolescence is a time of questioning and idealism, a time when the adolescent is curious and experiments with a number of new ideas. Because of the emergence of these hypothetical thinking abilities, the adolescent can envision the world as it could be and can imagine the so-called ideal self and compare his real self to it, resulting in increased self-awareness and sensitivity. He can perceive how others may perceive him, and become very sensitive to the audience he imagines is observing and evaluating him (Elkind, 1974).

Formal operational thinking also allows the adolescent verbal symbolic enjoyment so that he can act aggressively but in a socially acceptable way—with words. He can use the insult or double-entendre to hurt or "taste" forbidden fruit with minimal social sanction. He also can argue and "hold his own" in an argument with his parents since he now is operating on the same level of cognition as his parents. This obviously has the potential for creating greater strain in the home.

Kohlberg (1969) has felt that moral judgment as well is greatly dependent on cognitive capability. With the emergence of formal operations, moral judgments can be based on internalized ethical principles rather than external consequences such as fear of reprisal or personal gain. While adolescents do not necessarily attain an internalized level of moral reasoning (about 10% do on Kohlberg's scale of moral reasoning), without the higher levels of cognition one cannot operate at these internalized levels.

Cognitive changes also affect vocational planning and aspirations. Now the child is not limited to experiential options such as fireman and policeman, but many more hypothetical possibilities emerge.

If nothing else, an almost helpless sense of relativity begins to settle in. The child realizes that parenting styles, political systems, religious values, social rules, and many other institutions which provide structure are relative and subject to challenge. This realization is both exhilarating and troubling, and sometimes the reaction is to submit to some absolute for the stability it affords. This may explain why during adolescence a resurgence of interest in cults or even institutional religious affiliations occurs.

Autism and Cognition

There are two major aspects of cognitive functioning reported for autistic youth that depart from that of the normal population. First, while autistic children can be found at all levels of intellectual development, the majority exhibit some degree of intellectual impairment. As can be seen from the distribution of IQ scores depicted in Table 1, from 50% to 75% of autistic persons are reported typically to earn IQ scores within the mentally retarded ranges (DeMyer et al., 1973; Rutter & Lockyer, 1967). Second, the pattern of cognitive functioning departs from the normal distribution highlighting the cognitive and perceptual deficits common

Table 1
Intelligence Classifications and Incidence Rates for
the General and Autistic Populations

IQ	IQ classification	Percent of general population included[a]	Approximate percent of autistic population included[b]
130 and above	Very superior	2.3	
120–129	Superior	7.4	
110–119	High average (bright)	16.5	9
90–109	Average	49.4	
80–89	Low average (dull)	16.2	
70–79	Borderline intelligence	6.0	20
55–69	Mildly retarded	2.0	28
40–54	Moderately retarded		
25–39	Severely retarded	0.2	43
Below 25	Profoundly retarded		

[a]Adapted from Wechsler (1955).
[b]Adapted from Rutter, Greenfeld, & Lockyer (1967).

to the autistic syndrome. Generally the autistic person performs better on nonverbal tasks or on verbal tasks that require immediate memory. Poorest performances are registered on tasks requiring abstract verbal reasoning, sequential verbal problem-solving, or symbolization in general (Rutter, 1970; Tymchuk, Simmons, & Neafsey, 1977). Therefore for many autistic young people of "average" or near-average IQ, specific verbal weaknesses often combine with nonverbal strengths to result in an average IQ.

IQ scores obtained by autistic adolescents, however, have predictive properties similar to those obtained by other groups of children (Bartak & Rutter, 1976). For the Maudsley Hospital series, Rutter (1965, 1966) reported a correlation of .63 between initial IQ scores (5 years, 11 months) and Wechsler Full Scale scores 15 years later. As may be expected there is a high interrelationship between the autistic youngster's measured IQ and an estimate of his work and school capacity, *and* the severity of the autistic symptomology (DeMyer et al., 1973). In fact the most useful indices for prognostic purposes in childhood have been found to be IQ scores and speech and language development (DeMyer et al., 1973; Lotter, 1974; Rutter et al., 1967).

There does not seem to have been any systematic attempt to relate Piagetian conceptualizations to autism. Nevertheless it is interesting to speculate on the nature of the cognitive deficit common to the autistic syndrome in terms of a Piagetian understanding of adolescent development. As mentioned previously, as the normal adolescent enters the stage of formal operations, a "conceptual revolution" occurs that allows the ability to engage in a more complex understanding of the hypothetical, the abstract, and the relative. The level of retardation observed in a majority of autistic youngsters, and perhaps the nature of the cognitive deficit associated with autism, typically precludes reaching the stage of formal operations. With this assumption one would predict difficulty in judging the depth of relationships, in understanding innuendo and subtleties in verbal meaning, and in seeing themselves as others see them (Everard, Note 1). Yet it is possible to speculate that some autistic persons develop incomplete or inconsistent formal operational thinking. An ability for hypothetical reasoning in an area of, for example, mathematics may exist without generalization of logical operations across situations. For these youngsters there may be increased stress as teachers, employers, and peers may hold unreachable expectations. The difficulty with "inconsistent formal operational thinking" may be illustrated in the follow-up account of Jerry, originally diagnosed as autistic as a child by Dr. Kanner. When the report was written (Bemporad, 1979) Jerry was completing college, a task that presumably requires formal operational thinking. Yet Bemporad noted that "he cannot be relied upon to use 'common sense' as he cannot separate the trivial from crucial aspects of a problem" (p. 190).

The changes in normal adolescence resulting from newly developing cognitive potentials may widen the gap between the normal and the autistic. Because the cognitive dysfunction in the autistic adolescent affects social, personal, and academic progress, parents may find this developmental stage particularly distressing as differences between the normal and the exceptional solidify.

SOCIAL AND EMOTIONAL ASPECTS OF ADOLESCENCE

Peers and Parents

Next to physical changes the most cited popular characteristic associated with adolescence is an increased importance of peers and a decreased importance or influence of the immediate family. Whether by telephone, letter, or in person, social preening of one another seems to be an integral part of life of the American adolescent. Peer groups consist of *cliques* (three to eight members who share highly similar interests and are highly selective) and *crowds* (combinations of cliques and others with similar backgrounds and ages). Members of cliques are usually close friends whereas crowd interactions are more informal. The social structure of adolescence develops from separate single-sex cliques to interactions between these cliques. Later single-sex cliques join to form a number of heterosexual cliques that may then begin to interact in crowds. Finally, the crowd breaks up into loosely knit groups of couples (Dunphy, 1963).

Friendships within these groups become more stable the older the adolescent becomes. More stable friendships seem to be enjoyed by males although the intensity of the friendship is far greater for females. Of primary importance for establishing friendships among adolescent boys seems to be athletic skill, whereas scholarship is more important among girls (Friessen, 1968), although this no doubt is changing with the more recent merging of male–female sex roles. For both sexes perceived similarity, good looks, sense of humor, kindness, and unselfishness rate high on listings of traits associated with friendship and popularity. Breaking into established peer groups can be done, but seems to depend mostly on looks, clothing, and "ways of conducting oneself" (Littrell & Eicher, 1973). Despite the high value placed on having a close friendship, 25%–30% of college males and 20% of college females said they had not had a close same-sex friendship (Conger, 1977).

The influence of peer groups also changes during adolescence. It has been shown that conformity to peer group norms (e.g., hairstyles, clothing, music, and so forth) is greatest during early adolescence (11–13 years) and gradually decreases thereafter (Hartup, 1970), although it never entirely disappears, continuing even into adulthood for most people. While teens are influenced by peers, it seems that there is a high correspondence generally between parents and their adolescents with respect to basic value decisions. For attitudes of lesser consequence adolescent allegiances reflect both peer and parent views, depending on the particular issue. It is also of interest to note that the more extreme parenting styles (with respect to restrictive-permissive, and authoritarian–laissez-faire rearing styles) produce young people with more peer group conformity and less autonomy (Lefrancois, 1981).

Peer group interaction serves three important functions during adolescence:

Social. The peer group serves as a bridge between two very different social worlds. The predominant early childhood social relationship is one characterized by dependence, with the child viewing the parent as all-knowing and all-powerful. However, in order to function in most adult societies greater responsible independence must be acquired, and the peer group is a principal mechanism in this transition.

To bridge the two worlds one must learn new rules, how to keep them, how to bend them, and as well how and where to break them. The learning of these rules, unlike the alphabet or driving a car, is a rather informal process usually left up to an individual's incidental learning skills. The peer group has implicit rules almost as exacting as families or society, and to interact new roles are demanded. As self-confidence and experience are acquired the peer group takes on less and less importance. Group rules are next questioned and modified, and with maturity the safety of the peer and home nests are abandoned for more enriching though potentially more vulnerable encounters. In learning adult roles the peer group provides models and opportunities from which to learn.

Emotional. There is probably some similarity between the initial intense attachment and gradual relaxation of the child's desire to be with the mother and the young adolescent's group attachment which gradually lessens. The group is a "base" away from home in a territory which looks attractive yet scary. Peers serve as a home base where feelings and experience can be discussed and from which one can obtain the emotional salve which assures "I am normal, I am protected, I am accepted." In a very real sense the peer group and special people within the clique encourage "therapeutic" encounters to occur, forcing the adolescent to label and work through new feelings of heartbreak, anxiety, embarrassment, desire, self-doubt, and love.

Cognitive. A third function of the peer group is that of an educational center, that is, a setting where one can both receive and share information as well as perform "mini-experiments," trying new social ideas. For example, the peer group for many teenagers is a primary source of sex education (Athamasiou, 1973). Also, the group can serve as a sounding board to find one's own stand or can be used as a ready source for new positions; by explaining themselves to each other teenagers explain themselves to themselves (Osterrieth, 1969). Therefore with the emergence of formal operations the adolescent has a relatively structured and empathetic setting which fosters both cognitive challenge and experimentation as well as information and understanding.

Parental Changes

It is easy to conceptualize parents as rather constant pools of advice, services, and controls. These pools are neither constant nor tranquil, however, but the parental turbulence may not be noticed by the "egocentric" adolescent because so many other things in his own fast-changing world capture his attention. But many aspects of the parent's world other than the child are changing.

Like the adolescent the adult is experiencing physical changes which, although not as dramatic as those which usually characterize puberty, nonetheless make emotional demands. Problems surrounding the adult's own parents (failing health or death), reassessment of goals and values set years earlier, and an ever-changing youth-oriented society all contribute toward producing developmental stresses which probably equal those experienced by most adolescents. Add to these the parent's requirement to be therapist, friend, combatant, and advisor to the developing teenage son or daughter.

Dating

The first date usually occurs by age 13 for females and a bit later for males (Bell & Chaskes, 1970), and almost all adolescents have dated by 19. In date selection an initial encounter has as its major criterion physical appearance (Herold, 1974). Thereafter social and personal skills take on increased importance. Dating serves several functions in American adolescence. First, it is a socially accepted response to increased sexual feelings. In addition, increased attraction toward the opposite sex must be cognitively arousing as well since opposite-sex peers are partial unknowns physically, emotionally, and socially. Getting to know them is both an intriguing and yet fearful cognitive challenge.

Adolescents also date to claim or assert adult status. Interestingly, when nondating adolescents were asked about dating it was apparent that though each recognized the term and knew it as an appropriate adolescent behavior, most had little idea of such basic notions as where one might go on a date, the purpose of a date, or what one might do during the date (Jackson, 1975). Therefore it seems clear that expectations have been well developed and teens who want to be adult also know they must have opposite-sex companions; however, they are not always sure how to meet these expectations.

Dating can be its own reward in that it serves as an excuse for teens to go places and do things without having to do them alone or under the supervision of their parents. In fact it is this function that is most mentioned by teens when asked why they date (Lambert. Rothschild, Altland, & Green, 1972). Dating can also serve as an indirect reward, such as a basis of admiration from one's peers. For example, dating a certain person may bring status to oneself because of the date's status or reputation. Dating can also reward more "selfish" goals since having a date may ensure not being lonely or assure one of attention, friendship, and even affection.

Finally, dating might also be used to establish criteria for the ultimate selection of a mate or be the avenue of obtaining one. It is the information gained during dating which becomes the basis against which further comparisons are made. Courtship tactics are also learned and used when one wishes to decide whether to make a more serious commitment. Most early dating interactions occur without commitment or even emotional or interpersonal investment. But all that may change, and if used wisely dating can make that relatively permanent social allegiance and commitment a more fulfilling and meaningful one.

Adolescent Problem Areas

Although adolescence is a time of adjustment to new cognitive abilities, social expectations, and physical changes, a majority make the transition through this time without marked crisis. However, some do not. Particular forms of antisocial adjustment or expressions of dissatisfaction exist which, while not exclusive to adolescence, are associated with this particular development period.

Substance Abuse. The use of exotic drugs among adolescents increased during the 1970s but seems to have stabilized more recently, although it still presents a significant problem among U.S. teens. The most extensively used drug is alcohol. Approximately 10%–25% of young teenagers report drinking regularly. Among older teenagers 2% have a serious drinking problem (Bosma, 1976). The American Medical Association has declared that 1 out of 15 youths in the United States may become an alcoholic in the near future unless current practices change (*Boston Globe*, Jan. 26, 1974). Most adult alcoholics report having started drinking regularly by 15 years of age.

Estimates of marijuana use have ranged from 10% to 66% of high school graduates, depending on geographic location. While it is a drug used by a high proportion of teenagers, it does not appear to be as debilitating or habit-forming as alcohol (Zinberg, 1976). Like their parents, adolescents are using an increased amount of stimulants and tranquilizers to control mood states and energy levels. Use of inhalants (such as with glue or gasoline sniffing) to obtain "a high" is mostly a young adolescent practice. Use of hard drugs (e.g., heroin) seems to have stabilized in the last 10 years (about 1% of teens), although resultant fatalities from overdose and drug-related complications (such as hepatitis) are still alarming. Unfortunately rehabilitation efforts have not proved very effective in combating drug addiction (Achenbach, 1974).

Runaways. It is estimated that between 600,000 and 1,000,000 U.S.

adolescents run away from home each year. Many of these youths are from suburban middle-class homes, and are 15 years old on the average; about half are girls. Shelters and telephone hotlines have been established by groups in various cities to help with the problem (Ambrosino, 1971). As a symptom, running away may reflect a relatively mild reactive disorder or an expression of a significant psychological disturbance. Difficult home, school, and personal circumstances have all been identified as factors prompting running away.

Eating Disorders. Two types of eating disorders increase in frequency during the adolescent years. The first is anorexia nervosa, a serious medical and psychological condition characterized by excessive weight loss resulting from refusal and/or inability to eat. In the past as many as 10% of such cases resulted in death through starvation, although this fatality rate has decreased markedly through improved psychotherapeutic management. For unknown reasons anorexia nervosa is 10 times more prevalent among females than among males (Bruch, 1973).

The second eating disorder, and far more common, is obesity. Approximately 10% of today's teenagers are considered obese. The obese adolescent is at high risk for both medical and psychosocial problems, both during the teenage years and in those following, once this eating style has been established (Heald & Khan, 1976).

Crime. Individual crime and illegal gang activity among teenagers continues to increase dramatically. Persons under 21 account for 42% of the arrests for such serious crimes as rape and murder even though they comprise only 23% of the population (U.S. News and World Report, Sept. 6, 1976). It is estimated that 1 out of 10 of today's youth will be tried for criminal charges before he/she is 21 (Conger, 1977). The nature of the crimes committed has also worsened: street brawling and relatively minor offenses have given way to muggings, robberies, and the selling of protection. Because guns have replaced knives the number of killings has increased markedly. In large metropolitan areas the number of youths involved in gang activity runs into the tens of thousands (Miller, 1977). As with addictive drugs, rehabilitation efforts to curb further criminal activity of convicted teens has been shown to have minimal long-term effects (McCombs, Filipczak, Rusilko, Friedman, & Wodarski, Note 2).

Suicide. The rate of suicide among teenagers is approximately twice that of the population average (Lefrancois, 1981), making it the fifth leading cause of death among youth (Lavigne, Note 3). Although more females will attempt suicide, males are more likely to succeed. The most often cited reasons for suicide among adolescents include depression from feeling unwanted or unloved, difficulty in interpersonal relationships, and medical problems.

Autism and Social/Emotional Development

For the autistic child the lack of appropriate social relatedness is a cardinal symptom, and this difficulty with social perception and interaction continue into adolescence. The emphasis in this section will be on the mildly autistic child who interfaces with his community. It should be remembered, however, that approximately half of those children diagnosed as autistic are residing in long-term care facilities by middle adolescence (Lotter, 1974; Rutter, 1970).

While there is often a growing interest in reaching out to peers, the autistic teenager has difficulty with interpersonal skills, typically presenting barriers to establishing and maintaining friendships. Problems in judging the depth of relationship, in "social know-how," and in communication may result in rejection by an admired "in-group." The normal adolescent may be hesitant to jeopardize his or her own position in a clique or crowd by extending support to the autistic teenager. As Everard (Note 1) notes, "autistic young people are not necessarily 'loners' by choice; their attempts at sociability are poorly rewarded and they may find it easier not to try" (p. 4). At a time when sharing information to "check it out" becomes an integral part of the life of the normal adolescent, the universal communication problems of autistic persons may block access to peers. Expressive language may be marked by literalness, irrelevancy, repetition, and obsession with details. Baltaxe (1977) hypothesizes an impairment in speaker–hearer role relationship to account for the findings of difficulty in differentiating between old and new information, inadvertent rudeness, continued problems with the pronominal system, and difficulty in responding to questions of a personal or emotional nature found in analyzing the content of dialogues with autistic adolescents. Clearly the uniqueness in the communication style of the autistic adolescent would present a formidable barrier to breaking into a peer group when high value is placed on similarity and appropriate "conduct."

The exacting rules and roles that define adolescent peer groups also provide a roadblock to the autistic teenager who finds change so difficult. Often it is impossible for the autistic person to abandon his own set routines, and the frequently noted "lack of empathy" (Kanner et al., 1972; Rutter, 1970) shuts out the ability to understand and conform with groups norms. In later teen years, however, as the peer group takes on less importance, the better adjusted autistic person may find his or her way of interacting with others. As noted by Kanner et al. (1972) in their follow-up study, "they . . . discovered means of interacting by joining groups in which they could make use of their preoccupations . . . as shared 'hobbies' in the company of others. [They] . . . enjoy the recognition earned by the detail knowledge that they had stored up in years of obsessive rumination of specific topics" (p. 31).

The exclusion of the autistic adolescent from social cliques further shuts off a major source of social learning about the opposite sex. The poor prognosis for heterosexual friendships can be illustrated by the follow-up report from the Maudsley Hospital series that revealed only 1 of 64 autistic adolescents and young adults had a heterosexual friendship. Dewey and Everard (1974) conclude that the typical mildly autistic adolescent "learns by unfortunate experience that it is safer not to yield to the impulses to follow, touch, or speak to a person he finds attractive. When even tentative expressions of yearning cause trouble, it is no wonder that most autistic persons eventually decide sexual fulfillment is not for them" (p. 352). The most typical reaction to the emergence of sexuality is one of celibacy. Whether there is an increase in sexual tensions that is displaced onto other behaviors or whether there is truly a lack of sexual interest in the majority of autistic persons remains an avenue of exploration for future research.

In contrast to the developmental expectation of achieving emotional and social independence from parents, the lower- and middle-functioning autistic teenager who lives at home engages his or her caretakers in the task of "perpetual parenthood" (DeMyer, 1979). While parents of the normal adolescent are adapting to changes in their lives and those of their youngsters, the parents of autistic teens may be meeting the awareness of the life course of *infantile* autism with anger, disappointment, and sadness (Dewey & Everard, 1974). Parents of mildly autistic youngsters are also faced with uncertainties because of the continued awareness of the incompleteness of their son's or daughter's social repertoire necessary to function optimally in the world outside the sheltered home. The prognosis for emancipation from the home that comes with employment is poor for the autistic child. Generally not more than 5% of autistic persons are employed in their late teen and early adult years (Lotter, 1974; Rutter et al., 1967). Those same social adjustment problems that lead to their exclusion by their peers as young adolescents seem to contribute to their lower employability status compared to nonautistic persons matched for age, sex, and IQ. Seemingly for the reasons described above, antisocial behavior such as criminal involvement, substance abuse, running away, and suicide are rarely associated with autism. Adjustment difficulties centering around avoidance of social contacts rather than engaging in negative acts against their parents or the community seem to be more characteristic of autistic teenagers. Again, further research is needed before a clearer statement is possible.

THE AUTISTIC ADOLESCENT

Sociologist Robert Havighurst (1953) enumerated several "developmental tasks" which American teenagers need to master in order to bridge the gap between childhood and adulthood. In some ways one might define the social and emotional aspects of adolescence in terms of the events which each of these tasks focuses on. However, notice also how many of them draw on cognitive and physical aspects as well. The tasks include:

1. Achieving new and more mature relations with age mates of both sexes
2. Achieving a masculine or feminine social role
3. Accepting one's physique and using the body effectively
4. Achieving emotional independence of parents and other adults
5. Achieving assurance of economic independence
6. Selecting and preparing for an occupation
7. Preparing for marriage and family life
8. Developing intellectual skills and concepts necessary for civic competence
9. Desiring and achieving socially responsible behavior
10. Acquiring a set of values and an ethical system as a guide to behavior

If the successful mastery of Havighurst's tasks constitutes the social bridge from childhood to adulthood, the difficulties of the journey for the autistic adolescent are immediately clear if one considers the biological, cognitive, and social demands required. Even for those youngsters not residing in residential facilities by their late adolescence there is little expectation of true independence from the parental home. A detailed review of the literature reveals that only one or two youngsters with a diagnosis of early infantile autism were reported to develop a sufficient social repertoire by their early adult years to enter a marital relationship (DesLauries, 1978). The empathy necessary to establish friendships beyond a surface level is characteristically absent. As noted by Everard (Note 1) "[autistic young people] are apt to think of anyone who speaks kindly or who takes an interest in them as their friends" (p. 5). Their need for routine, their difficulty in adopting the flexibility required in a workplace, and their problems with communication combine to permit only a small percentage of autistic adults to be gainfully employed.

In short the social, emotional, and communication deficits that define the syndrome of autism in childhood continue, with some alteration, to impact on the adolescent to such a degree as to block, or in cases of lesser severity impede, the "rites of passage" that adolescence represents. In some respects adolescence may be the most difficult of developmental stages for the autistic person and his family. Although in childhood his being different from other youngsters is obvious, the community can be more accepting of the child. There may be special classes or schools available, and there is hope that with development will come change. As the autistic child moves through adolescence, his parents become acutely aware of the varying degrees of permanence of the cardinal symptoms of infantile autism, of the shortage or absence of appropriate programs, and of the dependency that is typical for the adolescent who cannot approach the goals of separation from his parents. While there are exceptions— youngsters who develop their particular musical talents, mathematical skills, or visual spatial exceptionalities—the majority of autistic adolescents are ill-prepared to "live in a world where no concessions are made and they are expected to conform" (Everard, Note 1). There is a great need to develop a range of sheltered living arrangements and meaningful work situations to preserve the hope and humanity of the exceptional adolescent and his family.

REFERENCES

Achenbach, T. M. *Developmental psychopathology*. New York: Ronald Press, 1974.

Ambrosino, L. *Runaways*. Boston: Beacon Press, 1971.

Ames, R. Physical maturing among boys as related to adult social behavior. *California Journal of Educational Research*, 1957, *8*, 69–75.

Athamasiou, R. A review of public attitudes on sexual issues. In *Contemporary sexual behavior: Critical issues in the 1970's* (J. Zubin and J. Money, eds.), Baltimore: Johns Hopkins University Press, 1973.

Baltaxe, C. Pragmatic deficits in the language of autistic adolescents. *Journal of Pediatric Psychology*, 1977, *2*, 176–180.

Bartak, L., & Rutter, M. Differences between mentally retarded and normally autistic children. *Journal of Autism and Childhood Schizophrenia*, 1976, *6*, 109–120.

Bayley, N. Development of mental abilities. In *Carmichael's manual of child psychology* (P. Mussen, ed.), New York: Wiley, 1970.

Bell, R. R., & Chaskes, J. B. Premarital sexual experience among co-eds, 1958 and 1968. *Journal of Marriage and the Family*, 1970, *32*, 81–84.

Bemporad, J. R. Adult recollections of a formerly autistic child. *Journal of Autism and Developmental Disorders*, 1979, *9*, 179–197.

Bosma, W. G. Adolescents and alcohol. In *Medical care of the adolescent*, 3rd ed. (R. Gallagher, F. P. Heald, & D. C. Garell, eds.), New York: Prentice-Hall, 1976.

Bruch, H. *Eating disorders*. New York: Basic Books, 1973.

Campbell, M., Petti, T. A., Greene, W. H., Cohen, I. L., Genieser, N. B., & David, R. Some physical parameters of young autistic children. *Journal of the American Academy of Child Psychiatry*, 1980, *19*, 193–212.

Cavior, N., & Dokecki, P. R. Physical attractiveness, perceived attitude similarity and academic achievement as contributors to interpersonal attraction among adolescents. *Developmental Psychology*, 1973, *9*, 44–54.

Cole, L., & Hall, I. N. *Psychology in adolescence*, 7th ed. New York: Holt, Rinehart and Winston, 1970.

Conger, J. J. *Adolescence and youth: Psychological development in a changing world.* New York: Harper & Row, 1977.

DeMyer, M. K. *Parents and children in autism.* Washington, D.C.: Winston, 1979.

DeMyer, M. K., Barton, S., DeMyer, W. E., Norton, J. A., Allen, J., & Steele, R. Prognosis in autism: A follow-up study. *Journal of Autism and Childhood Schizophrenia*, 1973, *3*, 199–246.

DesLauries, A. M. The cognitive-affective dilemma in early infantile autism: The case of Clarence. *Journal of Autism and Childhood Schizophrenia*, 1978, *8*, 219–232.

Dewey, M. A., & Everard, M. P. The near normal autistic adolescent. *Journal of Autism and Childhood Schizophrenia*, 1974, *4*, 348–356.

Deykin, E., & MacMahon, B. The incidence of seizures among children with autistic symptoms. *American Journal of Psychiatry*, 1980, *10*, 1310–1312.

Dunphy, D. C. The social structure of urban adolescent peer groups. *Sociometry*, 1963, *26*, 230–246.

Elkind, D. *Children and adolescents: Interpretive essays on Jean Piaget.* New York: Oxford University Press, 1974.

Friessen, D. Academic-athletic-popularity syndrome in the Canadian high school society. *Adolescence*, 1968, *3*, 39–52.

Gordon, S. *The sexual adolescent.* North Scituate, Mass.: Wadsworth, 1973.

Hartup, W. W. Peer interaction and social organization. In *Manual of child psychology.* (P. H. Mussen, ed.), New York: Wiley, 1970.

Havighurst, R. J. *Human development and education.* New York: Longmans, Green 1953.

Heald, F. P., & Khan, M. A. Disorders of adipose tissue. In *Medical care of the adolescent,* 3rd ed. (J. R. Gallagher, F. P. Heald, & D. C. Garell, eds.), New York: Prentice-Hall, 1976.

Herold, E. Stages of date selection: A reconciliation of divergent findings on campus values in dating. *Adolescence*, 1974, *9*, 113–121.

Inhelder, B. *The diagnosis of reasoning in the mentally retarded.* New York: Chandler, 1968.

Jackson, D. W. The meaning of dating from the role perspective of non-dating preadolescents. *Adolescence*, 1975, *10*, 123–126.

Kanner, L. Autistic disturbances of affective contact. *Nervous Child*, 1943, *2*, 217–250.

Kanner, L., Rodriguez, A., & Ashenden, B. How far can autistic children go in matters of social adaptation? *Journal of Autism and Childhood Schizophrenia*, 1972, *2*, 9–33.

Kinsey, A. C., Pomeroy, W. B., & Martin, C. E. *Sexual behavior in the human male.* Philadelphia: Saunders, 1948.

Kinsey, A. C., Pomeroy, W. B., Martin, C. E., & Gebhard, P. H. *Sexual behavior in the human female.* Philadelphia: Saunders, 1953.

Kohlberg, L. Stage and sequence: The cognitive developmental approach to socialization. In *Handbook of socialization theory and research.* (D. Goslin, ed.), Chicago: Rand McNally, 1969.

Lambert, G. B., Rothschild, B. F., Altland, R., & Green, L. B. *Adolescence: Transition from childhood to maturity.* Monterey, Calif.: Brooks/Cole, 1972.

Lefrancois, G. R. *Adolescence.* Belmont, Calif.: Wadsworth, 1981.

Liberman, D. A., & Malone, M. B. *Sexuality and social awareness*. New Haven, Conn.: Benhaven Press, 1979.

Littrell, M. B., & Eicher, J. B. Clothing opinions and the social acceptance process among adolescents. *Adolescence*, 1973, *8*, 197–212.

Livingston, S. Epilepsy in infancy, childhood, and adolescence. In *Manual of child psychopathology* (B. Wolman, ed.), New York: McGraw-Hill, 1972.

Lotter, V. Social adjustment and placement of autistic children in Middlesex: A follow-up study. *Journal of Autism and Childhood Schizophrenia*, 1974, *1*, 11–32.

Lowrie, S. H. Early marriage: Premarital pregnancy and associated factors. *Journal of Marriage and the Family*, 1965, *27*, 48–57.

Luckey, E. B., & Nass, G. D. A comparison of sexual attitudes and behaviors in an international sample. *Journal of Marriage and the Family*, 1969, *31*, 364–379.

Masters, W., & Johnson, V. I. *Human sexual response*. Boston: Little, Brown, 1966.

McClelland, D. C. Testing for competence rather than for "intelligence." *American Psychologist*, 1973, *28*, 1–14.

Mead, M. *Coming of age in Samoa*. New York: Morrow, 1928.

Miller, W. The rumble this time. *Psychology Today*, 1977, *10* (12), 52–59, 88.

Offer, D., Marcus, D., & Offer, J. L. A longitudinal study of normal adolescent boys. *American Journal of Psychiatry*, 1970, *126*, 917–924.

Osterrieth, P. A. Adolescence: Some psychological aspects. In *Adolescence: Psychosocial perspectives* (G. Caplan & S. Lebovici, eds.). New York: Basic Books, 1969.

Piaget, J. *The psychology of intelligence*. Totowa, N.J.: Littlefield, Adams, 1966.

Reitan, R. M. Psychological effects of cerebral lesions in children of early school age. In *Clinical neuropsychology: Current status and applications*. (R. M. Reitan & L. A. Davison, eds.), Washington, D.C.: Winston, 1972.

Reynolds, E. L., & Wines, J. V. Individual differences in physical changes associated with adolescent girls. *American Journal of the Diseases of Children*, 1951, *82*, 529–547.

Rutter, M. The influence of organic factors on the origins, nature and outcome of childhood psychosis. *Developmental Medicine and Child Neurology*, 1965, *7*, 518–528.

Rutter, M. Prognosis: Psychotic children in adolescence and early adult life. In *Childhood autism: Clinical, educational, and social aspects* London: Pergamon Press, 1966.

Rutter, M. Autistic children: Infancy to adulthood. *Seminars in Psychiatry*, 1970, *2*, 435–450.

Rutter, M., & Lockyer, L. A five to fifteen year follow-up study of infantile psychosis. *British Journal of Psychiatry*, 1967, *113*, 1169–1182.

Rutter, M., Greenfeld, D., & Lockyer, L. A five to fifteen year follow-up study of infantile psychosis. II. Social and behavioural outcome. *British Journal of Psychology*, 1967, *113*, 1183–1199.

Salamy, A. Commissural transmission: Maturational changes in humans. *Science*, 1978, *200*, 1409–1501.

Shipman, G. The psychodynamics of sex education. *Family Coordinator*, 1968, *17*, 3–12.

Simon, G. B., & Gillies, S. M. Some physical characteristics of a group of psychotic children. *British Journal of Psychiatry*, 1976, *110*, 104–107.

Sorenson, R. C. *Adolescent sexuality in contemporary America*. New York: World, 1972.

Tanner, J. M. Physical growth and development. In *Textbook of pediatrics*, Vol. 1, 2nd ed. (J. D. Forfar & G. C. Arneil, eds.), New York: Churchill Livingstone, 1978.

Tymchuk, A. J., Simmons, J. Q., & Neafsey, S. Intellectual characteristics of adolescent childhood psychotics with high verbal ability. *Journal of Mental Deficiency Research*, 1977, *21*, 133–138.

Walster, E., Aronson, V., Abrahams, D., & Rottman, L. Importance of physical attractiveness in dating behavior. *Journal of Personality and Social Psychology,* 1966, *4,* 508–516.

Weatherley, D. Self-perceived rate of physical maturation and personality in late adolescence. *Child Development,* 1964, *35,* 1197–1210.

Wechsler, D. *Wechsler intelligence scale for children—Revised.* New York: Psychological Corporation, 1974.

Zelnick, M., & Kanter, J. F. The resolution of teenage first pregnancies. *Family Planning Perspectives,* 1974, *6,* 74–80.

Zinberg, N. E. Marijuana, fact and fiction. *Psychology Today,* 1976, *10,* 45–52ff.

REFERENCE NOTES

1. Everard, M. *Mildly autistic young people and their problems.* Paper presented at the International Symposium on Autism, St. Gallen, Switzerland, July, 1976.
2. McCombs, D., Filipczak, J., Rusilko, S., Friedman, R. M., & Wodarski, J. S. *Long-term follow-up of behavior modification with high-risk adolescents.* Paper presented at the meeting of the Association for Advancement of Behavior Therapy, New York, 1976.
3. Lavigne, J. *Disorders among adolescents, II.* Unpublished manuscript, 1977. (Available from John Lavigne, Ph.D., Children's Memorial Hospital, 2300 Children's Plaza, Chicago, Illinois   60614).

3

Current Perspectives and Issues in Autism and Adolescence

GARY B. MESIBOV

Though somewhat neglected until recently, the topic of autism has received considerable attention from investigators in the last 10–15 years (DeMyer, 1979; Rutter & Schopler, 1978; Wing, 1972). Most of this research has involved children. However, despite the tremendous increase in research, there remains a large gap in our understanding of autistic people as they become adolescents and adults (Sullivan, 1977). Until recently this gap did not represent a major problem for service providers because such a high percentage of autistic adolescents and adults were living in residential institutions where few learning opportunities were available (Lotter, 1978). However, more successful intervention programs have resulted in more autistic adolescent and adult people functioning in community-based programs with increased learning opportunities and an accompanying need for more information. The purpose of this chapter is to help meet this increased need by reviewing the current understanding of autism in adolescents and adults and by making suggestions for future clinical and research efforts.

LITERATURE REVIEW

A major difficulty confronting those interested in adolescents and adults with autism is a lack of empirical data. The meager existing data

GARY B. MESIBOV ● Adolescent and Adult Services, Division TEACCH, Department of Psychiatry, University of North Carolina School of Medicine, Chapel Hill, North Carolina 27514.

come primarily from outcome studies, usually done 5–15 years after an initial evaluation, which are designed to determine the outcome of specific treatments or the natural outcome of autism in general. Because most autistic children were originally identified between the ages of 5 and 15, most of the outcome studies are done during their adolescent and early adult years. Although these studies are not designed to study older autistic people per se they do provide some useful information about the major problems of the older group. However, the focus on outcome rather than on adolescence and adulthood sometimes leads to an incomplete picture of the autistic adolescent or adult and his/her family.

The outcome literature on autistic adolescents and adults describes various aspects of their skills and needs including behaviors, social and interpersonal skills, seizures, cognitive status, and speech and language.

Behavior

The behavior of autistic people is of primary concern because it represents one of the most frequent difficulties associated with this disorder and is the major factor interfering with successful community placement (McCarver & Craig, 1974; Mesibov & Shea, Note 1). Behaviors that have been studied in autistic adolescents and adults include activity level, aggression, rituals, self-help skills, group participation, initiative, and self-control.

Activity level is one behavior that appears to improve as autistic children grow older. Ando and Yoshimura (1979) compared two groups of children, ages 6–9 and ages 11–14, on their activity levels and found significantly less activity in the older group. Rutter (1970) supports this finding, stating, ''Marked hyperkinesis is a common characteristic of autistic children in early childhood, but during middle and later childhood it is often gradually replaced by an inert underactivity in which the children appear lacking in any drive or impetus to do anything. Unless prodded to act, they tend to just sit'' (p. 440). Rutter argues that this reduction in activity level is physiological, perhaps related to some aspect of brain maturation. This finding of decreased activity during adolescence is supported by parent observations as well.

Changes in aggressive and self-injurious behaviors during adolescence are harder to assess than changes in activity level. Some investigators have reported increases in these behaviors while others have reported decreases. It does not appear that any general pattern has emerged as yet (Ando & Yoshimura, 1979; Rutter, 1970). Some of the controversy over this issue might result from the destructive potential of aggressive and self-injurious behaviors in autistic adolescents and adults. Even in situations where these behaviors have not increased from childhood to adolescence, but have in fact decreased, the effects of these behaviors can be much more dramatic because of the size and strength of older autistic people. Those arguing that aggression increases during adolescence might be responding to the greater effects of each aggressive action while those arguing that it decreases might be responding to the frequency with which aggressive actions occur.

Ritualistic and compulsive behaviors appear to improve somewhat during adolescence and adulthood. Several investigators (Rutter, 1970; Rutter, Greenfeld, & Lockyer, 1967) describe these behaviors as most intense during middle childhood and tending to decrease during adolescence and adulthood. Mesibov and Shea (Note 1) noted the same trend in higher functioning autistic people in community-based programs.

Ando, Yoshimura, and Wakabayashi (1980) have recently reported improved self-help skills, group participation, initiative, and self-control in a group of 11- to 14-year-old autistic people as compared with a group of 6- to 9-year-olds. The self-help skills of toileting and feeding were superior in the older group, which is consistent with the findings of other studies (Rutter, 1970; Rutter et al., 1967). Improvements in group participation and initiative were determined by the respective items on the AAMD Adaptive Behavior Scale (Grossman, 1973). The differences in group participation resulted because fewer younger children participated in group activities, even with considerable encouragement. Differences in initiative resulted because fewer older autistic people refused to do assigned activities. The authors designed their own self-control scale, and on this measure group differences resulted from a higher number of older autistic children who could stay in their seats and concentrate in class.

Social and Interpersonal Skills

The literature on social and interpersonal skills has similar trends to the behavior literature: these skills generally improve during adolescence and adulthood, although with certain qualifications and exceptions.

Rutter's (1970) report is representative of the findings in this area. Describing his Maudsley Hospital sample, he stated that interpersonal relationships improved in 50% of the cases as the children got older. In 15% of these improvement was so marked that the children no longer "appeared autistic" in adolescence. However, even though marked improvement was noted, Rutter (1970) cautions, "usually the children remained reserved, without social 'know-how' and seemingly unaware of the feelings in others. Warmth in interpersonal relationships continued to improve in a few children even after adolescence, but difficulties remained'' (pp. 438–439).

DeMyer, Barton, DeMyer, Norton, Allen, and Steele (1973) and Brown (1969) have reported similar improvements in social and interpersonal skills during adolescence. In describing Brown's Putnam follow-up and his own Maudsley sample, Rutter (1970) has written, ''Among those who had made the most progress, about half showed an interest, friendliness and involvement with other people: but they lacked the skills in interpersonal relationships needed to proceed from acquaintance to friendship. In these children the failure to make friends was a source of distress and unhappiness, showing that at least in them, the lack of friends was the result of a lack of social skill, not of social interest. Other autistic children had become generally more friendly and interested in people but still remained reserved and socially isolated outside the family'' (p. 439).

The findings of Ando and Yoshimura (1979) are somewhat different from those already described. Comparing 6- to 9-year-old children with 11- to 14-year-olds they found no differences on their measures of social and interpersonal skills, which consisted of eye contact and withdrawal. There appear to be two possible explanations for these discrepant findings. First, the IQs of the Ando and Yoshimura group were much lower than the IQs of the children in the other studies. Their data could therefore simply represent another instance of the already-documented finding (Rutter, 1970) that autistic children with IQs of less than 70 improve more slowly than those functioning at higher levels. Another explanation could be the global measures of social skills employed by Ando and Yoshimura, consisting only of eye contact and withdrawal. Perhaps more specific measures assessing a wider range of skills would have demonstrated greater improvement.

Seizures

There is accumulating evidence that many autistic children develop seizures for the first time during adolescence or early adulthood (Creak, 1963; Kanner, 1949; Rutter et al., 1967). Creak (1963) noted the occurrence of seizures in seven cases during adolescence and Kanner (1949) described a similar phenomenon.

Several investigators (Bartak & Rutter, 1976; Deykin & MacMahon, 1979) have carefully documented the onset of seizures in adolescence and early adulthood. They found that these seizures occur in one-quarter to one-third of the autistic children who were seizure-free in childhood, but rarely in those with IQs greater than 70. As with the decrease in activity level noted earlier, Rutter argues that the adolescent onset of seizures is related to the physical maturation process occurring during that time.

Cognitive Status

Several outcome studies have focused on IQ changes and academic progress during adolescence. The IQ data suggest that changes occurring in autistic persons during adolescence are similar to changes in their nonhandicapped peers. In general scores remain relatively stable during this period and are usually consistent with scores obtained during middle childhood. As with nonhandicapped children, significant changes of up to 15 points are sometimes reported (DeMyer et al., 1973; Rutter, 1970); however, these are the exceptions rather than the general trend. When changes occur they can be upward as frequently as downward. The one exception to this trend is the finding (Rutter, 1970) that several of the Maudsley children who developed seizures during adolescence showed a marked deterioration in their intellectual ability.

Bartak and Rutter (1976) observed greater academic progress for higher functioning autistic adolescents (IQs greater than 70) than for those functioning at lower levels of ability. In the higher functioning group they reported modest academic gains in reading accuracy, reading comprehension, and arithmetic, with larger gains in arithmetic than in reading (Rutter & Bartak, 1973).

Ando et al. (1980) also found larger academic gains for autistic adolescents in arithmetic as compared with reading. Although there were some small gains in reading and writing, these did not achieve statistical significance. According to Ando et al. (1980), the greater improvement in arithmetic skills resulted from the older group's abilities with number concepts. There were no differences between the two groups in arithmetic computational skills such as addition and subtraction.

Speech and Language

The literature suggests that the language skills of autistic people improve very slowly, but consistently, up to adolescence and perhaps even beyond (Ando & Yoshimura, 1979; Rutter & Schopler, 1978). Except for this trend there appear to be few discernible patterns; however, consistent observations have been reported.

First, about half the children diagnosed as autistic are still without functional speech at adolescence. This figure has been reported by the Kanner group (Eisenberg, 1956), the Maudsley study (Rutter et al., 1967), the Smith Hospital study (Mittler, Gillies, & Jukes, 1966), and DeMyer's group (DeMyer et al., 1973).

Second, of the 50% of autistic people who do develop speech by the time they are adolescents, a significant percentage acquire it after the age of 5. In the Maudsley group 22% of those children without functional expressive language at age 5 developed it later on; the figure was 17% in the DeMyer et al. (1973) group. Most of the late language developers had relatively high nonverbal IQs.

Third, even those autistic children who have good language skills at adolescence tend to evidence some irregularities of delivery, usage, and understanding (Rutter & Schopler, 1978). Difficulties in delivery include a flat monotone with little lability of emotional expression and staccato speech, lacking cadence and inflection. The main problem with usage includes a formality of language, lacking ease in use of words and leading to a pedantic mode of expression. In addition many autistic adolescents and adults tend to converse by a series of obsessive questions related to their particular preoccupation at that time (Mesibov & Shea, Note 1). The main difficulty with understanding is the problem of abstract concepts. Ricks and Wing (1975) noted the example of an autistic child who became terrified when his mother said she had "cried her eyes out."

LITERATURE REVIEW SUMMARY AND DISCUSSION

The outcome literature is encouraging in that autistic children generally improve in specific skill areas during adolescence and adulthood. Studies have shown that activity level generally decreases, behavior becomes more manageable, self-help skills improve, speech and language show continual development, the IQ remains relatively stable, and the children generally become more sociable. The only major problem developing during adolescence is the onset of seizures, although aggressive and self-injurious behaviors become more problematic if not more frequent.

In direct contrast to the relatively bright picture emerging from the literature on specific skills are the realities of adolescence and adulthood for most autistic people. Most parents report increasing difficulties in managing their older children, and the overall outcome figures are not very encouraging. For example, the Maudsley study found fair to good outcomes in only 17% of their autistic adolescents (Rutter, 1970); Eisenberg (1956) reports only 27% of the Kanner sample with good outcomes;

Brown (1969) reports 27% of her sample with fair or better outcomes; and DeMyer et al. (1973) reports 16–25% with fair to good outcomes. Moreover the frequency of institutionalization among this group is extremely high (Lotter, 1978).

Why this discrepancy? Why do the data on general skills suggest increasing difficulties? One possibility is that although autistic children show some improvement in specific skills during adolescence, their rate of improvement is not sufficient to accommodate the increasing demands placed upon them as they grow older. Normally the development of a person must keep pace with the accelerating demands of his/her environment. For example, a 5-year-old boy who behaves like a normal 3-year-old will find this behavior problematic because a kindergarten classroom will be less able to accommodate him than a preschool program would be. Available programs are much more demanding and less individualized for autistic adolescents and adults than programs for younger children. In order to function successfully in these programs older autistic people need greater skills than was previously the case. Although autistic people do improve as they get older, they do not appear to improve enough to meet the increased demands of available programs.

Another possible explanation relates to the physical growth that accompanies adolescence and adulthood. A child who weighs 195 pounds needs much better behavior than a child weighing only 45 pounds. Mildly unpleasant behaviors like pushing or shoving in a small child can become destructive and dangerous in a full-grown adult. Perhaps the improved behaviors noted in the literature are not sufficient to accommodate increased demands related to a larger physical stature.

PROGRAMMATIC NEEDS

For these reasons, efforts must be expanded to improve outcomes for autistic adolescents and adults by not only continuing to develop their existing skills but also by further structuring their environments with more appropriate programs and services. If community programs are to be successful for older autistic clients, more must be done in skill areas related to successful community functioning as well as in developing more appropriate programs.

There have been numerous discussions of what is needed for severely handicapped people to function successfully in the community (NARC, 1975). These discussions and the continuing experiences of community-based programs suggest that the following issues must be addressed if we are to improve the outcomes of autistic adolescents and adults: improvement of social and interpersonal skills, development of vocational training and employment opportunities, management of aggression and sexuality, and definition of the role of the family.

Social and Interpersonal Skills

If the outcomes in community-based programs are to be significantly improved autistic people must receive more intensive and effective training in social and interpersonal skills. Kanner, Rodriguez, and Ashenden (1972) have cited social skill as the most crucial ability for those with positive outcomes. They observed that autistic persons with positive outcomes during adolescence "became uneasily aware of their peculiarities and began to make a conscious effort to do something about them. This effort increased as they grew older. . . . Again and again we note a felt need to grope for ways to compensate for the lack of inherent sociability" (pp. 29–30). According to these investigators, autistic persons' understanding of their differences and a desire to overcome them were the main factors differentiating successful from unsuccessful outcomes.

Other investigators have made similar observations, noting an increased desire for social contact among autistic adolescents able to express their needs. For example, Rutter (1970) claims, "In these children the failure to make friends was a source of distress and unhappiness, showing that at least in them, the lack of friends was the result of a lack of social skill, not of social interest" (p. 439). Bemporad's case study (1979) also noted an expressed desire to be involved with peers, but a tendency to be rejected by them. Katharine Stokes (1977), a parent of an autistic adolescent, poignantly describes the social needs of her son, "Yet Sam needs other human beings who not only care about him but who enjoy sharing with him in reciprocally satisfying human contact. Sam does not need a sexual partner in the adult sense, but he needs someone to hug occasionally as well as someone to comfort him when he is troubled" (p. 292). Apparently there is agreement that as autistic children become adolescents and adults at least some of them develop an increased desire for contact with others but maintain an inability to meet this need effectively.

Given this apparent desire for social interaction, the importance of social exchanges in our society, and the difficulties that autistic people have in this regard, a major priority must be given to social skills training. A highly structured, very specific social skills training program is required, given the nature of the difficulties and the ways in which autistic people learn best. Specific behavioral social skills training programs have been described using modeling, behavioral rehearsal, and extensive feedback (Kanner, 1946; Rutter, 1978). A program applying similar principles has been used with learning-disabled children (LaGreca & Mesibov, 1979), and has shown some promise for use with autistic people as well. Though promising, most of these programs are designed for higher functioning, verbal autistic adolescents and adults. Until proven otherwise it may be assumed that those without verbal skills have similar social needs and desires. Social skills programs developed for more verbally oriented autistic people should be adapted to those persons without expressive language as well.

Although the already-described process for teaching autistic people social and interpersonal skills shows considerable promise, it does not specify what skills should be taught. However, there is literature on social problems of autistic people suggesting that developing empathy, lessening rigidity, and decreasing social distance might be important skills to emphasize. DesLauriers (1978) has written on the lack of empathy in autistic adolescents and adults, using the example of an autistic adult describing his feelings at a funeral: "I stood there . . . and I knew that I should feel sadness and compassion, but I couldn't really feel it!" (p. 222). The rigidity often characterizing older autistic people makes it hard for them to meet people's needs and also for others to adjust to them. Although there is some indication that community-based programs help reduce this rigidity, more specific training in this area is needed. The social distance that autistic adults maintain is another concern. They often focus on themselves, appearing to be in a world of their own. Their tendency to obviously exclude others interferes with satisfying social contacts.

Any social skills training efforts should take into account characteristic difficulties with empathy, rigidity, and social distance. In addition, common behavior problems must also be addressed if these efforts are to be effective.

Vocational Training and Employment Opportunities

Community-based programs for autistic adolescents and adults can not be successful unless the employment picture improves dramatically. In order to function in a community autistic adolescents and adults need worthwhile and productive daytime activities which can only be provided through increased employment training and work opportunities. Presently the employment prospects for autistic people are somewhat bleak. The Maudsley (Bartak & Rutter, 1976), Creak (1963), and Kanner (1949) populations each found only about 15% of their clients in competitive employment, suggesting that appropriate vocational opportunities are not being provided for about 85% of the autistic population.

A major problem seems to be the U.S. government's main agency for training handicapped people, the Department of Health and Human Services' Vocational Rehabilitation Division. Although efforts are being made to change this agency's system, it is presently designed for people needing only short-term help to become fully employed. Unfortunately this is not an appropriate model for autistic people who need long-term training to achieve their maximum potential which, even after extensive training, is not always full employment. A change in the system is certainly needed to provide long-term training to help people progress as far as their capabilities allow.

Rutter (1978) described several other changes that are needed as well. These involve meeting the employment needs of autistic people more appropriately by providing specific training and making adjustments in certain employment situations. Appropriate training should include teaching older autistic people to adhere to work routines, adapt to changes, and avoid socially embarrassing behaviors. Accommodations in the work situation should include the establishment of predictable routines, day-to-day contact with a limited number of people, supervisors who are willing and able to assert personal guidance and control, and many more on-the-job training experiences. The final point is particularly important because even successful autistic people usually have a series of failures prior to their employment successes (Rutter, 1978).

Finally, another important vocational need is for staff to accompany autistic clients into employment situations in order to help them make all the necessary adjustments. One model describes these staff as trainer-advocates (see Chapter 7), who first learn a job and work routine themselves and then teach these to an autistic client. The trainer-advocate remains with the autistic client in the employment setting until the client has learned to perform the routines. This appears to be an especially effective model for higher level autistic people because of their ability to follow relatively complex routines once having learned them.

Aggression

As noted earlier, aggression in autistic adolescents and adults shows no apparent increase over childhood aggression; however, the problem of aggressive behaviors becomes much more compelling as autistic people grow older. The major reasons for this are that as adolescents and adults autistic people are physically larger and their aggressive outbursts can be much more destructive. In addition the school and vocational settings where autistic adolescents and adults typically spend their days are much less able or willing to cope with aggressive behaviors.

Bemporad (1979) suggests that aggressive outbursts in autistic adolescents and adults might be motivated by their inability to understand and successfully master their environments. As an example he quotes one higher functioning autistic adolescent: "According to Jerry, his childhood experience could be summarized as consisting of two predominant experiential states: confusion and terror. A recurrent theme that ran through all of Jerry's recollections was that of living in a frightening world presenting painful stimuli that could not be mastered. Noises were unbearably loud, smells overpowering. Nothing seemed constant; everything was unpredictable and strange. . . . He was also frightened of other children, fearing that they might hurt him in some way. He could never predict or understand their behavior" (p. 192).

Although we might understand the incredible frustrations that lead to aggressive behaviors in autistic adolescents and adults, we must still develop more effective ways of working with aggression. Successfully coping with the problem of aggressive behaviors in autistic adolescents and adults requires managing aggressive behaviors, reducing the frequency of occurrence, and developing greater understanding of these behaviors by the community.

Behavior-modification techniques, applying basic principles of learning (Hilgard & Bower, 1966), have been effective in managing aggressive behaviors in severely handicapped people. When applied systematically and consistently these techniques have generally been able to control the aggressive behaviors of autistic people. However, when working with autistic adolescents and adults greater use of positive reinforcement techniques is needed (Favell, 1977). This is important because of the difficulties involved in punishing physically large clients, and also the well-documented drawbacks of punishment procedures including negative public reactions, aggression, and therapist unwillingness to use these procedures (Foxx & Azrin, 1972; Hughes & Davis, 1980; Ulrich & Azrin, 1962).

Although not as widely known as techniques for managing aggressive behaviors, some ways of reducing aggression have proven useful as well. Because one source of aggression in autistic people is their constant confusion and resulting anxiety, efforts to structure their environments should reduce these feelings and consequent aggressive behaviors. Biofeedback techniques also appear promising for reducing aggression. Schroeder, Peterson, Solomon, and Artley (1977) showed that EMG feedback can reduce self-injurious behaviors by inducing relaxation in a severely handicapped, nonverbal client. They suggest that muscle relaxation is incompatible with self-injurious behaviors. A similar incompatibility should occur between muscle relaxation and aggression. Hughes and Davis (1980), using biofeedback with a higher functioning client, also saw improvement in aggressive behaviors. They suggest that more verbally oriented, structured relaxation procedures might be effective with verbal autistic people.

Finally, a better understanding of aggressive behaviors in autistic people on the part of nonhandicapped citizens is also necessary. Although several techniques hold much promise for managing and reducing aggression these behaviors will still occur to some extent, and therefore nonhandicapped citizens must learn more about them. They must learn that in the rare instances in which aggression occurs it is not motivated or representative of hostility or irrationality, but is rather a part of the frustration of autism and the terrible anxiety and confusion that accompanies it. Communicating this understanding along with applying the positive management and relaxation techniques hold the most promise for dealing with aggression in community-based programs.

Sexuality

The development of community-based programs following the principle of normalization (Wolfensberger, 1972) has produced an increased emphasis on questions of sexuality for autistic adolescents and adults. Major concerns have come from two sources: communities fearing the sexuality of autistic people, and advocates wanting to assure that autistic people are allowed to exercise their sexual rights. Balancing community and individual rights has been very difficult indeed.

Communities' fears that the sexuality of autistic people will disrupt their neighborhoods and endanger their children is a most important issue. These fears, plus concerns that group homes for handicapped people will lower property values, are the major reasons why many communities oppose these programs (Keating, 1979). Advocates for autistic people must confront these concerns because, ultimately, community-based programs will not succeed without community support and assistance. There are some effective strategies for enlisting community support. First, it is important to maintain a continual dialogue with members of the community as a means of educating them and providing a forum when problems arise. Participating in civic groups, having open-houses, and organizing a neighborhood advisory group are ways of starting and maintaining such a dialogue. Second, specific behaviors can be taught to residents to minimize possible conflicts with the community over sexuality. These include appearing in public only when fully dressed, masturbating only in the privacy of one's room, and learning to touch and hug only people whom one knows very well. Obviously there are many other important behaviors that must be taught as well.

The problem of teaching autistic adolescents and adults how to handle and enjoy their own sexuality is also important. To date most of the literature on sexuality and handicapped people has not been directly applicable to autistic people (Fischer, Krajicek, & Borthick, 1973; Kempton, 1975). More recently a program for teaching sex education to autistic people has appeared (Lieberman & Melone, 1979), and this represents an encouraging beginning. However, much more is needed, addressing a wider variety of concerns and problems which would be applicable to the total range of autistic people.

In addition to working with communities and developing more programs, the issue of sexuality and handicapped people requires us to reexamine our personal values and how they might or might not apply to autistic people. Because most autistic people will not form our society's traditional sexual unions consisting of marriage and a family, we must evaluate our feelings about possible alternatives, weighing the needs of autistic people for appropriate sexual outlets against the values and morals of society. For example, one issue of concern in several group homes involves homosexual relationships among clients. While some people do not want to further alienate the handicapped from the mainstream of society by allowing these relationships to continue, others are reluctant to force these residents to give up one of the few relationships available to them (Mesibov, Note 2). How we react to the alternative sexual behaviors that will surely emerge from community-based residential programs is another issue of great importance.

Role of the Family

A clearer description of the family's role in the treatment of autistic adolescents and adults is also needed. Recent approaches (Schopler & Reichler, 1971) have emphasized the value of involving families in the treatment of their autistic children. Although the Schopler and Reichler model has been effective in working with parents of younger autistic children, it must be recognized that families of autistic children do not have the resources or energy to pursue such intensive treatment efforts throughout the lives of their children (Sullivan, 1977).

A less intensive, though meaningful, role for parents of autistic adolescents and adults should be delineated. This role might include planning and developing the resources their children will need, and monitoring these programs once established. Estate planning is one of the first tasks for families of autistic adolescents and adults in assuming this new role. The estate plan should provide for all monetary and material goods in a way that will not jeopardize the handicapped person's eligibility to participate in community-based residential and vocational programs. Parents will undoubtedly have to consult a lawyer who is experienced in these matters to carry out this task.

Families of autistic adolescents and adults can also help establish the community-based programs that will be needed for their children. This can involve work with local chapters of the National Society for Autistic Children or other groups which are developing these much-needed programs. Once these programs are established, parents must continually monitor them to be sure they remain consistent with their original mandates.

Finally, parents can assume the role of general advocate. Because all the necessary programs for autistic adolescents and adults will not be available in the foreseeable future there will be a continual need for advocacy on the local, state, and national levels. Parents have always been the most energetic and effective advocates that handicapped people have had, and will need to continue this work if their goals are to be achieved.

CONCLUSION

A review of the sparse literature on adolescents and adults with autism suggests that some improvement in their skills and behavior occurs during childhood. Unfortunately the improvement is unable to keep pace with the increasing demands that society places upon an individual as he/she approaches adulthood, especially when that individual has autism. The role of parents and professionals must therefore be twofold. First, we must continue to work on developing essential skills, using improved techniques and a greater understanding of what constitutes survival skills, as these become available. Second, we must continue to work in our communities, helping existing programs to make the accommodations necessary for autistic people to succeed and developing new programs when necessary. We hope the combination of improved skills and increasingly flexible and innovative programs will allow autistic adolescents and adults to live more productive and rewarding lives in their communities.

REFERENCES

Ando, H., & Yoshimura, I. Effects of age on communication skill levels and prevalence of maladaptive behaviors in autistic and mentally retarded children. *Journal of Autism and Developmental Disorders*, 1979, *9*, 83–93.

Ando, H., Yoshimura, I., & Wakabayashi, S. Effects of age on adaptive behavior levels and academic skill levels in autistic and mentally retarded children. *Journal of Autism and Developmental Disorders*, 1980, *10*, 173–184.

Bartak, L., & Rutter, M. Differences between mentally retarded and normally intelligent autistic children. *Journal of Autism and Childhood Schizophrenia*, 1976, *6*, 109–120.

Bemporad, J. R. Adult recollections of a formerly autistic child. *Journal of Autism and Developmental Disorders*, 1979, *9*, 179–197.

Brown, J. L. Adolescent development of children with infantile psychosis. *Seminars in Psychiatry*, 1969, *1*, 79–89.

Creak, E. M. Childhood psychosis: A review of 100 cases. *British Journal of Psychiatry*, 1963, *109*, 84–89.

DeMyer, M. K. *Parents and children in autism*. Washington, D.C.: Winston, 1979.

DeMyer, M. K., Barton, S., DeMyer, W. E., Norton, J. A., Allen, J., & Steele, R. Prognosis in autism: A follow-up study. *Journal of Autism and Childhood Schizophrenia*, 1973, *3*, 199–246.

DesLauriers, A. M. The cognitive-affective dilemma in early infantile autism: The case of Clarence. *Journal of Autism and Childhood Schizophrenia*, 1978, *8*, 219–229.

Deykin, E. Y., & MacMahon, B. The incidence of seizures among children with autistic symptoms. *American Journal of Psychiatry*, 1979, *136*, 1310–1312.

Eisenberg, L. The autistic child in adolescence. *American Journal of Psychiatry*, 1956, *112*, 607–612.

Favell, J. E. *The power of positive reinforcement: A handbook of behavior modification*. Springfield, Ill.: Charles C Thomas, 1977.

Fischer, H. L., Krajicek, M. J., & Borthick, W. A. *Sex education for the developmentally disabled: A guide for parents, teachers, and professionals*. Baltimore: University Park Press, 1973.

Foxx, R. M., & Azrin, N. H. Restitution: A method of eliminating aggressive-disruptive behavior of retarded and brain-damaged patients. *Behavior Research and Therapy*, 1972, *1*, 305–312.

Grossman, H. J. *Manual on terminology and classification in mental retardation*. Washington, D.C.: American Association on Mental Deficiency, 1973.

Hilgard, E. G., & Bower, G. H. *Theories of learning*. New York: Appleton-Century-Crofts, 1966.

Hughes, H., & Davis, R. Treatment of aggressive behavior: The effect of EMG response discrimination biofeedback training. *Journal of Autism and Developmental Disorders*, 1980, *10*, 193–202.

Kanner, L. Irrelevant and metaphorical language in early infantile autism. *American Journal of Psychiatry*, 1946, *103*, 242–245.

Kanner, L. Problems of nosology and psychodynamics of early infantile autism. *American Journal of Orthopsychiatry*, 1949, *19*, 416–426.

Kanner, L., Rodriguez, A., & Ashenden, B. How far can autistic children go in matters of social adaptation? *Journal of Autism and Childhood Schizophrenia*, 1972, *2*, 9–33.

Keating, R. The war against the mentally retarded. *New York*, Sept. 17, 1979, pp. 87–94.

Kempton, W. *A teacher's guide to sex education for persons with learning disabilities.* North Scituate, Mass.: Duxbury Press, 1975.

LaGreca, A. M., & Mesibov, G. B. Social skills intervention with learning disabled children: Selecting skills and implementing training. *Journal of Clinical Child Psychology*, 1979, *8*, 234–241.

Lieberman, D. A., & Melone, M. B. *Sexuality and social awareness.* New Haven, Conn.: Benhaven Press, 1979.

Lotter, V. Follow-up studies. In *Autism: A reappraisal of concepts and treatment* (M. Rutter & E. Schopler, eds.), New York: Plenum Press, 1978.

McCarver, R. B., & Craig, E. M. Placement of the retarded in the community: Prognosis and outcome. In *International review of research in mental retardation (Vol. 7).* (N. R. Ellis, ed.), New York: Academic Press, 1974.

Mittler, P., Gillies, S., & Jukes, E. Prognosis in psychotic children: Report of follow-up study. *Journal of Mental Deficiency Research*, 1966, *10*, 73–83.

National Association for Retarded Citizens. *Educating the 24-hour retarded child.* Arlington, Tex.: National Association for Retarded Citizens, 1975.

Ricks, D. M., & Wing, L. Language, communication, and the use of symbols in normal and autistic children. *Journal of Autism and Childhood Schizophrenia*, 1975, *5*, 191–221.

Rutter, M. Autistic children: Infancy to adulthood. *Seminars in Psychiatry*, 1970, *2*, 435–450.

Rutter, M. Developmental issues and prognosis. In *Autism: A reappraisal of concepts and treatment.* (M. Rutter & E. Schopler, eds.), New York: Plenum, 1978.

Rutter, M., & Bartak, L. Special educational treatment of autistic children: A comparative study. II. Follow-up findings and implications for services. *Journal of Child Psychology and Psychiatry*, 1973, *14*, 241–270.

Rutter, M., & Schopler, E. (Eds.), *Autism: A reappraisal of concepts and treatment.* New York: Plenum Press, 1978.

Rutter, M., Greenfeld, D., & Lockyer, L. A five to fifteen year follow-up study of infantile psychosis. II. Social and behavioral outcome. *British Journal of Psychiatry*, 1967, *113*, 1183–1199.

Schopler, E., & Reichler, R. J. Parents as co-therapists in the treatment of psychotic children. *Journal of Autism and Childhood Schizophrenia*, 1971, *1*, 87–102.

Schroeder, S. R., Peterson, C. R., Solomon, L. J., & Artley, J. J. EMG feedback and the contingent restraint of self-injurious behavior among the severely retarded: Two case illustrations, *Behavior Therapy*, 1977, *8*, 738–741.

Stokes, K. S. Planning for the future of a severely handicapped autistic child. *Journal of Autism and Childhood Schizophrenia*, 1977, *7*, 288–297.

Sullivan, R. C. Parents speak. *Journal of Autism and Childhood Schizophrenia*, 1977, *7*, 287–288.

Ulrich, R. E., & Azrin, N. H. Reflexive fighting in response to aversive stimulation. *Journal of Experimental Analysis of Behavior*, 1962, *5*, 511–520.

Wing, L. *Autistic children: A guide for parents and professionals.* New York: Brunner/Mazel, 1972.

Wolfensberger, W. *The principle of normalization in human services.* Toronto: National Institute on Mental Retardation, 1972.

REFERENCE NOTES

1. Mesibov, G. B., & Shea, V. *Social and interpersonal problems of autistic adolescents and adults*. Paper presented at the meeting of the Souteastern Psychological Association, Washington, D.C., March 1980.
2. Mesibov, G. B. *Protecting the rights of mentally retarded citizens in community-based settings*. Paper presented at the conference on Legal Trends and Issues in Developmental Disabilities, Jackson, Miss., September 1979.

II

Individual Needs

4

Language and Communication Needs of Adolescents with Autism

CATHERINE LORD and PATRICIA J. O'NEILL

Adolescence is a time of transition for youngsters with autism as well as for others. Greater interest in social interaction, acquisition of basic self-care behaviors, and familiarity with the requirements of being in a group and in a school classroom place autistic adolescents in a different position in terms of "readiness to learn" than they could have taken 4 or 5 years earlier. In addition increasing concern about vocational skills and potential for community living often influence the goals and expectations set for autistic adolescents by families and professionals.

Changes in expectations and concerns about language and communication may occur gradually as the child becomes an adolescent. The usual period of transition is between the ages of 10 and 15, when previously established perspectives on goals and methods used in language teaching are reassessed. This shift may occur for language programming in particular because communication is a necessary activity for everyone. Unlike riding a bicycle or handling money, communication cannot be avoided or carried out for the autistic adolescent by someone else, no matter how difficult language is for the youngster.

In addition so little is understood about how normally developing children learn to communicate that much of the early years of language

CATHERINE LORD ● Department of Psychology, Glenrose Hospital, Edmonton, Alberta, Canada T56 0B7. PATRICIA J. O'NEILL ● St. Paul Program for Autistic Children and Social Development, St. Paul, Minnesota 55119.

training is often spent in a search for the "trigger" that will set off the nearly miraculous sequence of language acquisition that occurs for most young children as infants and toddlers. By the time a child with autism has reached older school age or adolescence it is generally clear whether or not the autistic child has entered this sequence. This is not to say that after adolescence autistic children stop learning communication skills. Rather, by the time an autistic child reaches adolescence parents and professionals are faced with the knowledge that in most cases what the youngster has already learned is all that he will learn. By adolescence there is less hope that stimulation will at that point set off a self-perpetuating process of language development. With the recognition of these limitations, priorities in communication training often shift from teaching linguistic elements and hoping that a flexible language system capable of conveying complex ideas to a wide audience (i.e., spoken and written English) will emerge, to helping individual youngsters communicate as readily and clearly as possible with familiar people in whatever ways they can. Hence programming becomes much more pragmatic in terms of immediate needs. Often more functional goals might have been appropriate even earlier, but for many different reasons they were not put into operation.

On the other hand, in the case of the small proportion of autistic children who acquired a truly productive, flexible language system by adolescence, the youngsters will usually have already learned much of the content of most language programs. In this case programming for language may shift from using a normal developmental sequence of grammar to more academic instruction in reading and writing or to emphasizing social goals concerning the use of language in a variety of situations or to both academics and social skills.

The particular focus of this chapter, communication and language in adolescents with autism, concerns how to make decisions about appropriate programs to meet the needs of this particular age group. First we present a brief review of research concerning the language skills of adolescents with autism, followed by three case studies. This section concludes with suggestions of criteria for evaluating the appropriateness of a communication program for individual children, given what we know about the communication skills of autistic adolescents in general. Second, general approaches taken by language training programs are described, with a discussion of several representative programs and the extent to which each satisfies our proposed criteria for autistic adolescents. The third, concluding section contains a discussion of several new directions in the study of language and autism.

CHARACTERISTICS OF LANGUAGE AND COMMUNICATION IN ADOLESCENTS WITH AUTISM

Fewer than 10% of autistic individuals have language skills approximating those of normally developing children of the same chronological age (Wing, 1976). In fact most autistic children and adolescents have language skills that are significantly below their mental as well as chronological ages. Since the greatest proportion of autistic individuals are moderately to severely retarded, one could therefore infer that the language skills of most adolescents with autism are more limited than most normally developing preschool children. In fact epidemiological studies typically describe about half the population of individuals with autism as being mute or having no communicative speech (Lotter, 1966, 1967). While "communicative speech" is itself an ambiguous term, at the least this statement implies that most autistic children do not readily and clearly communicate in conventional ways outside of very specific situations.

Language performance below that of nonverbal cognitive skills and a limited ability to participate in social relationships are two deficits relating to communication that are shared by all autistic adolescents. However, how these deficits are manifested differs greatly across individuals. While language ability is not perfectly predicted by intelligence, performance on nonverbal or verbal intelligence tests is highly related to eventual or current use of language. Autistic children with IQs above 70 have a much greater chance of acquiring useful language than autistic children with IQs below 50 (Bartak & Rutter, 1976). The language of autistic children with IQs below 50 is typically very limited. Wing and Gould (1979) found that 63% of severely retarded autistic youngsters had language comprehension ages below 20 months. The language of children with IQs between 50 and 70 is more variable in level, but even some adolescents who perform in the "normal" range of intelligence on nonverbal intelligence tests may have more restricted use of language than normally developing 3- or 4-year-olds.

When autistic youngsters do learn to speak or to sign, they typically follow normal patterns of learning in their use of word order and different grammatical structures, at least as can be measured in cross-sectional studies (Bartolucci, Pierce, & Streiner, 1980). However, the age at which these aspects of language are learned is typically much later than for other children. By older school age or adolescence some autistic youngsters have learned grammatical inflections and morphemes (such as past tense -*ed* or the preposition *in*), though autistic children show greater variability both over time within an individual child and between children than typically occurs in other populations (Pierce & Bartolucci, 1977). In an unpublished study (O'Neill & Lord, Note 1) we found that even severely retarded autistic adolescents produced a surprising variety of semantic relations (e.g., agent, action, recipient) during their relevantly infrequent attempts at spontaneous speech. Though these adolescents used a very limited number of grammatical structures in their sign or speech to serve only a few communicative functions, they varied the semantic relations they used from 10 to 20 different meanings. For higher functioning adolescents use of semantic and syntactic aspects of language can be quite complex. One study found that the language of a group of autistic adolescents with normal or close to normal nonverbal intelligence was virtually indistinguishable from the language of a group of dysphasic teenagers matched in age, though presumably both groups were more limited than normal controls (Cantwell, Baker, & Rutter, 1978).

Autistic youngsters of all levels of intelligence may echo words and sentences they have heard, though there is some evidence that echolalia is often outgrown by adolescence (Rutter, 1977). Echolalia can occur with varying degrees of communication intent. It can follow immediately after the sentence it repeats or occur days later, as in a child repeating a commercial. It can be exact or "modified" by changes in words or structure. Echolalia can be problematic for a number of reasons. Autistic adolescents may actually use echolalic phrases that they themselves do not understand, which can cause others to overestimate the youngsters' comprehension abilities. On the other hand echolalia is not always completely meaningless. An adolescent may use an echolalic or memorized phrase such as "Come on down" in an almost appropriate way to ask someone to come to him quickly. During adolescence echolalia may become less a linguistic problem and more a social or vocational one. A person who loudly repeats television commercials to himself is not very welcome in a sheltered workshop or a movie theater. Sometimes adolescents with autism will have complicated, though often concrete, fantasies (e.g., about building elevators, being a pharmacist) that they will talk about at great length. When echolalic phrases are mixed in to these self-directed conversations, echolalia may be misinterpreted as evidence of auditory hallucinations or delusions.

In some ways the language deficits associated with autism may be more apparent in comprehension, where the listener has to anticipate what the speaker intends, than in production. Sometimes echolalia and the use of rote phrases can mask the extent to which a child really possesses different language structures, but all except a few of the more high-functioning autistic children show comprehension deficits. In a recent study (Lord & Allen, Note 2) we found that autistic adolescents ranging in age from 12 to 16 years and in nonverbal IQ from 35 to 65 typically performed less well on a task requiring comprehension of simple sentences (e.g., "Roll the apple to the dog") than nonautistic retarded children matched on chronological and mental age who in turn performed less well than a group of normally developing 2-year-olds. Sentences with more than four elements (i.e., action–attribute–object–recipient, "Push the big truck to the frog") were more difficult for most of the autistic subjects. Scores on the Peabody Picture Vocabulary Test, a measure of receptive vocabulary, were also lower, on the average, for the autistic adolescents (mean score = 3.8 years) than for their nonautistic retarded schoolmates (mean score = 4.9 years), though higher than those of the 2-year-old normal control group.

Language comprehension in autistic individuals has also been shown to be affected by their limited use of semantic or knowledge factors about the probability of events (i.e., that "the mother is changing the baby's diapers" is more likely than "the baby is changing the mother's diapers") (Tager-Flusberg, in press). Most normally developing children would find it easier to identify a picture depicting the first than the second sentence. For autistic youngsters one might expect less difference. Whether this pattern occurs because of limited knowledge (e.g., autistic children may not know that mothers as opposed to babies typically change diapers), or because of the children's failure to apply their knowledge about everyday events to the particular task at hand, is not clear.

In this same vein autistic children have been described as literal and concrete, that is, as failing to move beyond the meaning of specific words to use social context to understand colloquial expressions or metaphors (e.g., they might take expressions like "Hold on" or "Keep it down" literally). One secondary result of these difficulties in both using immediate context and applying general knowledge to facilitate comprehension is that the vocabularies of autistic adolescents may often be quite limited and quite spotty. One cannot assume because an autistic youngster knows the words "ambulance" and "snowmobile" that he necessarily knows the more general terms "truck" or "bus."

One could ask how specific to spoken language are the deficits of autistic children. Communication is by definition a social behavior as well as a cognitive skill. Unfortunately autistic adolescents have difficulty with nonverbal social aspects of language as well as with the more cognitive or linguistic structures. Bartak and his colleagues (Bartak, Rutter, & Cox, 1975) found that when compared to dysphasic youngsters, autistic 4- to 10-year-olds used and understood gestures less well than the other children. Autistic children have been shown to use different strategies for recognizing faces than other children (Langdell, 1978). Such studies suggest that there may be very basic differences in the ways autistic children process nonverbal messages as well as language.

Occasionally autistic children are shown to have significantly greater abilities in an alternative communication mode such as writing or signing than in speech. Yet in most cases comprehension and production remain limited. Only 6% of the children studied by DeMyer (1979) were described as performing at age level on paper-and-pencil tasks. Those children who could write at all tended to be much better at copying or writing from memory than in generating novel communicative sentences. In another study high-functioning autistic children had better word recognition skills than dysphasic children, but had greater difficulty in reading for comprehension (Bartak et al., 1975). Some autistic adolescents are very adept at phonetic reading, but like other autistic youngsters their comprehension tends to be limited (Cobrinik, 1974). Similarly, sign language has given some autistic children a method of communicating in addition to or instead of speech (Bonvillian & Nelson, 1976; Fulwiler & Fouts, 1976; Creedon, Note 3). However, both vocabulary and sentence structure tend to remain limited even for children who create their own novel utterances using signs (Shaeffer, Kollinzas, Musil, & McDowell, 1977; Creedon, Note 3). Word boards and picture systems have also been useful in providing essentially mute autistic children with ways of initiating communication (LaVigna, 1977; Schopler, Reichler, & Lansing, 1975); however, there is no evidence that in most cases they radically *alter* the level of the adolescents' basic understanding of language. One implication of this finding is that alternative systems need to be evaluated very carefully to make sure that the child is using them in ways that add to his use of speech and gestures. Sometimes progress in learning an alternative system consists simply of a child's working to reach the level he has already attained using more conventional methods. If this progress allows him more opportunity or flexibility to communicate, then it is worth working toward; if not, even clear acquisition curves do not prove the usefulness of the program.

Case Studies

In order to illustrate the preceding brief review of the characteristics of language in autistic adolescents, three youngsters, whose abilities might be considered representative of the varying abilities and needs of autistic adolescents, are described below.

Sally is a 13-year-old girl with autism. She has no speech at all and cannot imitate or produce speech sounds on demand. She is severely retarded and has extremely limited motor skills. Sally understands oral speech up to about three-term directions or statements (e.g., "Get the raincoat for John"). She can nod or shake her head yes or no when prompted. Sally has a wordboard (with a 20- to 30-word vocabulary) which she uses to communicate such things as "water," "wagon," and "bathroom." She uses this board at home to ask for food and at school if she is specifically directed to go get a word. Nevertheless, at school at least, her primary method of communication is to attract a teacher's attention by standing nearby and shaking her head and torso back and forth violently. Once an adult is watching her, she glances back and forth at the teacher and the desired object or location until he guesses what she wants. She also attempts to communicate with other children by grabbing their clothing and placing her face immediately in front of theirs and making soft grunting sounds. Sally lives at home with her parents and two sisters. Because of her developing sociability, Sally will be transferred out of the autism class and into a class for moderately retarded adolescents next year.

Johnny is a 16-year-old moderately retarded boy with autism. He speaks only rarely. When he does talk, it is in a monotone with very poor articulation so that even people who know him well find it very difficult to understand him. His utterances vary from single words to longer, often routinized sentences such as "Could I please have a drink of water?" His language is repetitive, primarily consisting of sentences built around three or four sentence frames such as "Could I please have . . ." and "I want X, please." Like Sally, Johnny's comprehension is limited to three- or four-term sentences; however, his receptive vocabulary is somewhat higher and similar to that of most 3-year-olds. Unlike Sally, however, Johnny clearly has some productive speech and can use his language system for communication. On the other hand self-initiated language is still quite rare for Johnny. Very seldom does he speak to anyone except his primary teacher and even then he usually makes requests in a very circumscribed situation (e.g., asking for food during snack time). Johnny lives in a group home with four autistic adolescents. His group home managers feel that he is too withdrawn; they would very much like to see him talk more.

Michael is a 15-year-old boy with autism who performs in the borderline range of mental retardation on nonverbal intelligence tests. Michael speaks clearly and in quite sophisticated sentences. He uses grammatical inflections and complex structures such as relative clauses, though he occasionally leaves off plurals and makes errors in the use of pronouns. He has the receptive vocabulary of most 10-year-olds, and can understand quite long (five- to six-term) directions. However, Michael still has some difficulty in comprehending language when he is in a group and when a series of directions is given rapidly. He can read and write at about the fourth-grade level. He spends part of his day in a class for mildly retarded adolescents and part in a class for generally lower-functioning autistic adolescents. Michael's language problems relate more to academic and social issues than to linguistic structure. He has a great deal of difficulty understanding his fourth-grade science and social studies texts. He has difficulty with any but the most concrete, fill-in-the-blank written work. Socially, Michael is interested in several topics (e.g., game shows, bus routes) and questions (e.g., "Where do you keep your . . ?") that becomes very repetitious for familiar people and are not viewed as very appropriate by strangers. Michael has difficulty judging the appropriateness of his social behavior and in initiating interaction in ways that are suitable given his age and size. He occasionally launches into song during conversation and has recently begun to ask friends and acquaintances rather naïve but embarrassingly personal questions that seem to relate to sexual interests. Michael lives at home with his mother and 11-year-old sister. He enjoys the freedom of the neighborhood and spends the late afternoons, when his mother is still at work, hanging around the local shopping center.

Criteria for Language Programs

How would one evaluate potential language programs for these three youngsters who represent typical autistic adolescents? The goal of the programs is increased communication, so in a way success should be measured purely on whether the program allows the adolescents greater flexibility in conveying their needs and ideas to other people and a better understanding of others' needs and ideas. Learning a particular communication task is not enough. In addition, how this communication is achieved is relatively unimportant. One primary criterion for evaluating potential might then be that whatever is taught should be a behavior that can be acquired quickly. For the two lower-functioning youngsters there is simply too much for them to learn in too short a time to spend 6 months teaching a single word or sign. For Michael, the more highly skilled adolescent, there is already evidence that he can learn relatively quickly and so there is no reason not to select methods that use his strengths to help him communicate.

As shown in Table 1, a second criterion could be whether the behavior

Table 1
Criteria for Language Programs

---

1. Can the behavior be acquired relatively quickly?
2. Is the behavior immediately useful to the child or to the people with whom he spends his time?
   a. Does it allow the adolescent to express his own ideas, to express his needs and preferences, or to learn new things?
   b. Does the modality of the communication system fit into the adolescent's established pattern of behaviors and preferences?
   c. What social factors influence the possible usefulness of the communication method?
3. Does the adolescent *use* the behavior *to communicate?*
   a. Does he use it in his own spontaneous communications or only when prompted to do so? How specific a prompt is required to elicit the behavior?
   b. Does the behavior occur outside the situation in which it was taught?
   c. Can the adolescent use the behavior flexibly, modifying it slightly across situations?

---

taught is immediately useful to the child. Will it allow him to express ideas he already possesses? Will it allow him to express his needs or wants? Will it allow him to learn? For Johnny, who has very little interest in the weather or group sports, teaching him the names of favorite objects or their locations (e.g., kitchen, closet, bathroom) may be much more useful in terms of his needs than learning weather conditions or verbs to describe different motor movements that he has no interest in making. For Michael, who would like very much to be able to talk to other teen-agers, helping him extend the topics of his sentences to appropriate sub-jects such as group sports or even the weather may be more important than changing his grammatical structure or teaching him new words.

We can ask if the modality of the communication system is appro-priate given an adolescent's other abilities. For Michael and Johnny the modality of speech is already established. For Sally, however, modality is still an open question. Picture systems may not be used productively by highly distractible youngsters such as Sally, who would have difficulty sorting through a group of pictures to select the correct one. Sally may be able to learn signs that her teacher could identify in a one-to-one teaching situation, but her extremely limited motor skills make it unlikely that others would understand her signs. Very general gestures may be the modality that allows her to communicate with the greatest number of people. Nevertheless, pictures and signs may be worth using as well in specific situations with different demands.

In addition we can ask what changes will enhance the usefulness of the communication modality the adolescent already uses. Increasing the length of Johnny's sentences theoretically would make it somewhat easier for him to communicate clearly, except that his poor articulation is much worse with lengthy sentences. In the long run several single words, one at a time, plus backup gestures may prove much more useful to others who want to understand Johnny's speech than will lengthening his sentences.

Social factors also contribute greatly to the potential usefulness of a communicative behavior. For Michael, understanding the social consequences of some of his inappropriate questions may be a far more significant thing for him to learn than correct use of verb forms. Johnny may need systematic exposure to social situations in which he can use the language he already has, far more than he needs to learn more language to be used in situations that rarely occur. For Sally, who has become increasingly social and peer-directed in the last few years, one might want to help her shift from clothes grabbing to handshaking while also teaching some social behaviors to follow up her initial attempts to get a classmate's attention.

The final criterion in Table 1 is an empirical one: Does the new behavior work? Is it used by the adolescent to increase his understanding of others' communications? Does he use it in his spontaneous communications? If so, does he use it flexibly; does he combine it with other familiar behaviors? If not, will he use the behavior reliably if prompted to do so? Teaching Michael to begin a conversation with a stranger by introducing himself has little value if he requires a teacher's prompting to keep him from talking about buses. If Sally uses her wordboard regularly and effectively at home to indicate her choice for a snack, the finding that she rarely gets above 75% correct in classroom word-to-food picture matching may not be very important. One implication of this criterion is clear: in order to assess changes in communication the behavior must be measured before, during, and after in the context in which it is supposed to occur. Knowing that Johnny can label 50 foods on Peabody cards can be useful information, but this measure is not a substitute for knowing if anyone ever refers to those foods in conversations with Johnny, and if so how he responds, or if Johnny ever uses the food names spontaneously outside the teaching situation.

CURRENT APPROACHES TO LANGUAGE INTERVENTION

Existing approaches to language intervention with autistic and other severely language-impaired individuals generally follow either nondevelopmental or developmental models. Nondevelopmental approaches emphasize teaching those aspects of language that will be particularly useful to the individual and will most quickly improve his or her communication skills (Goetz, Schuler, & Sailor, 1979; Schuler, 1980). Such approaches are less biased than other views on determining cognitive prerequisites to language learning. They may not necessarily follow the sequence of language acquisition found in normally developing children.

Nondevelopmental approaches are typically associated with the use of operant conditioning techniques to teach specific elements of adult language (Sulzbacher & Costello, 1970). In an effort to simplify learning, adult language is usually broken down into specific elements such as morphological rules or language concepts (e.g., size, color, possession) and taught in a sequence of steps (Guess, Sailor, & Baer, 1978; Lovaas, 1977). Intervention often consists of teaching targeted language elements in blocks of training trials within a highly structured teaching situation. Once mastery has been achieved on a specific target, attempts can then be made systematically to transfer or generalize its use to more natural settings.

Developmental approaches to language intervention often make some use of operant conditioning techniques, but within the pattern of language acquisition found in normally developing children (MacDonald & Horstmeier, 1978; McLean & Synder-McLean, 1978). Developmental approaches may emphasize various aspects of language for teaching. The primary psycholinguistic intervention has been to teach syntactical and grammatical rules used in language (Stremel & Waryas, 1974). Other interventions view language acquisition as closely linked to overall cognitive development (MacDonald, Blott, Gordon, Spiegel, & Hartmann, 1974; Miller, 1977). Such approaches emphasize the role of experience or knowledge that the individual brings to the language learning process. Like the processes of assimilation and accommodation in cognitive development, language intervention can be thought of as teaching new language skills that directly stem from the communication skills and knowledge the child already possesses (Morehead & Morehead, 1974).

A wide variety of nondevelopmental and developmental interventions have been used to teach both understanding and use of verbal language, as well as nonverbal alternatives, to autistic youngsters. Space does not allow an extensive review of these different interventions so we have selected a few representative programs to discuss in more detail.

Nondevelopmental Approaches

Over a 10-year period Lovaas (1977) used prompting and reinforcement techniques within a discrimination format to teach specific language skills to 20 nonverbal or echolalic autistic children. The first step of training involved establishing imitative speech in previously nonverbal children. The children were then taught to understand and use labels and more abstract concepts (e.g., pronominal relations and temporal cues) followed by the development of conversation, questioning, and grammatical skills.

The Functional Speech and Training Program (Guess et al., 1978) is designed to teach five dimensions of language: (1) reference or labeling; (2) control (requesting items, e.g., "I want X"); (3) self-extended control (requesting information about unknowns, e.g., "Where is X?"); (4) integration (spontaneous and conversational use); and (5) reception or understanding. These dimensions are taught in a series of 60 sequenced steps broken down into five content areas: labels for people and things, action, possession, color, and size and relation/location.

Data from selected subjects who have received intervention using either the Lovaas or Guess, Sailor, and Baer programs indicate that the rate of progress can vary greatly with individuals and that some steps are far more difficult (i.e., take more time to learn) than others. In some steps reported by Lovaas, thousands of trials were needed for children to learn concepts such as colors.

Given the time investment usually needed to establish speech and the age of the autistic adolescent, such programs may be of relatively little benefit to low-functioning or mute autistic adolescents like Sally, the girl described earlier, who do not already possess some formal language. Such intervention programs can be of value, however, in teaching autistic adolescents with some basic language skills to use and respond to specific language elements within a highly predictable, structured teaching situation.

Autistic adolescents like Michael and Johnny, who possess good rote memory skills or who have fairly sophisticated language concepts, can often progress rapidly through some steps of such programs, particularly those steps that deal with more concrete aspects of language such as labeling. However, other steps of the program that teach more complex or abstract concepts may have little real meaning for many adolescents with autism. For example, one step of the functional language program involves answering yes/no questions such as "Is this a X?" The ability to answer such questions correctly first requires that the individual know the name of the object and then be able to make a judgment about the validity of the question. Even though the answer requires only a simple one-word response, the ability to answer yes/no questions involves an understanding of more complex concepts than some later steps such as labeling colors. Some thought also needs to be given as to when (or ever) such questions are asked. Thus this aspect of the program may be appropriate (though perhaps unnecessary) with a verbal youngster like Michael but far less successful and useful for an adolescent like Johnny.

The importance of clear articulation should also not be underestimated. Some language-impaired adolescents whose speech is poorly articulated have reportedly had difficulties being understood by others even when they move through the sequence of such language programs. On the other hand in some cases improvement has been noted as the children progress through the program.

Neither of the programs incorporates any steps for transfering or generalizing the language elements taught to other settings. Only general instructions are available to facilitate the use of the language learned to more natural situations. Thus it is not at all clear that the programs would necessarily have any immediate use to the adolescents. A careful needs assessment might allow selecting those parts of programs relevant to the child's interests and environments. For high-functioning autistic adolescents with more language, like Michael, such intervention strategies may end up teaching very little he does not already know. The programs do not automatically address the autistic individual's fundamental problem in learning to use language for social communication. However, the programs do offer carefully thought-out, tried-and-tested series of behaviors that provide a place to start assessing social needs and usefulness.

Developmental Approaches

Psycholinguistic. Stremel and Waryas (1974) have developed an intervention program using behavioral learning strategies to teach syntactic and grammatical rules to individuals with minimal language skills. The program begins with one-to-one instruction to teach the understanding and use of nouns and verbs. The words are then combined to teach different syntactical rules, e.g., noun + verb, verb + object. Increasingly complex grammatical aspects of language are then taught such as pronouns, wh- questions, auxiliary verbs, and noun/verb tense agreement.

Even for the autistic adolescent with fairly developed language skills, the learning of syntactic and grammatical rules can be a difficult task. Such complex abstract rules may be useful primarily to those autistic individuals who can be expected to participate independently in the mainstream of society and who will need to be able to communicate with a wide range of different people. Grammatical inflections and complex rules probably do little to make oral communication itself much more efficient or clear when the communication describes immediate contexts or needs. However, an adolescent who leaves out word endings or makes obvious grammatical errors may be socially conspicuous and also have difficulty with language used outside of familiar contexts (i.e., writing and reading). Most autistic adolescents can rely on word order and the context provided by the immediate physical environment to help convey the meaning of his words to familiar people. The needs of the autistic individual can be communicated just as well with "drink water, please" (spoken as he stands near the sink) than by teaching the child elaborate grammatical rules to express in a complete sentence such as "I would like a drink of water, please." The primary value of the longer sentence is social, so that it becomes important only when the need to be polite is as great as the need to communicate.

Cognitive. The Environmental Language Intervention Program (MacDonald et al., 1974) was designed to teach young, language-delayed children to use semantic rules found in the early stages of language development in normal children (Bloom, 1970; Brown, 1973). Imitation, cued conversation, and play strategies are used to teach the understanding and use of semantic rules like action + object (e.g., "throw ball") and agent + action (e.g., "Daddy throw") within the context of the activity (i.e., as Daddy throws the ball). The program has been used with a variety of language-impaired individuals including autistic persons, who ranged in age from 1 to 30 years. Data from the program's use with six Down's syndrome preschool-age children indicates that the MLU (mean length of utterance) and the frequency and range of semantic relation increased following intervention in a clinic and at home. Parent reports and anecdotal records also indicate that the children spontaneously used the semantic relations they were taught.

O'Neill and Lord (Note 1) also used Stage I semantic relations (Brown, 1973) along with functions expressed in the early stage of normal language development (Halliday, 1975) as a basis for language intervention with six autistic individuals, four of whom were adolescents. Within the context of a familiar event, individual children were taught to express a new meaning (i.e., semantic relation) or function (i.e., social purpose), or were taught a new word to express a semantic relation or function already possessed. For example, one autistic adolescent was taught to express a new semantic relation (i.e., describing his own action) using a word ("open") and function (get permission) that he already used spontaneously. The youth was taught to use the new semantic relation by saying "open" as he asked if he could open his milk carton at lunch.

Following 4–8 weeks of intervention the specific aspects of language taught (i.e., words, semantic relations, or functions) were learned by all the children in the contexts in which they were presented. In addition the frequency of spontaneous utterances in general increased as measured by language samples obtained prior to intervention and at regular intervals during interventions. We hypothesized that the interventions had measurable effects rather quickly since the individuals were not required to learn an elaborate series of steps prior to using language within a communicative context.

Even though cognitively oriented approaches have been primarily designed for young children, such programs may be of some value to autistic adolescents with emerging language. The underlying strategy of using old knowledge to teach new knowledge can be used for autistic children and adolescents who function at any level. For the nonverbal, severely retarded, autistic adolescent like Sally this might mean taking a form of communication she already possesses (e.g., pulling the clothing of other children to attract their attention) and teaching her a "new" or more acceptable form of communication derived from that behavior (e.g., tapping another child on the shoulder). For those autistic adolescents like Johnny and Michael who already exhibit varying degrees of some formal language skills this might mean teaching more varied meanings or functions for the words they already possess, or teaching words that better express some familiar meanings or functions. Teaching adolescents with autism to use the aspects of language they already possess can help make their often rote, rigid use of language more flexible.

Teaching language within a context or activity that has meaning for the youngster facilitates spontaneous use of language. Contextual cues may provide useful information to help the child both understand and use language in a variety of settings. Directly teaching the child to use language within a meaningful context also helps those people to whom he is trying to communicate better understand his intent. Furthermore the child's parents and family can learn rather easily how to arrange activities that are part of the child's daily routine at home to teach important language skills.

ALTERNATIVE COMMUNICATION STRATEGIES

Many of the nondevelopmental and developmental intervention strategies already described have been adapted for use with autistic and other severely language-impaired children who do not speak at all. The development of nonspeech communication strategies becomes increasingly critical as the autistic child gets older and the likelihood of speech development lessens. Both manual and visual communication systems have been designed in an attempt to circumvent the complex processing requirements of spoken language.

The purpose of these systems is often to provide the mute youngster with an alternative to speech as a way of expressing himself. For many individuals, the adolescent's comprehension of the alternative system is no better than his understanding of speech, in which case comprehension of oral language provides access to far more people. On the other hand alternative modalities can allow a mute child a way of expressing his own needs or ideas. In some cases alternative systems (i.e., total communication) have also been used as a way of initiating or enhancing the acquisition of speech as well. Schaeffer et al. (1977) taught three 4- to 5-year-old autistic children signs and imitative speech in daily 4-hour sessions. Over the course of a year and a half the boys progressed from learning to produce spontaneous signs to producing spontaneous signed speech and finally to producing spontaneous speech.

Taking a different approach, LaVigna (1977) used errorless teaching procedures to train three 17- to 18-year-old nonverbal, severely retarded persons to discriminate three written word labels for foods. Following some 1,000–1,500 training trials these individuals learned to match the food word (e.g., "mint") to the appropriate food. Other investigators have reported teaching some higher functioning but mute individuals to communicate by typing or spelling out words with preformed letters (Schopler et al., 1975). The Non-Speech Language Intervention Program (Non-Slip) (Carrier & Peak, 1975) was developed to help severely retarded, nonverbal children communicate using abstract plastic shapes that represent syntactic structures such as articles, prepositions, and nouns. Following preliminary matching and discrimination training the individual is taught to arrange the symbols into a "sentence" string: article + noun + verb auxiliary + verb + preposition + article + noun. Finally, individuals are taught that specific symbols represent classes. Symbols within a class like nouns can be substituted to change the meaning of the sentence. Picture–symbol systems ranging from the more formalized Fokes' Sentence Builder or Bliss symbols to informal uses of photographs have also been used to augment or substitute for speech (Fokes, 1978; Vanderheiden & Harris-Vanderheiden, 1976).

For some rare autistic individuals an alternative to speech will provide the method that will trigger rapid acquisition of a flexible and communicative nonvocal language. Generally occurrence of such rapid progress has been reported in very young autistic children whose language comprehension was probably relatively good to start with (Schaeffer et al., 1977; Creedon, Note 3). What is probably more typical for autistic youngsters is that alternative systems are acquired slowly in a very concrete fashion. In our experience most children continue to understand speech and gestures better than any other modes even while relying on signs or pictures to express their own ideas (Schaeffer et al., 1977; Creedon, Note 3). In fact the extent to which alternative systems are always used productively is not clear. Calculator and Dollaghan (Note 4) found that seven nonverbal, developmentally delayed persons who were experienced users of communication boards more often relied on gestures and vocalizations for communication than the use of their boards.

The question then becomes one of whether the method allows the child to communicate something more effectively or appropriately than he already can. Thus if a wordboard allows a mute adolescent like Sally to identify the material she needs in a vocational activity or to ask about the absence of a classmate, its relatively long acquisition period may be worthwhile. However, for a youngster like Johnny who would probably not use the Non-Slip sequence away from the work table and would probably not generalize from it to speech, time might be better spent in other ways. Alternative systems can sometimes be more useful for the teacher or parent, who wants to give a mute or difficult-to-understand child a limited set of choices or to present a sequence of events, than the methods may be for the adolescent himself. Thus a picture system can give the autistic adolescent an opportunity to express preferences for meals in the coming week or a representation of the steps involved in packaging seeds. In these practical situations the alternative systems may have real value even though the adolescent may never use them independently or flexibly.

SOCIAL SKILLS TRAINING

For some autistic adolescents whose language skills are relatively strong, the concern goes beyond encouraging the youngsters to use their language to encouraging them to use language in a socially appropriate fashion. There is no simple answer to this difficulty. However, like the language programs discussed earlier, social skills training programs can provide a place to start. Both informal and formal training programs exist to teach social skills, though few are specifically aimed at either adolescents or autistic individuals. Though it was originally designed for younger normally developing children, we have elected to discuss here the cognitive approach to real-life problem-solving created by Spivack and Shure (1974) because of its detailed design and wide accessibility.

Spivack and Shure's training program consists of a script, a series of daily lessons, that begins with cognitive prerequisites of social problem-solving and then stresses discussions of alternative ways of dealing with social situations. The initial sessions contain discussions of such cognitive prerequisites as "same" and "different," "all" or "some," and the identification of facial expressions from pictures. Problems to be discussed later in the script include such situations as a girl wanting a boy at the bottom of the slide to get off so she can slide down and a girl wondering why her brother is crying. Suggestions are also made for use of the problem-solving techniques around specific issues such as aggression, sharing, and self-control.

Most higher functioning adolescents like Michael will already have most of the cognitive prerequisites of the program; if not, the concepts taught should be those that can be learned quite rapidly. The problem-solving technique may also be quite appropriate, although one would probably want to change the particular situations discussed to better match the needs and interests of adolescents.

For autistic adolescents with more limited intellectual and language skills, such as Sally, learning the cognitive prerequisites might be very time-consuming, and in some cases impossible. In addition one could not count on the youngster's ability to generalize from concrete tasks such as picture identification to recognition of the facial expression of classmates or teachers. This concern would be relevant for both Sally and for Johnny, where spontaneous generalization of skills has tended to be very limited. However, it may be possible to modify some of the informal problem-solving techniques and vignettes to reduce the cognitive requirements and create situations more relevant for these adolescents. For example, rather than discussing what a hypothetical boy should do if someone accidentally bumps into him, teachers or youngsters from another program could act out the event in question, role-play various solutions, and then have the less verbal adolescents show how they would respond to the same event rather than have them tell about it.

As in the language programs the most critical question is whether the program affects the youngsters' social communication skills outside the training sequences. The likelihood that this will occur is obviously much greater if the social problems "solved" during training are situations that occur in the youngsters' life and are important to them. Since the range of skills and living situations of autistic adolescents is great, social-communication training programs require just as much individualization as the language programs discussed earlier. While social skills training does not usually fall under the heading of language programming, the overlap between language use and social behaviors is great. The next few years should provide us with a better sense of how to address these needs for adolescents with autism.

SUMMARY AND CONCLUSIONS

By the time a person with autism reaches adolescence his individual pattern, in terms of abilities and preferences, interests and motivations, is absolutely critical to planning for communication. No longer can goals for communication be determined by the system (i.e., the spoken and written language of his culture) that provides access to the greatest number of people and ideas. Rather, plans need to consider the particular environment in which a youngster will live and the knowledge that he has that needs to be expressed. On the other hand environments can also be modified, often in very minimal ways, to allow the adolescent to use the communication skills he has.

In the past 15 or 20 years many methods of teaching autistic youngsters have been shown to be effective. Information has also accumulated concerning the developmental sequence of communication skills, giving us some insight into which tasks may be easier or more difficult for most children. As both developmental and nondevelopmental programs are disseminated, they appear less and less distinguishable from each other, with behavior programs building on developmental principles and developmental programs depending on behavioral training methods. From both perspectives the most serious problem appears to be shared: autistic youngsters often learn what we teach them but fail to use this learning to communicate about their own needs and interests. The question then becomes one particularly poignant for adolescents nearing the end of their education: Are we teaching them anything useful? For it to be useful, language has to provide an autistic adolescent with a way to describe something he wishes to communicate to another person or a way for that person to indicate to the youngster something that the autistic child needs or wishes to know. Facilitating this process requires careful consideration of with whom the adolescent is communicating and what he has to say. It is this kind of consideration that we have barely begun.

REFERENCES

Bartak, L. & Rutter, M. Differences between mentally retarded and normally intelligent autistic children. *Journal of Autism and Childhood Schizophrenia*, 1976, *6*, 109–120.

Bartak, L., Rutter, M., & Cox, A. A comparative study of infantile autism and specific developmental receptive language disorder. I. The children. *British Journal of Psychiatry*, 1975, *126*, 127–145.

Bartolucci, G., Pierce, S., & Streiner, D. Cross-sectional studies of grammatical morphemes in autistic and mentally retarded children. *Journal of Autism and Developmental Disorders*, 1980, *10*, 39–50.

Bloom, L. *Language development: Form and function in emerging grammars.* Cambridge, Mass.: MIT Press, 1970.

Bonvillian, J. D., & Nelson, K. E. Sign language acquisition in a mute autistic boy. *Journal of Speech and Hearing Disorders*, 1976, *41*, 339–347.

Brown, R. *A first language: The early stages.* Cambridge, Mass.: Harvard University Press, 1973.

Cantwell, D., Baker, L., & Rutter, M. A comparative study of infantile autism and specific developmental receptive language disorder. IV. Analysis of syntax and language function. *Journal of Child Psychology and Psychiatry,* 1978, *19,* 351–362.

Carrier, J., & Peak, T. *Non-Slip (Non-Speech Language Initiation Program).* Lawrence, Kan.: H & H Enterprises, 1975.

Cobrinik, L. Unusual reading ability in severely disturbed: Clinical observation and a retrospective inquiry. *Journal of Autism and Childhood Schizophrenia,* 1974, *41,* 163–175.

DeMyer, M. K. *Parents and children in autism.* Washington, D.C.: Winston, 1979.

Fokes, J. *Fokes' Sentence Builder.* New York: Teaching Resources, 1978.

Fulwiler, R., & Fouts, R. Acquisition of sign language by a noncommunicative autistic child. *Journal of Autism and Childhood Schizophrenia,* 1976, *6,* 43–51.

Goetz, L., Schuler, A., & Sailor, H. Teaching functional speech to the severely handicapped: Current issues. *Journal of Autism and Developmental Disorders.* 1979, *9,* 325–344.

Guess, D., Sailor, W., & Baer, D. Children with limited language. In *Language intervention strategies* (Vol. 2) (R. L. Schiefelbusch, ed.), Baltimore: University Park Press, 1978.

Halliday, M. Learning how to mean. In *Foundations of language development* (Vol. 1) (E. Lenneberg & E. Lenneberg, eds.), New York: Academic Press, 1975.

Langdell, T. Recognition of faces: An approach to the study of autism. *Journal of Child Psychology and Psychiatry,* 1978, *19,* 255–268.

LaVigna, G. W. Communication training in mute autistic adolescents using the written word. *Journal of Autism and Childhood Schizophrenia,* 1977, *7,* 135–150.

Lotter, V. Epidemiology of autistic conditions in young children. I. Prevalence. *Social Psychiatry,* 1966, *1,* 124.

Lotter, V. Epidemiology of autistic conditions in young children. II. Some characteristics of parents and children. *Social Psychiatry,* 1967, *1,* 163.

Lovaas, O. J. *The autistic child: Language development through behavior modification.* New York: Wiley, 1977.

MacDonald, J., & Horstmeier, D. *Environmental language intervention program.* Columbus, Ohio: Merrill, 1978.

MacDonald, J., Blott, J., Gordon, K., Spiegel, B., & Hartmann, M. An experimental parent-assisted treatment program for preschool language delayed children. *Journal of Speech and Hearing Disorders,* 1974, *39,* 395–415.

McLean, J., & Synder-McLean, L. *A transactional approach to early language training.* Columbus, Ohio: Merrill, 1978.

Miller, J. On specifying what to teach: The movement of structure to structure and meaning, to structure and meaning and knowing. In *Educational programming for the severely and profoundly handicapped* (E. Sontag, J. Smith, and N. Certo, eds.), Reston, Va.: Council for Exceptional Children, 1977.

Morehead, D., & Morehead, A. From signal to sign: A Piagetian view of thought and language. In *Language perspectives: Acquisition, retardation and intervention* (R. L. Schiefelbusch and L. L. Lloyd, eds.), Baltimore: University Park Press, 1974.

Pierce, S., & Bartolucci, G. A syntactic investigation of verbal autistic, mentally retarded and normal children. *Journal of Autism and Childhood Schizophrenia,* 1977, *7,* 121–134.

Rutter, M. Autistic children: Infancy to adulthood. *Seminar in Psychiatry,* 1970, *2,* 435–450.

Rutter, M. Infantile autism and other child psychoses. In *Child psychiatry: Modern approaches* (M. Rutter & L. Hersov, eds.), Philadelphia: Lippincott, 1977.

Schaeffer, B., Kollinzas, G., Musil, A., & McDowell, P. Spontaneous verbal language for autistic children through signed speech. *Sign Language Studies*, 1977, *17*, 287–328.

Schopler, E., Reichter, R., & Lansing, M. *Individualized assessment and treatment for autistic and developmentally disabled children. Vol. II.* Baltimore: University Park Press, 1980.

Schuler, A. L. Teaching functional language. In *Critical issues in educating autistic children and youth* (B. Wilcox & A. Thompson, eds.), Washington: U.S. Department of Education / Office of Special Education, Division of Innovation and Development, 1980.

Simmons, J., & Baltaxe, C. Language patterns of adolescent autistics. *Journal of Autism and Childhood Schizophrenia*, 1975, *5*, 333–351.

Spivack, G., & Shure, M. B. *Social adjustment of young children.* San Francisco: Jossey-Bass, 1974.

Stremel, K., & Waryas, C. A behavioral-psycholinguistic approach to language training. In L. McReynolds (Ed.), Developing systematic procedures for training children's language. *ASHA Monographs*, 1974, *18*, 96–130.

Sulzbacker, S. J., & Costello, J. M. A behavioral strategy for language training of a child with autistic behaviors. *Journal of Speech and Hearing Disorders*, 1970, *35*, 256–277.

Tager-Flusberg, H. On the nature of linguistic functioning in early infantile autism. *Journal of Autism and Developmental Disorders*, 1981, *11*, 45–56.

Vanderheiden, G. C., & Harris-Vanderheiden, D. Communication techniques and aides for the nonvocal severely handicapped. In *Communication assessment and intervention strategies* (L. L. Lloyd, ed.), Baltimore: University Park Press, 1976.

Wing, L., & Gould, J. Severe impairments of social interaction and associated abnormalities in children: Epidemiology and classification. *Journal of Autism and Developmental Disorders*, 1979, *9*, 11–30.

Wing, L. *Early childhood autism.* London: Pergamon Press, 1976.

REFERENCE NOTES

1. O'Neill, P., & Lord, C. *A functional and semantic approach to language intervention with autistic children.* Manuscript in preparation.

2. Lord, C., & Allen, J. *Comprehension of simple directives by autistic children.* Manuscript in preparation.

3. Creedon, M. P. *Language development in nonverbal autistic children using a simultaneous communication system.* Paper presented at the biennial meeting of the Society for Research in Child Development, Philadelphia, March 1973.

4. Calculator, S., & Dollaghan, C. *Communication boards in an institutional setting.* Paper presented at the Symposium on Research in Child Language Disorders, University of Wisconsin, Madison, Wisconsin, June 1980.

5

The Educational Needs of the Autistic Adolescent

H. D. BUD FREDERICKS, JAY BUCKLEY,
VICTOR L. BALDWIN, WILLIAM MOORE, and
KATHLEEN STREMEL-CAMPBELL

While significant strides have been made toward providing more effective techniques for teaching the autistic child and adolescent, and although the educational opportunities for these students have increased within the last 10 years, appropriate educational programs for the autistic population are not yet a reality. In this chapter we focus on the educational needs of the autistic adolescent and describe the characteristics of autistic children that determine what special education should offer. The characteristics of the educational environment and the specific curricular areas to achieve these overall objectives are outlined. We discuss the interaction of the parent with the school to help implement the curriculum, and indicate some considerations of classroom management that we feel must be present to accommodate the specific characteristics of autistic adolescents.

H. D. BUD FREDERICKS, JAY BUCKLEY, VICTOR L. BALDWIN, WILLIAM MOORE, AND KATHLEEN STREMEL-CAMPBELL • Teaching Research Infant and Child Center, Monmouth, Oregon 97361

CHARACTERISTICS OF AUTISTIC ADOLESCENTS THAT IMPACT ON EDUCATION

In considering the educational needs of the autistic adolescent we need to begin with the student and identify his* characteristics that will influence the education environment. Some major characteristics of the autistic population have been referred to in other chapters', and include the following:

1. The extreme range of levels of intelligence
2. Deficits in receptive and expressive language and communication
3. Deficits in social interaction
4. Deficits in responding to environmental stimuli
5. The failure to generalize and/or maintain trained skills or behavior, and
6. The occurrence of repetitive and/or inappropriate behaviors

Range of Intellectual Functioning

The autism syndrome has been found to occur in children at all levels of intelligence, ranging from the profoundly handicapped to the normal child, and can develop in children with quite heterogeneous conditions. Bartak and Rutter (1976) point out that the mentally handicapped and the normally intelligent autistic student may have rather different educational needs.

A summary of results of follow-up studies of diagnosed groups of autistic children completed by Lotter (1978) indicates that the most accurate predictions of likely social outcomes of autistic children are based on cognitive variables, such as IQ, language skills, and school performance. The results also showed that the different groups of autistic children vary widely. The majority of studies showed that autistic children with normal nonverbal intelligence made educational progress and approximately half of these individuals ended up employed. Those individuals with autism and severe global mental retardation remained severely handicapped and the majority ended up in some form of long-term institutionalization (Rutter, 1970).

However, the current research of Schopler and Mesibov (in press) indicates that the limited progress of the severely handicapped autistic

---

*We have used the male gender pronoun to refer to the student and the female gender pronoun to refer to the teacher/trainer. This selection of pronoun usage is not meant to reflect a discriminatory position, but rather to provide clarity for the reader.

child may be a consequence of our inability to provide effective educational intervention rather than their inability to learn. Schopler and Mesibov conducted a program evaluation of the TEACCH program in which a structured psychoeducational teaching approach and the use of parents as co-therapists are two significant components. These authors reported the rate of institutionalization for autistic adolescents seen in the TEACCH program as only 7%. This low rate of institutionalization was seen with the older, more severe autistic adolescents as well as with the higher functioning adolescents. Parents reported two of the areas of improved adaptation as being social skills and language. These results indicate that significant progress can be made with the more severely handicapped autistic child and adolescent.

Deficits in Receptive and Expressive Language. The majority of autistic children and adolescents demonstrate some level of deficit in receptive and expressive language skills. Lovaas and his colleagues have offered perhaps the most comprehensive long-term results of developing speech in severely handicapped autistic children. The results of specific research and training programs are overall optimistic, but Lovaas (1978) also points to the limitations of these results in that: (1) treatment gains were often situation-specific with limited generalization; (2) follow-up measures showed large differences depending on the environment; and (3) treatment proceeded slowly, with the nonverbal children demonstrating less progress than the echolalic children in acquiring some form of verbal responding (Lovaas, 1977).

The limited success of speech training with nonverbal children (both autistic and those with other developmental delays) leads to the use of nonspeech in nonvocal language intervention programs including manual signs (Fulwiler & Fouts, 1976; Miller & Miller, 1973; Stremel-Campbell, Cantrell, & Halle, 1977; Creedon, Note 1), simultaneous sign speech (Schaeffer, 1980), abstract symbolic language (Carrier & Peak, 1975; de Villiers & Naughton, 1974; McLean & McLean, 1974; Premack & Premack, 1974), and some form of written system (Hewett, 1965; Marshall & Hegrenes, 1972). While these nonspeech modes of language training have increased our potential to teach language to nonverbal children, decisions concerning the use of oral or nonoral methods of training and the use of individual selection of specific nonoral modes lack an empirical base. In addition, Churchill (1972) stresses that we must be cautious in defining gains that are reported in the development of "functional language." For even though it is possible to train previously nonverbal or echolalic children to use spoken, gestural, or written language to label objects, actions, and wants, to answer questions, and to follow instructions within highly controlled contextual settings, assessments and training procedures to determine the extent of the child's ability to generate spontaneous speech or to understand the component parts of sentences when they are not dependent on situational cues are still lacking.

Deficits in Social Interaction. Perhaps one of the most common characteristics of autistic children and adolescents is the severity and duration of the social handicap. The development of social interaction skills in the autistic student becomes critical if one considers the relationship of early social interactions and communication development. Howlin (1978) points out that the poor social interaction and poor communication skills evidenced by the autistic child may be a result of the child's inability to comprehend what is expected in the social situation rather than an unwillingness to do so. She also suggests that ways in which autistic children can be helped to cope more adequately in social situations, and ways to determine how social interactions are affected by environmental conditions, are necessary if we are to provide more appropriate educational programs.

Deficits in Responding to Environmental Stimuli. An additional characteristic was initially identified through studies by Kanner (1944) and Rimland (1964), who indicated that autistic children fail to respond to environmental stimuli. Experimental studies (Hermelin & O'Connor, 1970; Ornitz, 1974) supported the finding that the autistic child has difficulty integrating sensory data from different modalities. The majority of autistic children tend to respond to only a limited portion of cues when presented with a stimulus complex. This tendency is identified as stimulus overselectivity by Lovaas, Schreibman, Koegel, and Rehm (1971). A number of related studies employing a discrimination-learning paradigm were used to determine the response strategies of children who fail to learn. The first of these (Lovaas et al., 1971) found that autistic children responded predominantly to only one modality (usually either visual or auditory) while normal children responded similarly to all three stimuli (visual, auditory, and tactile). Similar results were obtained in a second study (Lovaas & Schreibman, 1971) when the complex stimulus consisted of only two components. Both studies found that the additional cue could be trained when it was presented separately, even though it remained nonfunctional when presented with other cues. A third study (Koegel & Wilhelm, 1973) attempted to determine if the overselectivity was a function of the presentation of simultaneous stimulation in different sensory modalities or a function of the multiplicity of the cues, even if they were in the same modality. The results demonstrated that stimulus overselectivity was present both when the stimulus complex was presented across modalities and also when the stimulus complex involved multiple cues within the same modality. This overselectivity of stimuli should be considered in planning the educational environment offered to the autistic child.

Failure to Generalize and Maintain Trained Skills. Browning (1971) and Lovaas, Koegel, Simmons, and Stevens-Long (1973) demonstrated that behavioral change in a one-to-one treatment situation did not adequately generalize to other situations. Rutter and Bartek (1973) evaluated different educational approaches and found that the behavioral movements observed in specific educational settings did not generalize to the home and other settings.

Lovaas et al. (1973) collected generalization and follow-up measures on 20 autistic children. Follow-up results that were recorded 1–4 years after treatment depended largely on the type of posttreatment in the environment. Those children whose parents were taught to carry out training continued to improve while institutionalized children regressed. Additional research data (Stokes & Baer, 1977; Walker & Buckley, 1972) support the overall finding that generalization does not take place without special intervention in the nontraining environment. Therefore we must expect that generalization of treatment gains to nontraining settings should be considered the exception rather than the rule, and that generalization should be planned or actively programmed (Kazdin & Bootzin, 1972; Stokes & Baer, 1977).

Repetitive and/or Inappropriate Behavior. The educational progress of the autistic child and adolescent is often further hampered by the frequent occurrence of inappropriate behaviors. These behaviors may include stereotypic or repetitive behaviors that interfere with teaching appropriate social, language, self-help, or vocational skills. A number of studies (Koegel & Covert, 1972; Berberich, Perloff, & Schaeffer, 1966; Lovaas, Freitas, Nelson, & Whelan, 1967; Wolf, Risley, Johnston, Harris, & Allen, 1967; Wolf, Risley, & Mees, 1964) employed operant approaches to eliminate a wide range of inappropriate behaviors with autistic children. In general the results of these studies showed that operant techniques were effective in decreasing or eliminating a number of inappropriate behaviors. However, the results of these studies were based on a small sample of children who were trained by skilled professionals on a one-to-one basis in highly controlled environmental settings. Additionally, follow-up and generalization to untrained settings were not measured or reported.

Wing (1978) suggests that the social deficits, the repetitive stereotyped behavior, the abnormalities affecting comprehension, the use of all forms of communication, and the development of symbolic functioning are facets of the same underlying impairment in autistic children. This suggestion would seem to imply that the relationship of inappropriate behaviors to social interaction skills and communication skills should be an important consideration in planning the educational environment for the autistic adolescent.

The preceding discussion has focused on identifying the characteristics of the autistic child or adolescent to which the educational environment must respond through organization and curricular arrangement. In addition, other considerations that relate to any adolescent must be made. These considerations include the selection of age-appropriate materials and activities, the physical and emotional changes that all adolescents experience, and the ultimate potential functioning of that adolescent in an adult society.

In addition to the characteristics of autistic children, certain characteristics of the educational environment must be considered. The research literature indicates that specific variables greatly affect the autistic child's ability to learn.

CHARACTERISTICS OF THE EDUCATIONAL ENVIRONMENT

A number of studies have examined the relationship of the educational environment and the treatment gains of the autistic student. Rutter and Bartak (1973) compared three different types of classrooms and found that all children had large amounts of unoccupied time; however, children in structured programs showed the least amount of unoccupied time, 41% compared with 71% in the least structured program. Fredericks, Anderson, and Baldwin (1979) examined programs for the severely handicapped containing a variety of handicapping conditions including autism, deafblindness, mental retardation, and cerebral palsy, and determined that the major factor in improved learning was in maximizing the amount of instructional time within the environment. In a study of preschools for developmentally disabled children, Fredericks, Moore, and Baldwin (in press) again found that maximizing instructional time was a key element in children's learning. Both studies conducted by Fredericks et al. (1979, in press) demonstrated that a combination of one-to-one and group instruction provided little unoccupied time for the student.

Two studies (Fredericks et al., 1979; Moore et al., 1981) have determined that the quality of consequences and a task-analyzed curriculum are other essential ingredients in a successful educational environment. The frequency with which programs are updated is also an important factor. Updating refers to data analysis of skill acquisition programs and the modification of those programs based on that analysis. Koegel, Dunlap, and Dyer (1980) found that short intervals, 1 second verses 4 seconds, between the termination of one trial and the commencement of the next greatly influenced successful learning.

ROLE OF SPECIAL EDUCATION

What should we expect from the educational environment? What should be the overall purpose of education of the autistic adolescent? Education offered to the autistic adolescent should be designed to help him function more independently in our society and to help him perform more normally by reducing the aberrant behaviors which make him appear different. We recognize that "independence" and "normalcy" are relative terms. With one student the independent behavior may be simple communication skills that will allow him to indicate his needs, whereas another student may be capable of living independently in his own apartment, managing his own money, fulfilling the requirements of a job, and taking care of his bodily and personal needs. The range of independence is wide for autistic students, and educational programs must be prepared to accommodate this range.

A central issue concerning the education of autistic children is whether the needs of these children can be more appropriately met in special schools or in more heterogeneous school settings with other handicapped and normal children (Callias, 1978). Wing and Wing (1976) discuss the need for specialized units and the possibility of admitting autistic children to other types of schools. While this approach represents one system of service delivery, Callias (1978) questions whether the special classrooms need to be solely for autistic children.

A limited number of educational programs and research studies have been directed toward a more integrated educational placement (Bartak & Rutter, 1973; Lansing & Schopler, 1978; Russo & Koegel, 1977). However, the educational environment of the majority of severely handicapped autistic children typically remains one of segregated classrooms (Halpern, 1970; Hamblin, Buckholdt, Ferritor, Kozloff, & Blackwell, 1971; Koegel & Rincover, 1974). It is evident from the literature that more direct, controlled evaluations of the results of educational programs for autistic children are necessary in order to determine more effectively the most appropriate educational environments for these children (Bartak & Pickering, 1976; Elgar, 1976; Wing & Wing, 1976). Bartak (1978) studied the outcomes of students educated in self-contained classrooms and students educated in classrooms in which autistic children were integrated with other handicapped children. These classrooms differed on a number of other variables, however, and although Bartak found no advantages to children in the more integrated classroom, no disadvantages were reported. Even though Bartak's study demonstrated some methodological limitations, it provides an impetus to examine more closely the effects of different service delivery models.

Although the issue concerning segregated versus integrated educational environments remains a controversy, today's movement toward "least restrictive environments" in educational placements is providing direction to efforts at designing integrated educational environments for the handicapped child. However, one of the major thrusts of the integration process must be determining how these environments can be utilized more effectively in meeting both the educational and social needs of autistic children and youth (Callias, 1978). The integrated environment, the skills of the resource teacher and regular education teacher, and the attitudes of the public school personnel and peers must be systematically assessed prior to the placement of the autistic or other handicapped child in the integrated environment. Additionally the training of personnel and peers should be directly related to the needs assessment. Therefore if successful mainstreaming is to occur, the integrated program must be well planned, well organized, and highly structured.

The characteristics of the autistic adolescent and the characteristics of optimal educational environments are only two of the components to consider in developing appropriate educational programs. Additional considerations involve the functionality of what we are teaching all handicapped students based on the demands and attitudes of the family, the school system, and the community. In part our education program will consist of changing attitudes, providing family support, encouraging family involvement, and training direct and nondirect school personnel to interact more adequately with and train the autistic adolescent. The remainder of this chapter focuses on two major discussions: arranging the educational environment; and determining what to teach—curriculum.

ARRANGING THE EDUCATIONAL ENVIRONMENT

The arrangement of the educational environment includes five major components, which are: (1) a focus on functional living skills; (2) parent involvement; (3) support services; (4) classroom management; and (5) teaching strategies. These components determine *how* we train the autistic adolescent and develop an effective educational program.

A Focus on Functional Living Skills

Many autistic children and adolescents seem to be able to learn isolated skills and may demonstrate these skills in a rather rote, nonfunctional manner. This restricted use of learned skills and lack of generalization may in part be a result of our educational programs rather than of the student's failure to coordinate learned skills and demonstrate functional sequences of behavior in appropriate contexts. Perhaps because of the autistic student's failure to respond to environmental stimuli, we have isolated his education and training objectives to the point that they are no longer related to his functional environment. Initially the autistic student's education may need to be very systematically arranged to include a limited number of stimuli. However, if he is to function at any level of independence our concept of education must gradually expand beyond isolated training settings and beyond the classroom. His educational environment must at some point include the home, the grocery store, the restaurant, or any environment in which we ultimately want the behavior to occur.

Parent Involvement

The first step in expanding the concept of educational programming beyond the classroom or school is to involve the parent actively in the student's education. Thus we anticipate the parent functioning in three roles in the education program for the autistic student: (1) teaching at home; (2) assisting with generalization; and (3) volunteering at school.

The first role is a modification of what is now the traditional role of the parent in the Individual Education Program (IEP) process. Not only must the parent help decide what the student should be taught at school, but the parent must also agree that she is going to teach certain skills in the home. The parent can teach certain practical living and leisure time skills, and may have more opportunities to do that than the school. It will be recognized rather early in the child's secondary career that there is no way in which the school can teach all the skills contained in the curricula discussed later in this chapter. Therefore the parent should be requested to undertake some of that teaching. The school probably should teach the parent how to do that teaching. It will have to teach the parent how to cue the student and how to provide the student feedback if the parent does not already have these skills.

In the second role, parents assist with the generalization of skills taught at school. It makes little sense to teach a child how to scramble eggs in school if he does not have the opportunity to scramble eggs at home; it does little good to teach the child to select his own clothes if his mother selects them for him at home. Thus the parent and the school must be in close coordination as the various curricular areas are taught. Without the opportunity to generalize, these skills will not be maintained by the student and will not become part of his natural repertoire of behaviors. Too frequently we have seen students who have been taught to tell time in school lose that skill because they are not required to tell time at home or at school.

In the generalization process one of the difficulties that both the parents and school need to discuss is allowing the student to risk. Risk comes in two forms. First, there are situations which are potentially dangerous, such as learning to run an electric lawn mower, use knives, cross busy streets, and use public transportation systems. Yet there may all be essential skills which the student must learn. Having been taught them, he must then have the opportunity to practice them. It is the practice which carries with it that element of potential danger.

The other type of risk is not of danger but a social risk, as the student perceives it. Many students faced with social situations such as ordering food in a restaurant or depositing money at the bank feel intimidated, shy, or paniky as they interact with the bank teller or waiter (who in fact may not be intimidating at all). Because the student is unsure of the procedures, the student feels himself at risk. There is still another aspect when considering social risk. Frequently the more severely handicapped student may have serious communication difficulties which will generate unpleasant situations for him when dealing with other people. The student needs to be taught how to respond when others indicate that they do not understand what he is saying. Consequently the parent and the school must be willing to role-play these risk situations for the student to put him at ease so that he can function comfortably in them. Again this program is closely coordinated between the school and the home.

The third role of the parent is an unusual one at the secondary level, yet one that is highly recommended—the parent's serving as a volunteer in the secondary program. Volunteers are needed to assist in monitoring vocational, practical living, and leisure skills programs. During the course of volunteering the parent learns some skills in interacting with the student, learns the scope of the curriculum that the student must learn, and develops a greater appreciation of the capabilities of his or her own child. Volunteering is an excellent way for the parents to develop the close coordination with the school that is necessary to achieve success for their handicapped adolescent. Techniques for using volunteers in this situation and a more detailed discussion of the parent can be found in Fredericks and staff (1979).

The Use of Support Services

Frequently a necessary element in the educational program of the autistic adolescent is the provision of support services such as speech or physical therapy. To have the therapist work individually with each student is often the least efficient use of this professional's time and provides an insufficient amount of time for the student who needs the services. An alternative method of using the professional specialist follows the consultant model, where the therapist teaches both the parent and the teacher how to teach the child, and then monitors the child's progress through continual data collection. These data are verified by frequent probes conducted by the therapist.

To achieve the consultant model, certain elements must be used by the therapist and must be in a form readily understood by the teacher and parent, with explanation and demonstration by the therapist. These elements include: (1) assessing parent and teacher skills and needs; (2) establishing priorities for training with the parent and teacher; (3) explaining long-term objectives; (4) role-playing; (5) demonstrating programs; (6) assessing parent/teacher training; (7) providing feedback; and (8) monitoring training and student data.

A data system compatible with the task-analyzed curriculum must also be in use. The data system must show the student's progress during the instruction by the parent or teacher. The advantage of such a data system is that it allows the parent and teacher to move the student to the next step of the curriculum if the student's performance meets a certain criterion level. An alternative to such a continual data system is for the therapist to see the student once or twice a week in order to probe the student's progress and then to prescribe a program to be followed until the next visit. The disadvantage of this alternative is that it does not allow movement of the student through the steps of curriculum in the interim between visits of the therapist, and thus may retain a student at a certain level of a curriculum longer than necessary. However, if the therapist is seeing the student once or twice a week, this will not be too great a disadvantage.

Classroom Management

We must consider how to put all of this together in an educational environment for the handicapped, autistic adolescent. Fredericks (Fredericks & the staff of the Teaching Research Infant and Child Center, 1979) describes a classroom management system that has the essential components for the education of mildly and severely autistic students. These are as follows:

1. Individualized programming
2. Group and individual instruction
3. Use of volunteers

4. Parent involvement
5. Behavior management
6. Use of support personnel
7. A system of supervision or quality control

First, each program is individualized for each student. This of course is based on the student's Individualized Educational Program. In addition to an initial assessment, data are maintained on the student's progress in each education program, ideally on a daily basis so that the program can be modified daily. Too frequently students are maintained at lower levels in programs when they could advance more rapidly, or they are having difficulties with programs where modification is needed to assist them to advance at their optimum rate. Without data, the teacher is unable to make timely decisions based on the student's performance. At the very least data maintained every second or third day is considered essential for the type of population we are considering. Programs should be modified daily based on those data. One of the major objections to this type of data system is that it takes too much time. Recording either a 1 for a correct response or a 0 for an incorrect response has been demonstrated to consume a negligible amount of time. Analyzing the data takes longer. If the data are maintained daily, however, the modifications usually required are slight and can easily be handled. Fredericks, Anderson, and Baldwin (1979) demonstrated that a teacher with 6 weeks' experience in their data-keeping system can update educational programs on the average of one program per minute. (Updating means examining the data gathered on that day, analyzing it, and modifying or maintaining the program based on that analysis.) This means that in a classroom with 10 severely handicapped students, each with six individual programs, the average time responding to the data is 60 minutes. One should realize that this time constitutes the bulk of the teacher's preparation time for the next day because during this updating process she is determining what is going to be taught to each student in each program for the following day.

Inherent within this data system is also a system that includes a check on the maintenance of learned skills over time. Follow-up data are gathered on each student 2 weeks, 1 month, 3 months, and 6 months after learning a skill to ensure that it has been maintained in the student's repertoire of abilities.

A second characteristic of the educational environment is that instruction should be delivered both within groups and individually. This does not negate the concept of individualized programming, for even within the group the types of instruction should be geared to the functioning level of the individual student. This combination of individual and group instruction is especially suited for the learning characteristics of autistic students. During individual instruction the characteristics of stimulus overselectivity can be focused on and stimuli can be altered systematically to facilitate the autistic student's learning. After he learns a specific behavior or skill in the individual instruction setting, it can be generalized in the group instructional setting.

To facilitate the classroom organization to allow for this intricate combination of individual and group instruction, we recommend using volunteers to provide some of the individual instruction. Volunteers provide extra hands and eyes for the classroom teacher and her assistant. They can monitor seatwork, monitor and teach the vocational program, and teach some of the practical living and leisure time skills programs. Using volunteers requires provision for their training and frequent checking on the quality of their performance. A simple system of written communication between the teacher and the volunteer is mandatory since the teacher will not have the time to brief each volunteer verbally as he or she enters the classroom. In addition a flexible system of scheduling volunteers is necessary. Such a system of communication and scheduling takes some time and a fair amount of effort to establish, but once in place it significantly enhances the quality of classroom education. Fredericks and staff of the Teaching Research Infant and Child Center (1979) described the essential elements of successful volunteer usage and provided details on how to implement and maintain such a program.

Another advantage to the use of volunteers is that it provides a more economical way to deliver educational services. If a school district had to pay for personnel to deliver the amount of individualized instruction which volunteers are capable of providing, the special education budget would be stretched to the breaking point.

Where can volunteers be obtained? As we have recommended, parents make excellent volunteers. At the high school level the peer group is a lucrative source of volunteers; we have yet to encounter a high school, once the administrator ascertained the role of the student volunteers, that did not encourage students to participate in this way. It also provides potential career exploration for those who think they might want to be teachers of the handicapped. Women's church groups and other service organizations in the community have also been found to be good sources of volunteers.

The role of the parent has already been discussed, but it is an integral part of the classroom management system. The teacher must have a system to communicate frequently with the parent so that the student's programs can be taught in both environments, home and school.

Another characteristic of the classroom should be attention to the remediation of inappropriate behaviors. This is part of the social/sexual curriculum, but needs to be emphasized, for too frequently this area is ignored or not sufficiently attended to so as to remediate those behaviors that make the student unacceptable to others in our society. The data on these programs should be gathered on a daily basis. For high-frequency behaviors time sampling is appropriate; low-frequency behaviors are usually counted all day long. Although the data are gathered daily, behavior programs, unlike skill acquisition programs, are modified based on the data gathered on a weekly basis. More frequent changes would create for the student the semblance of inconsistent response to the behavior on the part of the environment. Moreover more frequent alteration of the program does not allow sufficient data to be gathered to make an accurate assessment of the effectiveness of the program.

Another consideration within the classroom environment is the role of support personnel, such as physical therapists and language therapists, who may be essential for some autistic children. These need to be incorporated into the classroom management system used by the teacher. Their consultant role has been discussed above.

Finally, and very often neglected, the supervisors of the classroom should have checklists by which they can monitor the quality of instruction in these programs. Without that feedback, the classroom teachers of the mildly or severely handicapped begin to feel isolated in the educational setting; moreoever the school principal or other supervisor begins to withdraw from supervising an integral part of her educational programs. An example of one item of the checklist for the type of classroom described herein is shown in Table 1, and provides for the administrator specific features of the classroom to check. Further, it establishes criterion levels to determine if that aspect of the classroom is functioning adequately. Such measures not only provide vehicles for supervisors to check quality, but also give teachers standards of performance.

Teaching Strategies

One of the basic differences between the mildly handicapped autistic child and the more severely handicapped autistic child is the way in which they are to be taught. The mildly handicapped student may benefit from instruction presented to him in what is termed a "total task approach." The task is modeled for him; then he tries to perform it, receiving feedback on the parts with which he is having difficulty. Practicing the task a few times allows mastery. All that remains is generalization, which will be discussed later. The more severely handicapped adolescent student may

Table 1
A Sample of One Item of the Classroom Observation Checklist

Individual programs are established for handicapped individuals
___ Present   ___ Not present   ___ N/A
A. *Item:* Task-analyzed programs
    Procedure: Choose ten programs and divide the number of programs task-analyzed by
             the total number of programs.
    Criterion: 9/10 or 90%
    Score: ____%

B. *Item:* Content of communication tool, i.e., clipboard, notebook, etc.
    Procedure: Check 25% (¼) of the communication tools for the following components
             (look at one program on each communication tool checked). Record a slash
             mark (/) if component is correct, record a zero (0) if component is incorrect.
             Include comments if components are present but are incorrect.

Present Indicate if any part of component is present	*Present at Criterion* Indicate if all parts of component are present	*N/A*	
1. ___	___	___	Weekly cover sheet (lists all programs)
2. ___	___	___	Reinforcers to be used (lists both social and primary and schedule)
3. ___	___	___	Language level of student (Receptive and Expressive)
4. ___	___	___	General comments (how to deal with target behaviors)
5. ___	___	___	Cues (verbal and nonverbal)
6. ___	___	___	Correction procedure (contains: negative feedback, cue, assist, socially reinforce)
7. ___	___	___	Reinforcement procedure
8. ___	___	___	Materials
9. ___	___	___	Criterion level for advancement
10. ___	___	___	Task analysis of behavior
11. ___	___	___	Raw data sheet
12. ___	___	___	Baseline on raw data sheet (conducted from most difficult to easiest tests, all steps from Task Analysis)

    Criterion: Item present 90%, items at criterion 80%
    Score: Total items present ____% Items at criterion ____%

C. *Item:* Number of Programs Conducted
    Procedure: Sample 25% (¼) of the communication systems. Count the number of

Table 1 (*continued*)

programs it would be possible to run for one day and divide this number into the total number of programs actually run. If the result is less than 80%, sample a second day.

Criterion: 80% of programs run on first or second day.

Score: _____%

D. *Item:* Reviewing of Academic Programs

   Procedure: Use a sample of three communication tools looking at ten teaching sessions (one to two programs) on each (total of 30 teaching sessions). Determine if teacher is responding to raw data by making changes if student is not succeeding (probe, program change, reinforcement change, criterion change) or succeeding (next step, probe ahead, posttest). Give one point for each correct update. Indicate each correct update by recording a slash (/). Indicate each incorrect update by recording a zero (0). Include comments if update is assessed as incorrect. Begin with the most recent teaching session.

	Stu. Pro. _____	Stu. Pro. _____	Stu. Pro. _____	Stu. Pro. _____
Next Step				
Same Step				
Program Change (Branch)				
Baseline				
Probe				
Reinforcement Change				
Criterion Change				
Posttest				

   Criterion: 24/30 or 80%
   Score: _____%

E. *Item:* Type of Data Collected

   Procedure: Check raw data sheets 25% (¼) programs to determine type of data taken:
   _____Continuous
   _____Daily summary
   _____More than once weekly
   _____Weekly
   _____Less than weekly
   Criterion: 80% continuous data
   Score: _____%

require that the task be taught step by step using a task-analyzed approach. This may at times be necessary for the less severely handicapped students also, especially for those tasks that have a large number of steps. An example of an appropriate task analysis for the handicapped student is shown in Figure 1, one of the skills of a Personal Hygiene Curriculum.

Terminal Objective: Trainee cleans around the base of each tooth with dental floss.

Prerequisite Skills: Pincer grasp (unless using flossing tool).

Phase I   Get floss container.
Phase II   Open floss container.
Phase III   Grasp end of floss.
Phase IV   Pull floss from container (approximately 12" length).
Phase V   Cut floss by pulling against cutting blade.
Phase VI   Wrap floss around forefinger of one hand. Press thumb against wrapped finger to hold floss.
Phase VII   Wrap floss around forefinger of other hand.
Phase VIII   Press thumb against wrapped finger to hold floss.
to
Phase XXXIX

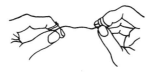

The following steps apply to Phases IX–XXXIX only.

Steps:
  1.   Position hands with thumbs pointing upward.

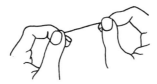

  2.   Position middle fingers at center of floss.

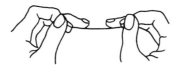

  3.   Insert floss between teeth at specified point by wiggling gently and pressing downward/upward (depending on which part of mouth is being worked on).
  4.   Push floss gently between gum and tooth to right.
  5.   Push floss gently between gum and tooth to left. Example of direction of floss for steps 4 and 5:

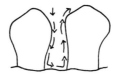

Phase XL   Throw away used floss.

Phase XLI   Replace floss container.

Suggested Materials: Floss.

Teaching Notes:
  1.   Teach Phases I through VIII, then teach Phase IX, steps 1–5; Phase X, steps 1–6, etc., through Phase XXXIX. Then teach Phases XL and XLI.
  2.   If trainee does not have pincer grasp, you may wish to use a flossing tool. If so, omit Phases I through VIII and add phases for use of a specific tool.

Figure 1. A sample task analysis of an oral hygiene skill—flossing teeth.

Training should include a number of "active generalization program-ming" techniques to facilitate generalization to new materials, new per-sons, and new settings. Stokes and Baer (1977) provide a number of basic techniques that can be used to increase generalization. First, it is impor-tant that generalization be measured prior to training, during training, and after the training criterion has been met. One of the first generalization programming techniques involves the use of multiple examplars. Initially more than one or two objects should be used in training. For example, if the student is learning to request an apple, then a green apple, a red apple, and a slice of an apple would be used in training so that the student's response to "apple" is not controlled by a specific color or shape. The student should also be trained in more than one setting (i.e., home, vo-cational setting).

A second technique would include selecting stimuli or physical and verbal cues that are common to the training setting and to settings in which we want the behavior to generalize. Peers, volunteers, and parents (involved in school and home programming) can serve as common stimuli. The stimuli or objects used for training should include those (actions or events) that are functional in a number of the student's environments.

A third technique includes concurrent training in which the student is learning more than one behavior at a time. In addition randomized cues are presented during training (i.e., "cut the bread," "cut the cheese," "open the bread") so that the student is learning the specific behavior and not responding in a rote fashion.

A fourth technique includes the gradual use of natural consequences and indiscriminable contingencies (at least in the last phases in the pro-gram). In this way the student learns what consequences will operate in nontraining environments. For example, if a student is being trained to greet peers appropriately, the final phases of training would include only the social consequences of a reciprocal greeting for an appropriate re-sponse.

CURRICULUM

What do we teach the adolescent autistic student to help him achieve normalcy at the most appropriate level? Our experience at the Teaching Research Infant and Child Center, where we have established programs for all types of handicapping conditions, has indicated that for all hand-icapped adolescents the overall curricular program areas are identical; however, the scope and sequence differs depending on the severity of the handicap and the individual needs of the student. Five curricular areas have been identified to be emphasized at the secondary level, which are, in order of priority: (1) social/sexual skills; (2) practical living skills; (3) leisure-time skills; (4) vocational education; and (5) functional academics.

A comprehensive curriculum involving each of these areas, giving students sufficient skills to function independently, is a vast undertaking. Educators have traditionally assumed that many of these skills are learned on the streets or in the home, yet our experience indicates that this is not the case.

Social/Sexual Skills

Considering the deficits in social interaction of autistic students, the major focus of the curriculum at the secondary level should be the social/sexual area. This curricular area emphasizes how to build relationships with other people, how to respond appropriately to other people in the home, in the community, and on the job, and how to initiate appropriate interactions with other people. This part of the curriculum focuses on the practical utilization of the language or communication system which in the early years of the student's training undoubtedly was the major focus of social skills training. This part of the curriculum teaches an adolescent how to protect himself against sexual exploitation and how to enjoy healthy sex habits. We feel that it is one of the most important curricular areas, since if the adolescent is unable to develop interpersonal skills he may ultimately fail in his vocational setting and in his interactions with others in the community. Without these skills he has little chance for a more complete and independent life.

Table 2 shows an example of a social/sexual checklist for a vocational setting. It provides an illustration of behaviors, some of which the student must learn ("greets others appropriately") and others which the student must avoid (aggression or self-stimulation). The example is by no means exhaustive nor ordinal in nature. This list of social behaviors would be appropriate for the mildly handicapped student. A similar list could be developed for appropriate social skills in a living environment or appropriate social skills in a restaurant or supermarket. Many of the same behaviors would appear on all lists (i.e. refraining from aggressive, self-stimulatory, and self-indulgent behaviors). Such a list for a restaurant might include how to respond appropriately to an intimidating waitress or waiter. These skills are best taught by placing the student in those situations, observing his behavior, taking a baseline on those behaviors, and then role-playing or otherwise correcting the behavior through a re-inforcement/feedback system. This entire social/sexual area must be highly

Table 2
Example of Social Skills Checklist for a Vocational Setting

Greets others appropriately
Discriminates who to talk to on the job
Initiates relevant conversation
Engages in conversation appropriately
Responds calmly to emotional outbursts of peers
Responds calmly to emotional outbursts of supervisor
Talks about emotional problems at appropriate time
Refrains from exhibiting inappropriate emotions on the job
Complies with work regulations
Discriminates when to comply with requests from peers
Contacts supervisor at appropriate times
Responds appropriately to critical feedback from supervisor
Responds appropriately to positive feedback from supervisor
Responds appropriately to change in routine
Moves about work setting appropriately
Refrains from bringing inappropriate items to work
Refrains from tampering with (or stealing) property of others
Responds appropriately to sexual advances from others
Refrains from inappropriate sexual activity at work
Laughs, jokes, and teases at appropriate times
Interacts with co-workers at appropriate times
Refrains from aggressive behaviors
Refrains from self-stimulatory behaviors
Refrains from self-indulgent behaviors
Complies with requests from supervisor

individualized so that the student comprehends what the social expectations are in each social situation.

An example of a sexual curriculum that is appropriate for all levels of handicapping children has been published by Alrick (1980). A sample of the behaviors to be taught with that curriculum are shown in Table 3.

Practical Living Skills

The second most important curricular area is practical living skills. Again we should assume that we are trying to teach the adolescent student to be independent, and therefore need to provide him with the skills that will allow him to take care of himself and his personal belongings, and to function appropriately in the community. Practical living skills include personal hygiene, care and maintenance of clothing, clothing selection,

Table 3

Example of Part of a Social/Sexual Curriculum (Psychological Emotional Implications)

A. Student identifies common feelings toward the opposite sex.

B. Student discusses the nature and purpose of the family unit.

C. Student demonstrates ability to cope with feelings rising from awareness of sexuality.

D. Student identifies flirting, its purpose and place.

E. Student identifies casual dating.

F. Student identifies steady dating.

G. Student identifies what being engaged may mean.

H. Student identifies what marriage is.

I. Student identifies possible physical consequences of sexual intercourse.

J. Student verbally or otherwise indicates stages that most permanent male/female relationships go through, i.e.,

> Dating casually
> Dating steadily
> Engagement
> Marriage

K. Student indicates ways a person may be able to spend time with another person that he/she wants to get to know:

> Asking a person out
> Going where the person is to talk
> Inviting them home, etc.

L. Given a list of specific behaviors, the student indicates which stage the relationship may be in:

> Refusing dates except with one person
> Talking about marriage
> Going out with the same person several times
> Having a baby
> Planning a wedding
> Deciding if he/she likes this person
> Having sexual intercourse

M. The student will define the following terms and their emotional implications:

> Sexual intercourse
> Menstruation
> Masturbation
> Pregnancy

---

care and maintenance of living quarters, cooking, shopping, storing food, money handling, budgeting, community mobility, and using facilities in the community.

Experience and conversations with parents indicate that the mildly handicapped student needs specific training in the area of practical living skills. Parents are able to teach some of these skills to their handicapped child, but as the child approaches the end of his educational years more and more parents complain that their adolescent is not ready to function independently in the community. Even elementary tasks such as clothing selection (i.e., choosing clothes that match and that are appropriate for the social occasion or season) are too difficult for many mildly handicapped students. Table 4 shows an example of a curriculum in the personal hygiene area, starting with basic personal hygiene skills such as washing hands and face, and moving through more complex personal hygiene skills such as shaving and menstrual care. This curriculum will accommodate both mildly and the more severely autistic population. However, the specific teaching strategies for the different levels of students may vary depending on the skills and individual needs of each student.

Leisure-Time Skills

The next most important curricular area is leisure-time skills. One could argue that vocational skills might be more important, but we are basing our ranking on the research data indicating that if we do not assist students to develop good social skills, care for their own needs, and provide for appropriate leisure time activities, they probably will not perform well in vocational settings.

The following reports are about mentally retarded individuals, but we may assume that the criteria for success are similar across handicapping conditions. Mithaug and Hagmeier (1978) and Johnson and Mithaug (1978) determined that social skills, language, and appropriate behavior were essential prerequisites for entry into sheltered workshops. Handicapped individuals often fail not because of their inability to do the work but because of an inability to adjust to the social demands of the world of work (Cronis & Justen, 1975; Pagel & Whitling, 1978). Through a time-sampling technique Nicklesburg (1973) found that the difference between 15 succeeding and 15 nonsucceeding trainees was that the nonsucceeding trainees spent more time standing idle, talking, joking, playing with others, laughing on the job, and being away from the assigned work station. Based on the preceding reports it is understandable that parents or guardians of 120 graduates of classes for the moderately retarded in a large southern California school district found a need for comprehensive postschool programming to meet the recreational and social needs of the retarded as well as to provide occupational and vocational training (Stanfield, 1973).

Again the argument is often presented that the mildly handicapped student does not need to be taught these skills. Our experience indicates

Table 4
Example of Personal Hygiene Curriculum

Bathing/Washing and Related Skills	Shaving
A. Washes hands	AA. Shaves underarms with safety razor
B. Dries hands	BB. Shaves underarms with electric razor
C. Washes and dries face	CC. Shaves legs with safety razor
D. Bathes or showers	DD. Shaves legs with electric razor
E. Adjusts water temperature	EE. Shaves face with safety razor
F. Cleans ears	FF. Shaves face with electric razor
G. Applies deodorant	GG. Replaces blade for injector, cartridges,
H. Applies hand and body lotion	etc.
I. Applies facial moisture cream	HH. Applies after shave lotion
J. Treats blemishes	
	Nail Care
Hair Care	II. Cleans nails with nail brush
K. Combs/brushes hair	JJ. Cleans nails with nail file
L. Washes hair	KK. Cuts nails
M. Blow-dries hair	LL. Files nails
N. Dries hair with portable hair dryer	MM. Applies nail polish
O. Hot-combs hair	NN. Removes nail polish
P. Makes two pincurls	
Q. Rolls hair	Use of Makeup
R. Curls hair using curling iron	OO. Applies perfume
S. Selects hair style	PP. Applies lipstick
	QQ. Applies blusher
Oral Hygiene	RR. Applies eye shadow
T. Brushes teeth	SS. Applies mascara
U. Flosses teeth	TT. Applies eyeliner
V. Uses mouthwash	UU. Applies eyebrow pencil
	VV. Removes makeup
Menstrual Care	
W. Puts on sanitary napkin	Miscellaneous
X. Changes sanitary napkin	WW. Blows and wipes nose
Y. Inserts tampon	XX. Cleans earmold of hearing aid
Z. Changes tampon	YY. Cleans eyeglasses

that the primary leisure-time skill of most mildly handicapped students is watching television. If they have additional leisure-time skills, these are limited in scope. In most cases the student has not been systematically exposed to other opportunities which would expand his leisure-time activities and provide him a more well-rounded and normal type of life.

The curriculum has two major divisions: (1) leisure-time activities that can be done at home; and (2) leisure-time activities that can be done in the community. Within each of those divisions there are three types of leisure-time activities: (a) participatory activities that can be done alone at home; (b) participatory activities that can be done with others; and (c) observational activities. Examples of solitary home participatory activities are shown in Table 5, which shows the wide scope of activities that can be found within each of these categories. Examples of at home participatory activities with other people include the entire range of cards, board games, ping-pong, and pool. The observational activities at home of course are watching television, listening to radio and records or tapes.

Activities in the community must be geared to the particular community where the student is living. Potential solitary activities include bowling, playing pool, swimming, jogging, and hiking. All of these can be done with others as well. In addition, throwing and catching a ball, playing basketball, pitching horseshoes, and badminton can be done with others. Observational activities in the community are usually those that are associated with watching team sports or going to the theater.

It is important that the student is exposed to leisure-time activities and taught how to use the facilities or how to participate. Frequently the lack of knowledge about the availability of such activities or how to perform them prevents the student from participating. The other consideration, especially with community activities, is transportation to and from the activity. We should not teach students to have expectations that they can attend events or participate in activities for which they are unable to obtain or use transportation.

Table 5
An Example of Leisure-Time Skills
(Solitary Participatory Activities, Home-Based)

Play Solitaire
Complete latch hook kit
Embroider
Paint by number
Color (adult coloring books)
Frame loom weaving
Knit squares (sew into afghans)
Coil basketry
Make beads
Model building
Drawing/sketching
Maintain scrapbook
Camera (film development)
Pet care
Picture puzzle
Garden (window boxes) plants

Vocational

The next curricular area is vocational. The Teaching Research Infant and Child Center has developed a three-stage vocational program that has been used with all types of severely and mildly handicapped children. The first two stages are conducted within or around the educational environment; the third stage is conducted in the community. The amount of time the student spends in each of these stages is similar for both the mildly and severely handicapped.

Stage 1 consists of brief exposures (4–6 weeks each) of five job opportunities found around the school building. These include janitorial and maintenance, food service, grounds-keeping/agricultural, office/clerical, and recycling. Each of these contains a variety of tasks that in most cases must be coordinated with the school administration or with various elements within the school. Our experience indicates that both the school cafeteria and the custodial force welcome students in a work experience situation as long as they do not have to do the training. The same holds true for the school secretarial force. Therefore a vocational trainer, the teacher, or the aide must provide the vocational teaching to the child. During Stage 1 the student is exposed to and assessed in all five work areas. The school year is divided into five parts and the student experiences part of each of the tasks required in each of the work areas. It is impossible to teach the student all the tasks required in any one area. For instance, a list of the essential skills in the food service area would be comparable to that contained in Table 6.

The recycling area requires some explanation because it is normally not part of school operations. In one community the school became a recycling collection center for cans and bottles when the student population was encouraged to bring them from home. The handicapped students separate the cans and bottles into appropriate containers. A paper-recycling project was also started when there was a great deal of paper that could be recycled and used again within a school. The students were taught to set up small cardboard boxes in each classroom and office, pick up the papers from the boxes, sort the papers to ensure that they were all of the correct size, and to stack them with the blank side up. These recycled papers were then placed in a press, glued on one end, and made into 8″ × 11″ pads or cut into memo pad size. These pads were then used by teachers and administrators within the school. Many business firms are willing to donate paper to a school for such a recycling effort. The expenses for the glue and for homemade presses are relatively small. In fact pads could even be sold for about 5¢ each. (In one government agency the use of pads made by special education students reduced the purchase of yellow lined pads by 75%).

Table 6
Essential Skills in the Food Service Area

- Setting serving trays
- Wrapping food in plastic wrap
- Wrapping food in aluminum foil
- Choosing utensils appropriate for food items
- Opening can with puncture-type can opener
- Opening can with top-removing can opener (manual)
- Opening can with electric can opener
- Delivering prepared food
- Busing trays
- Discriminating between food items that can legally be preserved and items that must be discarded
- Storing leftovers
- Rinsing dishes for dishwasher
- Loading dishwasher
- Cleaning food preparation tables
- Cleaning refrigerator
- Cleaning oven
- Slicing bagel horizontally in two
- Spreading butter
- Slicing cheese
- Dicing vegetables for salad
- Shredding lettuce
- Chopping onions
- Grating cheese
- Hard-boiling eggs
- Peeling hard-boiled eggs
- Setting up a salad bar
- Turning on burner
- Turning off burner
- Adjusting heat of burner
- Peeling garlic
- Crushing garlic in a garlic crusher
- Melting butter
- Making garlic butter
- Preparing garlic bread
- Serving garlic bread smorgasbord style
- Giving customer correct food item
- Offering customers napkins
- Preparing deep fryer
- Measuring
- Mixing dough
- Cutting doughnuts
- Packing doughnuts in boxes
- Cleaning deep freezer
- Discriminating when deep-fried foods are done
- Discriminating when foods being boiled are done
- Removing hot plates from oven
- Setting oven to correct setting
- Turning oven off
- Filling wash sink
- Filling rinse sink
- Filling sanitizing sink
- Washing pots and pans using three sinks
- Drying pots
- Putting pots in proper storage place
- Removing objects from kitchen cupboard to be cleaned
- Cleaning cupboard with sponge and cleaning solution
- Rinsing cupboard with clean sponge
- Cleaning sponge
- Replacing items to marked location
- Filling mop bucket
- Adding cleaning solution to bucket
- Wringing mop
- Mopping kitchen floor
- Emptying bucket
- Filling bucket with rinse water
- Discriminating between rinse mop and wash mop
- Rinsing floor
- Making coffee in coffee maker
- Making coffee in large coffee urn

The second stage of the vocational curriculum focuses on any two of the Stage 1 vocational areas. The student spends half a year in each. This is partially a result of the student's prior performance but also considers the student's preference. During this half-year stint in one of the job opportunities he is taught many more of the skills required in that particular type of work and gains proficiency in those skills. Proficiency was not a requirement for Stage 1. Stage 1 was designed primarily to orient the student to the world of work and various kinds of jobs. Some of the jobs required interactions with people, others required the ability to work alone;) (some required sedentary types of activities while others required a fair amount of physical labor. Thus the student was exposed to different types of work environments during Stage 1, and during Stage 2 he becomes proficient in two of the work areas.

Stage 3 involves placement in a community job and training that can lead to long-term employment. Some severely handicapped students for whom competitive community placement seems unfeasible may be placed in a sheltered workshop or activity center. One must be cautious about making that determination, however, for our experience has indicated that many of the more severely handicapped students can be placed in some community jobs if provided with adequate training and supervision. The vocational trainer must be the one who trains the student in that position in the local community. This means that the school district must have such a trainer on staff. This can be accomplished either through using existing vocational trainers and providing them with the skills to train handicapped students or by having a specially trained vocational trainer for handicapped students.

The entire purpose of the vocational program is to move the student from a sampling of jobs to a more intensive learning of vocational tasks and finally to placement in the actual world of work. In addition to the vocational elements, however, emphasis is placed on those skills which are listed in the social/sexual or practical living skill area where the student must interact with fellow workers, respond to employers, and make his way to and from the job. These are all part of the vocational training program and should be coordinated with the other parts of the curriculum.

Functional Academics

The final curricular area is functional academics. It is not academics in the traditional sense of the word. Certainly if the student is capable of writing, reading, and doing math, those skills are enhanced and built upon. Emphasis in this curricular area is on the practical use of such skills. Math skills are used to facilitate using money, telling time, and measuring. Reading skills are used to assist a student to follow directions or to provide the student essential information about his job or other activities in which he is engaged. Writing skills are used to assist the student to fill out applications, order books or magazines, or to communicate something meaningful to some other person.

The curriculum at the secondary level has been developed to include age-appropriate materials and activities that are geared to each individual student's developmental level. The curriculum has also been designed so that inappropriate behaviors are decreased while more appropriate behaviors (social or vocational) are being increased. Additionally the student's receptive and expressive language are not trained in isolation but as a part of the leisure or work activity. A severely handicapped student may be learning to ask for additional work materials by looking (eye contact) at the trainer and pointing to the place where the extra materials are stored while a mildly handicapped individual is required to use a four-word sentence to request needed materials.

SUMMARY

In this chapter we have attempted to describe the educational needs of the autistic child. We have offered a philosophy of special education as it pertains to these students. The arrangement of the educational environment was outlined to include these components: (1) the focus of where training occurs; (2) parent involvement; (3) supporting services; (4) classroom management; and (5) teaching strategies. We also presented specific curricular areas that we believe to be essential for the educational needs of the autistic adolescent and some examples of the implementation of those curricula.

Since the characteristics of the autistic individual include a deficit of social interaction, a strong emphasis was placed on the social curriculum. We feel that language and communication training should be an integral part of each training activity. Generalization strategies or techniques were discussed as being an important part of each training program.

REFERENCES

Alrick, G. Caring—an approach to sex education. Salem, Ore.: DAN Publications, 1980.
Bartak, L. Educational approaches. In Autism: A reappraisal of concepts and treatment (M. Rutter & E. Schopler, eds.), New York: Plenum Press, 1978.
Bartak, L., & Pickering, G. Aims and methods of teaching. In An approach to teaching autistic children (M. P. Everard, ed.), Oxford: Pergamon Press, 1976.
Bartak, L., & Rutter, M. Special educational treatment of autistic children: A comparative study. I. Design of study and characteristics of units. Journal of Child Psychology and Psychiatry, 1973, 14, 161–179.

Bartak, L., & Rutter, M. Differences between mentally retarded and normally intelligent autistic children. *Journal of Autism and Childhood Schizophrenia*, 1976, *6*, 109–120.

Browning, R. Treatment effects of a total behavior modification program with five autistic children. *Behavior Research and Therapy*, 1971, *9*, 319–328.

Callias, M. Educational aims and methods. In *Autism: A reappraisal of concepts and treatment* (M. Rutter & E. Schopler, eds.), New York: Plenum Press, 1978.

Carrier, J. K., Jr., & Peak, T. *Non-speech language initiation program*. Lawrence, Kans.: H & H Enterprises, 1975.

Churchill, D. W. The relation of infantile autism and early childhood schizophrenia to developmental language disorders of childhood. *Journal of Autism and Childhood Schizophrenia*, 1972, *2*, 182–197.

Cronis, T., & Justen, J. Teaching work attitudes at the elementary level. *Teaching Exceptional Children*, 1975, *7*(3), 103–105.

de Villiers, J. G., & Naughton, J. M. Teaching a symbol language to autistic children. *Journal of Consulting and Clinical Psychology*, 1974, *42*, 111–117.

Elgar, S. Organization of a school for autistic children. In *An approach to teaching autistic children* (M. P. Everard, ed.), Oxford: Pergamon Press, 1976.

Fredericks, H. D., Anderson, R., & Baldwin, V. The identification of competency indicators of teachers of the severely handicapped. *AAESPH Review*, 1979, *4*(1), 81–95.

Fredericks, H. D., & the Staff of the Teaching Research Infant and Child Center. *A data based classroom for the moderately and severely handicapped* (3rd ed.). Monmouth, Ore.: Instructional Development Corporation, 1979.

Fulwiler, R. L., & Fouts, R. S. Acquisition of American sign language by a noncommunicating autistic child. *Journal of Autism and Childhood Schizophrenia*, 1976, *6*, 43–51.

Halpern, W. I. The schooling of autistic children: Preliminary findings. *American Journal of Orthopsychiatry*, 1970, *40*, 665–671.

Hamblin, R. L., Buckholdt, D., Ferritor, D., Kozloff, M., & Blackwell, L. *The humanization process*. New York: Wiley, 1971.

Hermelin, B., & O'Connor, N. *Psychological experiments with autistic children*. London: Pergamon Press, 1970.

Hewitt, F. M. Teaching speech to an autistic child through operant conditioning. *American Journal of Orthopsychiatry*, 1965, *35*, 927–936.

Howlin, P. The assessment of social behavior. In *Autism: A reappraisal of concepts and treatment* (M. Rutter & E. Schopler, eds.), New York: Plenum Press, 1978.

Johnson, J., & Mithaug, D. A replication survey of sheltered workshop entry requirements. *AAESPH Review*, 1978, *3*(2), 116–122.

Kanner, L. Early infantile autism. *Journal of Pediatrics*, 1944, *25*, 211–217.

Kazdin, A., & Bootzin, R. The token economy: An evaluative review. *Journal of Applied Behavior Analysis*, 1972, *5*, 343–372.

Koegel, R. L., & Covert, A. The relationship of self-stimulation to learning in autistic children. *Journal of Applied Behavior Analysis*, 1972, *5*, 381–387.

Koegel, R. L., & Rincover, A. Treatment of psychotic children in a classroom environment. I. Learning in a large group. *Journal of Applied Behavioral Analysis*, 1974, *7*, 45–59.

Koegel, R., & Wilhelm, H. Selective responding to the components of multiple visual cues. *Journal of Experimental Child Psychology*, 1973, *15*, 442–453.

Koegel, R., Dunlap, G., & Dyer, K. Intertrial interval duration and learning in autistic children. *Journal of Applied Behavior Analysis*, 1980, *13*(1), 91–99.

Lansing, M. D., & Schopler, L. Individualized education: A public school model. In *Autism: A reappraisal of concepts and treatment* (M. Rutter & E. Schopler, eds.), New York: Plenum Press, 1978.

Lotter, V. Follow-up studies. In *Autism: A reappraisal of concepts and treatment* (M. Rutter & E. Schopler, eds.), New York: Plenum Press, 1978.

Lovaas, O. I. *The autistic child: Language development through behavior modification.* New York: Irvington, 1977.

Lovaas, O. I. Parents as therapists. In *Autism: A reappraisal of concepts and treatment* (M. Rutter & E. Schopler, eds.), New York: Plenum Press, 1978.

Lovaas, O. I., & Schreibman, L. Stimulus overselectivity of autistic children in a two choice situation. *Behavior Research and Therapy,* 1971, *9,* 305–310.

Lovaas, O. I., Berberich, J. P., Perloff, B. F., & Schaeffer, B. Acquisition of imitative speech in schizophrenic children. *Science,* 1966, *151,* 705–707.

Lovaas, O. I., Freitas, L., Nelson, K., & Whalen, C. The establishment of imitation and its use for the establishment of complex behavior in schizophrenic children. *Behavior Research and Therapy,* 1967, *5,* 171–181.

Lovaas, O. I., Schreibman, L., Koegel, R., & Rehm, R. Selective responding by autistic children to multiple sensory input. *Journal of Abnormal Psychology,* 1971, *77,* 211–222.

Lovaas, O. I., Koegel, R., Simmons, J., & Stevens-Long, J. Some generalization and follow-up measures on autistic children in behavior therapy. *Journal of Applied Behavior Analysis,* 1973, *6,* 131–165.

Marshall, N., & Hegrenes, J. The use of written language as a communication system for an autistic child. *Journal of Speech and Hearing Disorders,* 1972, *37,* 258–261.

McLean, L. P., & McLean, J. E. A language training program for non-verbal autistic children. *Journal of Speech and Hearing Disorders,* 1974, *39,* 186–193.

Miller, A., & Miller, E. E. Cognitive-developmental training with elevated boards and sign language. *Journal of Autism and Childhood Schizophrenia,* 1973, *3,* 65–85.

Mithaug, D., & Hagmeier, L. The development of procedures to assess prevocational competencies of severely handicapped young adults. *AAESPH Review,* 1978, *3*(2), 94–115.

Moore, M., Fredericks, H. D., & Baldwin, V. The long range effects of early childhood education on a TMR population. *Journal of the Division for Early Childhood,* 1981, *2,* 93–109.

Nicklesburg, R. Time sampling of work behavior. *Mental Retardation,* 1973, *11*(6), 29–40.

Ornitz, E. The modulation of sensory input and motor output in autistic children. *Journal of Autism and Childhood Schizophrenia,* 1974, *4,* 197–215.

Pagel, S., & Whitling, C. Readmissions to a state hospital for mentally retarded persons: Reasons for community placement failure. *Mental Retardation,* 1978, *16*(2), 164–168.

Premack, D., & Premack, A. J. Teaching visual language to apes and language-deficient persons. In *Language perspectives: Acquisition, retardation and intervention* (R. L. Schiefelbusch and L. L. Lloyd, eds.), Baltimore: University Park Press, 1974.

Rimland, B. *Infantile autism, the syndrome and its implications for a neural theory of behavior.* New York: Appleton-Century-Crofts, 1964.

Russo, D. C., & Koegel, R. L. A method for integrating an autistic child into a normal public school classroom. *Journal of Applied Behavior Analysis,* 1977, *16,* 579–590.

Rutter, M. Autistic children: Infancy to adulthood. *Seminars in Psychiatry,* 1970, *2,* 435–450.

Rutter, M., & Bartak, L. Special education treatment for autistic children, study II. Follow-up findings and implications for services. *Journal of Child Psychology and Psychiatry,* 1973, *14,* 241–270.

Schaeffer, B. Spontaneous language through signed speech. In *Nonspeech language and communication* (R. L. Schiefelbusch, ed.), Baltimore: University Park Press, 1980.

Schopler, E., & Mesibov, G. B. Multiple effects of treatment outcome for autistic children. *Journal of the American Academy of Child Psychiatry,* in press.

Stanfield, J. Graduation: What happens to the retarded child when he grows up? *Exceptional Children,* 1973, *39*(7), 548–553.

Stokes, T., & Baer, D. An implicit technology of generalization. *Journal of Applied Behavior Analysis,* 1977, *10,* 349–367.

Stremel-Campbell, K., Cantrell, D., & Halle, J. Manual signing as a language system and a speech initiator for the nonverbal, severely handicapped student. In *Educational programming for the severely and profoundly handicapped* (E. Sontag, ed.), CEC/MR Monograph, 1977.

Walker, H., & Buckley, N. Programming generalization and maintenance of treatment effects across time and settings. *Journal of Applied Behavior Analysis,* 1972, *5,* 209–224.

Wing, L. Social, behavioral, and cognitive characteristics: An epidemiological approach. In *Autism: A reappraisal of concepts and treatment* (M. Rutter & E. Schopler, eds.), New York: Plenum Press, 1978.

Wing, J. K., & Wing, L. Provision of services. In *Early childhood autism: Clinical, educational and social aspects* (L. Wing, ed.), Oxford: Pergamon Press, 1976.

Wolf, M., Risley, T., & Mees, H. Application of operant conditioning procedures to the behavior problems of an autistic child. *Behavior Research and Therapy,* 1964, *1,* 305–312.

Wolf, M., Risley, T., Johnston, M., Harris, F., & Allen, E. Application of operant conditioning procedures to the behavior problems of an autistic child: A follow-up and extension. *Behavioral Research and Therapy,* 1967, *5,* 103–111.

REFERENCE NOTE

1. Creedon, M. P. *Language development in nonverbal autistic children using a simultaneous communication system.* Paper presented at the meeting on Research in Child Development, Philadelphia, March 1973. (Available from EDRS, Leasco Information Products, 4827 Rugby Avenue, Bethesda, Maryland 20014; Reprint no. ED–78624 in microfiche and hard copy).

6

Recreation and Leisure Needs
A Community Integration Approach

PAUL WEHMAN

As more severely handicapped individuals are deinstitutionalized into the community (Gollay, Freedman, Wyngaarden, & Kurtz, 1978) or maintained in their natural families, the need for systematic program implementation of recreation skills has increased (Wehman, 1978; Wehman & Schleien, in press). The importance of recreational services has been observed frequently (Amary, 1975; Benoit, 1955; Stanfield, 1973; Wehman, 1977a). The critical nature of systematic assessment, skill selection, and instruction for leisure skills has only recently been noted, however (Snell, 1978; Wehman & Schleien, 1980; Ford, Brown, Pumpian, Baumgart, Schroeder, & Loomis, Note 1). Severely handicapped individuals usually include those with measured IQs between 0 and 40, and have been typically labeled as trainable mentally retarded, severely profoundly retarded, autistic, emotionally disturbed, deaf-blind, or multihandicapped. Most of these individuals exhibit substantial learning, behavior, and/or physical handicaps and therefore do not learn leisure skills without systematic instruction.

The purpose of the present chapter is to provide guidelines for systematic leisure skill training of autistic adolescents. First, a definition of leisure and a rationale for inclusion of play and leisure instruction into the educational curriculum are provided. Second, characteristics of an appropriate leisure skill program are outlined with supportive literature provided. Finally, guidelines for implementing a *trainer-advocacy* ap-

PAUL WEHMAN ● Division of Educational Services, Virginia Commonwealth University, Richmond, Virginia 23284.

proach to community-based recreation are delineated, along with illustrative case studies.

PLAY AND LEISURE: DEFINITION AND RATIONALE

Definition

We all enjoy engaging in leisurely activities which are a diversion from our daily work routine. Handicapped persons are no different; in fact they may have a stronger need for leisure and diversion due to living or working conditions that provide little joy in their lives. For example, in state institutions disabled individuals face an extremely drab existence in which ample free time may exist for play or leisure but little direction or guidance is available for channeling this time. Similarly, handicapped individuals who live alone in the community and hold jobs which may be dull and repetitious often find that these jobs provide minimal opportunities for cooperative interaction with co-workers. These individuals also require opportunity and direction in learning how to use leisure-time activities appropriately.

The elusiveness of defining play and leisure has been documented elsewhere (Ellis, 1973) and there is little need for extended discussion of this problem. Rather, an overview of several different efforts to define leisure might be more helpful in familiarizing the reader with the definitional complexities of this construct.

Ellis (1973) made perhaps the greatest effort in deciding on a theoretically and conceptually sound definition of play. He discussed in detail how a definition of play can be formulated depending on the perspective one takes in examining play. That is, the use of leisure may be defined by motive, it may be defined as voluntary behavior or content, or it may simply be considered undefinable. Ellis viewed leisure as a need to maintain an arousal level of activity, and eventually defined it this way: "Play is that behavior that is motivated by the need to elevate the level of arousal towards the optimal" (p. 110). He also made the critical point that pure play or leisure can occur only in the absence of all extrinsic consequences and when "the behavior is driven on solely by intrinsic motivation" (p. 110).

Hutt (1966) made another comparison in a discussion on specific versus diversive exploratory behavior. Similarly, Hurlock (1964) denoted play as "any activity engaged in for the enjoyment it gives, without consideration of the end result. It is entered into voluntarily and is lacking in external force or compulsion" (p. 442). Nunnally and Lemond (1973) presented play as only one component of a temporal sequence of exploratory behavior. These writers hypothesized that when an organism encounters a certain stimulus the following chain of behaviors occurs: (1) orienting behavior; (2) perceptual investigation; (3) manipulatory behavior; (4) play activity; and (5) searching activity. The chain ends as the organism becomes bored and must begin searching for new sources of stimulation. Play is viewed as the time when an organism engages in diversionary thinking or behavior.

In short, specific operational definitions of play and leisure have not been readily available in the literature. Perhaps a more cogent way of attacking the problem is to identify certain characteristics of leisure behavior, and then adapt these characteristics to operationalizing the salient variables which might be examined in play research or a play program. Beach (1945) presented certain qualities of play in animals which may be applicable here:

1. Playful behavior in animals as in man carries an emotional element of pleasure. Not all pleasurable activities are playful, but all play is assumed to be pleasurable.
2. Play is usually regarded as characteristic of the immature animal rather than the adult.
3. Play is customarily regarded as nonutilitarian (p. 524).

While attempts to define play have been a serious pedagogical exercise, it may be sufficiently elusive and irrelevant to warrant little continued effort. Identifying program variables which are critical measures of playful behavior or use of leisure time is probably of much greater utility. McCall (1974) used this strategy in his research on the exploratory behavior of infants through measuring variables such as latency (length of time) to respond to a newly presented toy, time of acting on or attending to a toy, and interaction or noninteraction with mother. Knapczyk and Yoppi (1975), in training cooperative and competitive play with developmentally disabled children, identified variables by operationalizing a hierarchy of social behaviors from onlooker or observer level through competitive play.

For the purposes of this chapter "leisure" and "play" activity are used interchangeably and may be considered as any action or combination of actions that the individual engages in for the apparent purpose of fun. These actions may not be harmful or consistently nonfunctional and repetitive.

Rationale for Leisure Instruction

Abundance of Leisure Time. All too often autistic individuals have an abundance of leisure time but have not developed the necessary skills to utilize their free time creatively or constructively. The actual amount of instructional time within the educational program may be for a relatively small part of the day with nothing to do during its remainder. The student's use of leisure time and his attitude toward recreation may determine the degree of success he will experience in other educational efforts; therefore appropriate free-time activities must be developed and systematically programmed. Unoccupied time must cease to be the dominant characteristic of an autistic individual's life.

Instruction Promotes Participating. Ford et al. (Note 1) have noted that recreation has been considered by many educators to be inappropriate for school instruction: "There seemed to be a general societal view which was also accepted by educators that recreation/leisure instruction should occur primarily after school, on vacations, weekends, etc. and valuable school-time should only be indirectly or peripherally devoted to such pursuits" (p. 1). This view unfortunately minimized recreation and leisure as viable instructional objectives on severely handicapped students' Individualized Education Plans.

Without systematic instruction in leisure skills, however, severely handicapped individuals will not learn the skills necessary to play appropriately (Wehman, 1977a). Even after the child has acquired a skill, without systematic instructional strategies he may never maintain, generalize, or self-initiate the skill into other environments (see Snell, 1978, for a detailed description of systematic instruction). Besides emphasizing the provision of activities that build on the present capabilities of the youth and prevent further disability, systematic instruction must be provided to foster engagement in appropriate leisure activity. Instruction of this sort may include assessing the leisure skill competencies of the individual, careful selection of materials and skills for instruction, and implementation techniques or specific training methods to assist in the acquisition, maintenance, and generalization of the skills.

Reduction of Inappropriate Social Behaviors. Individuals who are constructively using their leisure time are less likely to exhibit body rocking, head banging, violent actions, and social withdrawal. Autistic adolescents frequently engage in these inappropriate and unacceptable social behaviors. Research with autistic and other severely handicapped persons has clearly indicated that there is an inverse relationship between acquisition of play skills and self-stimulatory/abusive behavior (Favell, 1973; Koegel, Firestone, Kramme, & Dunlap, 1974). Recreational activities provide opportunities to the autistic person to learn to adjust to the social demands of society.

Means of Teaching Social, Motor, and Domestic Skills. The development of leisure skills in autistic youth will enhance social, motor, and domestic skill development. Leisure and recreational activities offer some of the most effective means for individuals to acquire and develop these skills.

Social skill development is facilitated through group activity (Marchant & Wehman, 1979). Children who fail to develop social skills are considered handicapped. The development of leisure behavior and participation in social activities will lead to making friends, getting along with others, learning to share, compete, cooperate, take turns, and in general make a more satisfactory social adjustment. An adequate social adjustment is required for successful daily living including time on the job, in the community, and with friends and family.

Recreation is also a vehicle for developing gross and fine motor skills. Inactivity usually results in *poor* eye–hand coordination, cardiovascular endurance, agility, dynamic and static balance, manual dexterity, and muscular strength. Because physical development is essential for a healthy body and self-concept, it is critical that autistic youth be given every opportunity to develop physically (Wehman, Renzaglia, Berry, Schutz, & Karan, 1978). Hill (Note 2) demonstrated how a cartoon box could be used to increase the purposeful arm movements and head control of a nonambulatory, profoundly retarded child. The student was taught to operate the device and look at the different cartoon sequences.

Eating in a fast-food restaurant is a domestically oriented leisure activity. One of the social activities enjoyed most frequently by a family is eating;* therefore it will be easier for autistic youth to participate with their families if appropriate eating skills are already present (Schleien, Kiernan, Ash, & Wehman, in press). Eating appropriately in a restaurant, using a vending machine, or preparing a snack at home are examples of leisure activities that require instruction and enhance social and domestic skills.

CHARACTERISTICS OF AN APPROPRIATE LEISURE SKILLS PROGRAM

When education and recreation professionals write leisure instructional objectives into autistic students' Individualized Education Plans,

*A 1978 Harris Poll documented eating as the most popular form of leisure for Americans.

they need an awareness of what characterizes an appropriate leisure skills instructional program. An optimal program should include: (1) a philosophical base of normalization that promotes the integration of handicapped with nonhandicapped persons; (2) modifications of equipment, rules, skill sequences, and facilities when necessary; (3) a behavioral approach to training; and (4) generalization of training.

The Role of Normalization and Integration in Leisure Program Planning

When applied to leisure skill programming, the philosophy of normalization (Wolfensberger, 1972) suggests several major concepts which need to be considered. For example, the criterion of chronological age-appropriateness as a means of skill selection (Brown, Branston, Hamre-Nietupski, Pumpian, Certo, & Gruenwald, 1979; Wehman & Schleien, 1980) is derived from normalization theory. Contemporary thinking in this area suggests that autistic and other handicapped students should be provided the opportunity to engage in leisure activities which are comparable to those engaged in by nonhandicapped peers. Wehman and Schleien (1980) have described procedures for selecting skills in this manner. Ford, Johnson, Pumpian, Stengert, and Wheeler (Note 3) have developed an excellent manual which lists numerous chronologically age-appropriate leisure activities.

Applying the normalization principle involves taking steps to reduce the "differentness" in both appearance and performance of disabled persons while simultaneously expanding the public's degree of acceptance for differentness. Leisure-education providers need to use "culturally normative" techniques with clients that facilitate acceptance from the public. For example, Wehman and Schleien (1980) describe modifications of equipment, rules, skill sequences, and facilities that enable severely disabled adults to participate in such normative leisure activities as bowling and photography. Such interventions both develop leisure skills which may generalize to other community settings and enable the general public to observe developmentally disabled persons participating *successfully* in normal leisure pursuits.

Another key to acceptance by nonhandicapped persons is the integration of only a limited number of handicapped participants in an activity. Handicapped people will be acceptable more readily by their nonhandicapped counterparts if their numbers in a particular setting do not exceed a proportion which could reasonably be expected to occur through normal interactions. Often-cited examples of special camps, large numbers of mentally retarded persons occupying several blocks of bowling lanes, and the inclusion of masses of handicapped individuals in swimming pools illustrate the negative effect such practices may have in leisure settings. It is important to keep the number of handicapped small because non-handicapped individuals will be more likely to exhibit a greater tolerance.

Successful involvement of disabled persons with nondisabled individuals, not other disability groups, is the ultimate goal of the normalization process. Therefore instructional or purely recreative pursuits such as horseback-riding programs for the handicapped, special-events days catering exclusively to disabled members of a community, and leagues and tournaments for handicapped participants do *not* achieve the ultimate goal of providing normative recreational environments. It serves no meaningful purpose, other than administrative convenience, to mass group handicapped individuals by their presumed category.

The techniques and procedures described later in two case studies can be implemented directly to promote participation by handicapped persons in appropriate activities in the community. For example, leisure skill instruction should be conducted in settings and time frames typical of society at large. Also related to the concept of appropriate recreation is the motivation underlying participation. As the ultimate impetus for leisure skill, instructional techniques should provide progressive success and achievement by the learner.

A cooperative approach is needed when involving handicapped persons in community settings. Potential resource persons who can exert a significant influence on the leisure lifestyle of a disabled person include family members, education and recreation personnel, volunteers and staff of advocate associations, and municipal recreation and social service personnel. The approach to leisure skill development illustrated in this chapter requires involvement from *all* persons concerned with this process. While the assessment procedures and certain adaptation techniques lend themselves naturally to formal education recreative settings, family members, peers, and others could readily become involved in supplementing and reinforcing leisure skill instruction in home and community settings.

Participation Made Possible Through Modifications

Another major characteristic of an appropriate recreation program for severely handicapped individuals is *participation*. Brown, Branston, Baumgert, Vincent, Falvey, and Schroeder (1979) have expressed a principle of partial participation, that is, the need to modify or adapt materials or activities to allow the individual to enjoy some degree of participation.

A major problem with many leisure activities for autistic youth has been that the activities are too passive in nature and that the individual is not included.

Fortunately there are a number of adaptations that can be utilized to facilitate partial participation by severely handicapped individuals. Wehman & Schleien (in press) have categorized these into *equipment, rules, skill sequence,* and *facility* modifications. The section below describes examples of each of these modifications in more depth. It should be noted, however, that adaptations are only used when necessary for participation and should be faded out as quickly as possible. The suggested adaptations may be considered as "lead-up" skills for those who consistently fail at the unadapted skills.

Equipment Modification. The equipment used in a recreational activity is frequently a barrier to participation because it usually has been designed by and for nonhandicapped individuals. Equipment can be adapted. For example, it can be modified to permit bowling by individuals with difficulties in fine and gross motor coordination, balance, and muscular strength required to lift and roll a bowling ball down an alley. The bowling ball could be placed on top of a tubular steel ramp. The bowler then "aims" the ramp at the pins and releases the ball. Or a bowling ball pusher similar to a shuffleboard stick could be used to push the ball down the alley. The pusher can be adjusted to various lengths, allowing ambulatory, non-ambulatory, short, and tall individuals to play. A third device, modified for use by a person unable to lift a conventional ball, is a handle-grip bowling ball. A simple palmar grasp and basic gross motor arm movements are required to manipulate this device. Once released, the handle snaps back flush into the bowling ball, allowing the ball to roll toward the pins. These modifications can permit many severely physically handicapped persons to enjoy bowling.

Rule Modifications. Most activities have a standard set of rules. If an individual's physical condition makes following a particular rule difficult, it may cause the participant to become a spectator instead. These difficulties need not be insurmountable, and may be overcome by changing the original rules of activities. Rules can also be modified or simplified when teaching a game and then later shaped to conform to the rules used by nonhandicapped peers.

Basketball requires a player to bounce or dribble the ball every time a step is taken. A change that permits one dribble for several steps down the court would permit an individual with difficulty in eye–hand–foot coordination to become an active member of the team. Perhaps with practice coordination will improve.

Pool has several variations, making it a flexible leisure-time activity. One can play 8-ball, which requires designating either stripes or solids to each player, or straight pool, which has a number of variations. In straight pool the players can call their shots, or can hit the balls in numerical sequence, or can shoot at any ball on the table and whoever pockets the most balls wins. Before choosing a pool game one must consider whether the handicapped person has difficulty discriminating numbers, or stripes from solids, and choose a game of pool accordingly.

Rule changes in card games may also be made. For example, "Concentration" requires the players to draw two cards consecutively in search of pairs. Difficulty in discriminating between numbered and picture cards can be decreased by assigning the same value to all picture cards (jacks, queens, kings).

A seemingly impossible task can be converted into an enjoyable recreational pursuit when rules are modified. Changing the rules allows an adolescent or adult to participate in an age-appropriate game or sport, rather than being forced to play with an age-inappropriate toy or participate in a child's game.

Skill Sequence Modifications. One of the most effective ways to teach a severely handicapped individual a recreational activity is to break the skill down into small component steps. These actions are identified through an analysis of the task itself and then sequenced in a logical order. However, often a sequence of steps applicable to a nonhandicapped individual's abilities may prove too difficult or impractical for a severely handicapped person to follow.

A hobby such as cooking illustrates the problem clearly. When boiling an egg, a nonhandicapped person might put the egg into a pot of water as the water is heating. It is obvious that this could be a hazardous problem for an individual with physical and/or intellectual limitation (it's easy to scald one's hand). The remedy is to rearrange the sequence of the component steps by training the cook to place the egg in the saucepan and then fill the pan with cold water. The saucepan is then placed on a stove burner, the burner turned on, and the water brought to a boil. This procedure does not alter the final results (a boiled egg) when a few minutes are added to the cooking time, but provides a safe and practical method of performing the task.

A modified skill sequence can also be applied to taking a picture. Typically one raises the camera to eye level and then places an index finger over the shutter-release button. However, individuals lacking sufficient fine motor coordination could be trained to position their finger over the shutter-release button prior to lifting the camera. In this way the individual would merely have to depress the button once the camera was in place.

Modifications of Community-Based Facilities. The community itself offers many age-appropriate recreations that nonhandicapped individuals enjoy regularly. The local swimming pool, museum, restaurant, library, or church are all public facilities available to handicapped people. Unfortunately many severely handicapped individuals are denied access to these places and consequently cannot utilize their leisure time in these environments. This problem is most evident for nonambulatory individuals who are unable to enter public buildings because of narrow doors, inadequate toileting facilities, and imposing staircases. In addition transportation to many of these facilities is inadequate. Many of the architectural barriers, however, have been overcome by the installation of wheelchair ramps leading to buildings, enlarged doorknobs, extended handles on drinking fountains, and other equipment modified for those with severe motor impairments.

While these physical modifications reduce barriers to utilization, there is one principle that must be seriously considered. The person using the equipment or facility must not at the same time be separated from interacting with the community in general. Those modifications should blend in with the standard equipment so no person would stand out as being very different. For example, pier fishing could be made accessible to severely physically impaired individuals and yet retain its normal qualities. Guidelines require:

1. An access walk to the pier of at least a 5-foot width to allow for turning of the wheelchairs
2. The provision of a handrail around the entire pier that, according to the Virginia Commission of Outdoor Recreation, must be 36 inches high and have a 30° angle sloping top for arm and pole rest
3. A kick plate to prevent foot pedals of wheelchairs from going off the pier
4. A smooth, nonslip surface on the access walk and pier

The adaptations described above represent the primary ways in which a creative teacher or therapist can reduce failure and frustration for severely handicapped persons. Although it is imperative that these adaptations be *individualized*, i.e., not provided for the group as a whole, and *temporary* in as many situations as feasible, it is certain that without the above-described modifications recreational involvement by many autistic handicapped individuals will be nonexistent or minimal at best.

A Behavioral Approach to Training

The methods component of instruction programs refers to the *procedures* and *activities* used to train in the desired skills. It must be emphasized that *training* and specific leisure skill *instruction* must take place for the severely handicapped to learn. It cannot be assumed that individuals with severe behavior and/or learning deficits will simply "pick up" leisure activities. Leisure skills must be trained. Numerous training procedures have been used with severely handicapped individuals. For example, specific reinforcement strategies have been used with severely retarded children to develop cooperative leisure actions (Favell, 1973; Morris & Dolker, 1974; Wehman & Marchant, 1978). Reinforcement has also been used with severely retarded adults in a changing criterion strategy which emphasized the behavior shaping of dart-throwing skills (Schleien, Wehman, & Kiernan, 1981). An extension of this shaping strategy was used in combination with weekly leisure counseling sessions with higher functioning retarded adults in a group home (Schleien, Kiernan, Ash, & Wehman, 1981).

The time-sampling measure, on the other hand, allows the teacher to assess the individual's leisure activity at different intervals of the day for brief time periods (30 seconds to 5 minutes). Assume the teacher is interested in documenting how much constructive leisure activity is taking place versus how much self-stimulatory stereotyping is occurring. The strategy would involve defining each behavior and then observing the occurrence or nonoccurrence of each behavior at designated time periods throughout the day. The time-sampling approach has been described in detail by Kazdin (1975) and Sulzar-Azaroff and Mayer (1977), and lends itself well to assessing leisure activities in an efficient way.

Generalization of Training

To special educators, a popular setting for teaching leisure and recreation skills is the classroom. There is an implicit assumption made that severely handicapped students will automatically *generalize* the skill to home or community environments. Yet we know that this inference cannot usually be made (Stokes & Baer, 1977). Therefore leisure instruction must actually take place in the community—in recreation centers, movie theaters, fast-food restaurants, parks, and Scout groups. Programming must also occur in the individual's home.

For example, Johnson and Bailey (1977) and Schleien, Wehman, and Kiernan (1981) both taught chronologically age-appropriate leisure skills to mentally retarded adults in group home settings. Hill, Wehman, and Horst (Note 4) provided training to severely retarded youth in the use of an electronic pinball machine in several community settings on a weekly basis. In each of these efforts the participants learned the skills and generalized them quickly.

The concept of training in leisure skills outside the classroom does not always mesh well with administrative concerns and the traditional public school service delivery system. Yet to accommodate the needs of severely handicapped students, teachers and administrators must adapt their usual means of service delivery. It is vital that students receive specific instruction in settings other than the classroom if parents are to consider these instructional efforts truly credible. Furthermore, generalization objectives should be included in the student's Individualized Education Plan when appropriate. Once teachers have established a routine for teaching leisure skills in the community they will also know which behaviors the community will not tolerate in severely handicapped students. This finding will help shape future curriculum selection.

A TRAINER-ADVOCACY APPROACH TO COMMUNITY-BASED RECREATION

From characteristics of a leisure program, an approach is planned for helping autistic youth participate in community-based recreation programs. The focus is not on the specific details of how to teach a leisure skills but rather on how to assist the integration of severely handicapped and nonhandicapped participants.

A trainer-advocacy approach is suggested for facilitating this integration. Such a service delivery system requires (a) instructional guidance by a staff person for the handicapped client at the place where the recreational activity occurs and (b) advocacy on behalf of the client to the group leader and the nonhandicapped participants in the group. This approach has been used with great success in placing and maintaining moderately and severely handicapped persons in competitive employment (Wehman, 1981). Once the individual has received a reasonable degree of acceptance by the members of the group (that is, some people in the group will take a special interest in the student), then the trainer-advocate staff person can reduce his or her involvement at the setting. There are six aspects of this approach which highlight its utility. They are:

1. The number of handicapped participants should be small for individualization.
2. Emphasis is on social acceptability and enjoyment by the client.
3. Social feedback from nonhandicapped participants.
4. Parental involvement in planning activity.
5. Ongoing nature of activity.
6. Appropriate matching of client leisure interest to program.

As a general rule of thumb 1–3 severely handicapped individuals are sufficient for integration into a nonhandicapped group of 8–10. Essentially the staff person directly assists in the initial adjustment process. Nonhandicapped people are usually somewhat uncomfortable during their first encounters with the severely handicapped. A small group makes it easier for the staff person to individualize the effort and help the nonverbal client communicate and thus be accepted more easily. This approach is in direct contrast to the practice of taking large busloads of severely handicapped people into town.

The social acceptance of the individual will play a major factor in how well the autistic individual adjusts, more so than a high degree of leisure skill proficiency. The essence of leisure is to participate and have fun; different individuals, whether handicapped or not, will experience enjoyment in spite of limited ability in an activity. It is far more important that the student minimize antisocial or inappropriate and bizarre behaviors, i.e., self-stimulatory motor actions or strange verbalizations. These types of behaviors tend to make most nonhandicapped individuals very uncomfortable, and hence, willingly or not, exclude the severely handicapped person from participation in the activity.

In a community activity such as going to a fast-food restaurant inappropriate social behaviors will effectively "turn-off" clerks and other consumers in the restaurant. Therefore it is imperative that a goal of social acceptability be paramount in leisure program planning. One example of an instructional goal is this area might be to keep one's hands at his sides when not engaged in an activity. Another goal would be to reduce or eliminate inappropriate verbalizations. It should be remembered, however, that these social skills are often best taught in the natural setting; hence there will probably be some initial adjustment problems.

The trainer-advocate must establish a dialogue with the nonhandicapped participants or consumers in the area. As the student participates in a formal social group it is vital to receive regular feedback as to how the student is being accepted. Ongoing evaluation throughout the weeks during which the activity takes place will let the staff and student know how the rest of the group feels about the severely handicapped person.

Evaluation can take the form of verbal communication or even written survey forms.

Since participation in a predominantly nonhandicapped group may be threatening to parents of autistic youth, it is necessary whenever possible to involve parents in planning the activity. Issues to consider include: transportation; location of setting; type of activity; age, sex, race, etc., of nonhandicapped participants; and the student's interest and preference. When parents can observe their son or daughter participating in an enjoyable activity with nonhandicapped peers there is a greater likelihood that they will encourage further involvement in normal community recreation programs. Without parental support it is highly improbable that the program will work.

Another feature of a trainer-advocacy approach is that the community activity should be ongoing in nature. For optimal learning and experience for both the severely handicapped and nonhandicapped participants, repeated exposure is an essential element. One-time-only field trips tend to have a fleeting impact on the student and do not allow for full sampling of the reinforcing aspects of selected leisure activities.

The individual's specific strengths and preferences must also be carefully considered in designing a community recreation program. Bates and Renzaglia (1978) have outlined several points which address the importance of matching the individual's interests with selected recreational activities available in the community. The reader is referred to their 1978 chapter for instructional strategies for community-based recreation programming. An initial assessment of a client's strengths and weaknesses must be made at this time and then matched to what the community has available.

Case Study Illustration of Leisure Skill Training

In order to demonstrate a number of the guidelines and principles discussed in this chapter, it will be helpful to highlight two case studies which were conducted with severely handicapped adolescents.* The leisure skills presented were selected to demonstrate an expanded range of leisure options for severely handicapped individuals. Students were taught use of a Frisbee and how to operate an electronic pinball machine in a community setting.

---

*Portions of these case studies were presented in "Instructional Programming for Severely Handicapped Youth" (Wehman & Hill, Note 4).

Program I: Use of a Frisbee

Participants and Setting. The two participants, Ron and Ralph, are males, 21 and 19 years old. They have been classified as severely retarded with IQs measuring below 30. Their expressive vocabulary is very limited, i.e., Ralph exhibits echolalic speech; Ron, however, is presently in a picture communication program. Both participants engage in high rates of inappropriate activities during free time. The setting was a public school for severely and profoundly handicapped students in Richmond, Virginia.

Rationale for Skill Selection. Frisbee was selected as an activity for several reasons. First, it was portable and could be played in a number of places. Second, it was an inexpensive object to purchase. Third, the motor actions required were quite simple to perform once they were carefully coordinated. Finally, Frisbee can be a two-part skill usually requiring a second person; the interdependent nature of the activity was viewed as desirable since the participants engaged in minimal cooperative leisure.

Task Analysis. The task analysis was initially drawn from the leisure curriculum developed by Wehman and Schleien (1981). It was then modified by the instructor for use with the participants in this program, i.e., catching and throwing skills were both utilized. The following task analysis formed the basis for initial assessment and instruction:

Throwing the Frisbee:

1. Hold Frisbee in throwing position, fingers curled on underside, thumb topside, index finger on edge.
2. Raise dominant arm, lifting Frisbee to shoulder level.
3. Bend elbow, bringing Frisbee inward toward chest.
4. Continue bending elbow until rim on Frisbee makes contact with nondominant shoulder.
5. Quickly extend elbow outward away from body.
6. When elbow is fully extended, release grasp on Frisbee.
7. Throw Frisbee 3 feet (keeping underside of Frisbee parallel to ground).
8. Throw Frisbee 6 feet (keeping underside of Frisbee parallel to ground).
9. Throw Frisbee 10 feet (keeping underside of Frisbee parallel to ground).
10. Throw Frisbee 15 feet (keeping underside of Frisbee parallel to ground).

Catching the Frisbee:

1. Stand away from (at least 5 feet) and facing other player.

2. Extend both arms outward toward other player, palms outward, fingers extended.
3. Follow path of Frisbee through the air (using eyes and hands).
4. When Frisbee approaches, grasp in hands firmly.

Teaching Procedures. From the initial baseline data a step was selected for instruction. Ron began instruction on step 1 of Frisbee throwing and Ralph's training started on step 4 of catching. These steps were the target behaviors that each individual was unable to complete independently.

A staff person initially modeled the entire skill prior to a 15-minute training session. Instruction was then begun on the specific training step in the Frisbee-throwing task analysis. A four-step hierarchy of (a) independent response, (b) verbal prompting, (c) modeling, and (d) physical guidance was used for purposes of training and subsequent data collection. The trainer would initially provide a verbal cue to Ron and then Ralph to complete the step. If the student performed it correctly he was socially reinforced. If not, then the verbal cue was repeated and a model was presented. If the response was correct then social reinforcement was provided. This sequence of graduated guidance was repeated throughout the training session. Training trials were alternated between the two students, and took place inside and outside the school.

Behavior Observation. Five training trials on the target steps were given during 15-minute instructional sessions daily. Data were collected dependent on which step of the cue hierarchy was necessary for performance by the student. Nonreinforced probe data were then collected weekly on the skill to monitor progress. These data were collected when a trainer gave the general cue (i.e., "Ron, throw the Frisbee"). At a later point in the program it was decided to collect nonreinforced probe data at the end of each session instead of weekly. This was done for more regular feedback on student progress.

Results. Baseline data in Figure 1 indicated that Ron did not exhibit any Frisbee skills whereas Ralph's data showed a minimum of steps he was able to complete independently, i.e., Ron functioning at 0-step proficiency level of throwing, Ralph averaging 61% on catching. Once systematic instruction was provided, both participants' Frisbee-playing skills increased to 100%. After criterion was met, a maintenance program was initiated so Ron and Ralph would sustain this particular skill, and when given the opportunity would generalize playing Frisbee to different settings. The maintenance program provided intermittent reinforcement for Ron and Ralph to throw the Frisbee for gradually extended lengths of time.

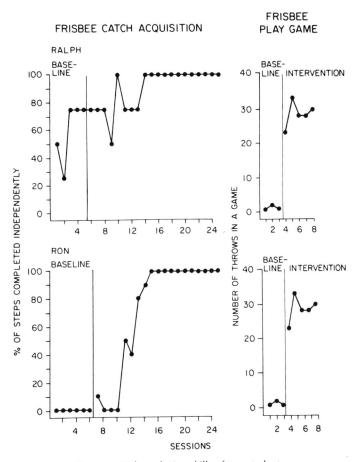

Figure 1. Frisbee-playing skills of two students.

Program II: Playing Pinball

Participants and Setting. Sam is a severely retarded nonverbal 15-year-old male. He is severely spastic, has limited use of one hand, and exhibits an uncoordinated gait. Sam exhibits simple eating and dressing skills. His social behavior is frequently characterized by shrieks and non-compliance. Much of Sam's pinball training took place in the same public school setting described in the previous study; however, in order to increase the amount of training in the community, instructional sessions alternated between the school and a local bowling alley which had pinball machines. This community training was also completed during school hours.

Instructional Procedures. The training procedure utilized was identical to that described in Program I. The graduated cue hierarchy of verbal cue, model and demonstration, and physical guidance were used depending on Sam's response level. Social reinforcement was delivered immediately upon successful completion of steps. Sam received approximately 10–15 minutes of training prior to a posttest on each step called a nonreinforced probe. As stated above, training and data collection occurred in school and in a community setting on an alternating basis (i.e., one training day occurred in school and the next training day in the community).

Behavior Observation. Progress in pinball performances was assessed using nonreinforced probe data after a stable baseline of preintervention pinball skill was established. As in Study I, nonreinforced probe data consisted of observing which steps in the task analysis Sam could complete independently following the verbal cue "Sam, play pinball." Data were collected after training in school and community setting. A percentage of steps completed independently was calculated after each session. Interrater reliability coefficients with a second rater once weekly ranged from .96 to 1.00.

Experimental Design. An alternating treatment design (Hersen & Barlow, 1977) was used to evaluate the instructional program. This design has rarely been used to assess treatment variables across different environments but it lends itself to assessing generalization.

Results. Figure 2 shows data collected on Sam's pinball performance in each separate environment. Circled dots are school probes; uncircled dots are community probes. Sam demonstrated steady improvement in operating the electronic pinball machine in both environments as revealed in Figure 2 by an increasing proficiency over a total of 17 instructional sessions. It is of note, however, that both baseline sessions in the community and the first four community generalization probes after intervention showed *lower* performance on the pinball steps than seen in the school baseline sessions or the first five probes after instruction at school. Mean percentage of steps completed independently in both settings over all sessions also show higher performance in the school setting, ($\overline{X}$ School Baseline: 47%; $\overline{X}$ Community Baseline: 42%; $\overline{X}$ School Performance: 71%; $\overline{X}$ Community Performance: 70%). This trend appears less conspicuous as instruction in the two settings continues in that, out of the final six probes, three at school and three in the community, the three community probes are equal to or higher than the school probes.

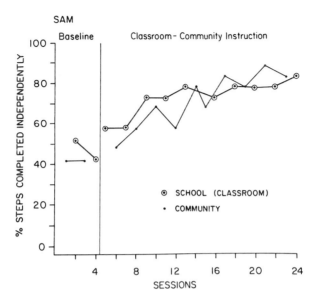

Figure 2. Pinball performance at school and in the community.

General Discussion

The results of these two programs provide support for severely hand-icapped adolescents' ability to acquire chronologically age-appropriate leisure skills. It is incumbent upon teachers and the professionals who work with the handicapped youth to include leisure education objectives into the students' Individual Education Plans. Furthermore these objectives must be taught in a *sequential* and *systematic* manner; it cannot be assumed that they will simply evolve into the student's repertoire of free-time behaviors.

An optimal service delivery model, which was unfortunately not re-flected in this program, would employ skilled therapeutic recreation specialists who could serve as consultants to teachers in assessment and skill selection, activity adaptation, instruction, and community integration. The present programs did not demonstrate the critical linkage into the community and homes. Although these objectives were discussed with family members of the participants, there was not a systematic follow-through for generalization and maintenance.

CONCLUSION

If we are to reverse the perpetual cycle of parent reluctance to involve severely retarded youth in normal community activities, then it is crucial for teachers and administrators to lead the way in prompting community integration. To combat this cycle we must first understand it. Parents who show a long history of isolating a handicapped child within the home often express fear of embarrassment with their child in public and the consternation of previous rejection by the community in general. In addition generally low expectations are held regarding the benefits to their child or to nonhandicapped people from greater community integration. The need to reverse these attitudes increases as more severely handicapped individuals are deinstitutionalized into the community.

ACKNOWLEDGMENTS: The author gratefully acknowledges the help, insight, and comments of Janet Hill and Stuart Schleien in developing this chapter.

REFERENCES

Amary, I. *Creative recreation for the mentally retarded*. Springfield, Ill.: Charles C Thomas, 1975.

Bates, P., & Renzaglia, A. Community based recreation programs. In *Recreation programming for developmentally disabled persons* (P. Wehman, ed.), Baltimore: University Park Press, 1978.

Beach, F. Current concepts of play in animals. *American Naturalist*, 1945, *79*, 523–541.

Benoit, E. P. The play problem of retarded children: A frank discussion with parents. *American Journal of Mental Deficiency*, 1955, *60*, 41–45.

Brown, L., Branston, M., Baumgart, D., Vincent, L., Falvey, M., & Schroeder, J. Using the characteristics of current and subsequent least restrictive environments in the development of curricular content to severely handicapped students. *Journal for the Association of the Severely Handicapped*, 1979, *14*, 4.

Ellis, M. *Why people play*. Englewood Cliffs, N.J.: Prentice-Hall, 1973.

Favell, J. Reduction of stereotypics by reinforcement of toy play. *Mental Retardation*, 1973, *11*(4), 24–27.

Gollay, E., Freedman, R., Wyngaarden, M., & Kurtz, N. *Coming back*. Boston: Little, Brown, 1978.

Hersen, D., & Barlow, D. *Single subject experimental designs*. New York: Pergamon Press, 1977.

Hurlock, E. *Child development*. New York: McGraw-Hill, 1964.

Hutt, C. Exploration and play in children. *Symposium of the Zoological Society of London*, 1966, *18*, 61–81.

Johnson, M., & Bailey, J. The modification of leisure behavior in a half-way house for retarded women. *Journal of Applied Behavior Analysis*, 1977, *10*, 2.

Kazdin, A. E. Behavior modification. Homewood, Ill.: Dorsey Press, 1975.

Knapczyk, D., & Yoppi, J. Development of cooperative and competitive play responses in developmentally disabled children. *American Journal of Mental Deficiency*, 1975, *80*, 245–255.

Koegel, R., Firestone, P., Kramme, K., & Dunlap, A. Increasing spontaneous play by suppressing self-stimulation in autistic children. *Journal of Applied Behavior Analysis*, 1974, *7*, 521–528.

Marchant, J., & Wehman, P. Teaching table games to severely retarded children. *Mental Retardation*, 1979, *17*, 150–152.

McCall, R. Exploratory manipulation and play in the human infant. *Monograph of the Society for Research in Child Development*. Chicago: University of Chicago Press, 1974.

Morris, R., & Dolker, M. Developing cooperative play in socially withdrawn children. *Mental Retardation*, 1974, *12*(6), 24–27.

Nunnally, J. C., & Lemond, L. Exploratory behavior and human development. In *Advances in child development and behavior*, Vol. 8 (H. W. Reese, ed.), New York: Academic Press, 1973.

Reid, D., Willis, B., Jarman, P., & Brown, K. Increasing leisure activity of physically retarded persons through modifying resource availability. *AAESPH Review*, 1978, *3*(2), 78–91.

Schleien, S., Kiernan, J., & Wehman, P. Evaluation of an age appropriate leisure skills program for mentally retarded adults. *Educational Training of the Mentally Retarded*, 1981, Feb., 13–19.

Schleien, S., Kiernan, J., Ash, T., & Wehman, P. Developing independent cooking skills in a profoundly retarded woman. *Journal of the Association for Severely Handicapped*, 1981, *6*(2), 23–29.

Schleien, S., Wehman, P., & Kiernan, J. Teaching leisure skills to severely multihandicapped adults. *Journal of Applied Behavior Analysis*, 14, *4*, 513–520.

Snell, M. (Ed.), *Systematic instruction for the moderately and severely handicapped*. Columbus, Ohio: Merrill, 1978.

Stanfield, J. Graduation: What happens to the retarded child when he grows up? *Exceptional Children*, 1973, *39*, 1–11.

Stokes, T., & Baer, P. An implicit technology of generalization. *Journal of Applied Behavior Analysis*, 1977, *10*, 349–367.

Sulzar-Azaroff, B., & Mayer, L. *Applied behavior analysis procedures with children and youth*. New York: Houghton Mifflin, 1977.

Wehman, P. *Helping the mentally retarded acquire play skills: A behavioral approach*. Springfield, Ill.: Charles C Thomas, 1977a.

Wehman, P. (Ed.), *Recreation programming for developmentally disabled persons*. Baltimore: University Park Press, 1977b.

Wehman, P. *Competitive employment: New horizons for the severely disabled*. Baltimore: Paul Brookes, 1981.

Wehman, P., & Marchant, J. Improving free play skills of severely retarded children. *American Journal of Occupational Therapy*, 1978, *32*(2), 100–172.

Wehman, P., & Schleien, S. Assessment and selection of leisure skills for severely handicapped persons. *Education and Training of the Mentally Retarded*, 1980, *14*(3), 36–42.

Wehman, P., & Schleien, S. *Leisure and handicapped individuals: Adaptations, techniques, and curriculum*. Baltimore: University Park Press, 1981.

Wehman, P., Renzaglia, A., Berry, G., Schutz, R., & Karan, O. Developing a leisure skill repertoire in severely and profoundly handicapped persons. *Journal of the Association for Severely Handicapped*, 1978, *3*(3), 162–172.

Wolfensberger, W. *Principles of normalization*. Toronto: National Institute of Mental Retardation, 1972.

REFERENCE NOTES

1. Ford, A., Brown, L., Pumpian, I., Baumgart, D., Schroeder, J., & Loomis, R. *Strategies for developing individualized recreation/leisure plans for adolescent and young adult severely handicapped students*. Unpublished manuscript, University of Wisconsin at Madison, 1981.
2. Hill, J. W. Use of an automated recreational device to facilitate independence leisure and motor behavior in a profoundly retarded male. In *Instructional programming for severely handicapped youth* (P. Wehman & J. Hill, eds.), Richmond, Va.: Virginia Commonwealth University, 1980.
3. Ford, A., Johnson, F., Pumpian, I., Stengert, J., & Wheeler, J. *A longitudinal listing of chronological age appropriate and functional activities for school-aged moderately and severely handicapped students*. Madison, Wisc.: Madison Public Schools, 1980.
4. Wehman, P., & Hill, J. *Instructional programming for severely handicapped youth*. Richmond, Va.: Virginia Commonwealth University, 1980.
5. Hill, J., Wehman, P., & Horst, G. Acquisition and generalization of leisure skills in severely and profoundly handicapped youth: Use of an electronic pinball machine. *Journal of the Association for Severely Handicapped* (in press).

7

School Doesn't Last Forever; Then What? Some Vocational Alternatives

SIDNEY M. LEVY

In industrial societies such as the United States participation in the labor force, job status, and earning power are critical factors in determining an individual's value in that society. Unfortunately people with physical and mental handicaps have been discriminated against vocationally either by total exclusion from the labor force or by employment in jobs not commensurate with their skills or potential.

Recently attempts to rectify that injustice have begun. Federal legislation guaranteeing the rights of all handicapped people to participate in the mainstream of society has been passed (1973 Rehabilitation Act and P.L. 94–142).

Still, the passage of laws alone does not resolve the problem unless they are effectively implemented and enforced. Although most people would accept the idea that handicapped people should have the same vocational options and opportunities as do other members of society, current findings do not show that this is happening. In a 1978 report the U.S. Department of Labor stated that only 41% of all disabled people are employed (Federal Register, 1978). If a focus is made on moderately, severely, or profoundly handicapped people, the percentage decreases greatly. The Greenleigh Associates (1975) report found that only 13% of sheltered workshop clients were engaged in competitive employment. Stanfield (1973), surveying a trainable mentally retarded population, found that many were not participating in any programs at all but remained at

SIDNEY M. LEVY ● Department of Special Education, George Peabody College, Vanderbilt University, Nashville, Tennessee 37203.

home after public school graduation. Without the advocacy of professionals and the determined effort of the families of handicapped citizens to secure their rights, the laws will continue to be unimplemented or ineffective.

Of all the types of handicapping conditions people are afflicted with, those indiviuals classified as autistic have received the least consideration for vocational participation. A possible explanation for this exclusion from programs might be the types of behaviors autistic people frequently display. As a group they are described as having great difficulty relating to people, being unresponsive to social stimuli, engaging in self-stimulating behavior, and having language problems (Kauffman, 1977). These kinds of behaviors greatly affect an individual's employability. This chapter is an attempt to establish the concept that in spite of these problems autistic people do have vocational potential, to discuss the current types of vocational alternatives available to them, to offer ways to enhance their vocational viability, and to discuss how their participation in the labor force might be facilitated in the future.

The potential of handicapped people at all functioning levels to learn job skills has been demonstrated through recent advances in training and behavioral technology (Bellamy, Peterson, & Close, 1975; Levy, Pomerantz, & Gold, 1977). Techniques such as task analysis, systematic training, and behavior modification have proved to be highly effective. Through the use of those techniques severely and profoundly handicapped people, including autistic individuals have learned such difficult industrial tasks as assembling bicycle brakes (Gold, 1972), cam switches (Bellamy et al., 1975), and electric circuit boards (Levy et al., 1977). Although these people have demonstrated the potential to learn and perform difficult tasks, they have not had the opportunities to do so. Almost all of their work activities in current vocational programs have been restricted to highly simplified repetitive tasks that require minimal training (Greenleigh Associates, 1975). In fact it appears, given the limited opportunities handicapped people have to learn and use higher level vocational skills in existing work settings, that the training technology may have surpassed its application (Levy, 1980). While it is essential for professionals and other concerned people to continue to develop the teaching technology, they must at the same time work toward providing appropriate vocational opportunities for handicapped people to apply their skills.

AVAILABLE VOCATIONAL OPTIONS

There are presently two basic vocational alternatives available to handicapped people—sheltered work facilities and competitive job settings. Traditionally most people who are classified as moderately, severely, or profoundly handicapped, if they are place in a work program at all, are considered appropriately placed in sheltered work programs. More mildly handicapped people are directed toward competitive jobs.

Sheltered Work Programs

Sheltered work programs consist of two basic types, the work activity program and the sheltered workshop. The work activity program is designed to meet the needs of lower functioning people. The program is designed to provide very basic prevocational training in a work setting as well as training in other skill areas such as self-help and recreation. To be eligible for a work activity program an individual must have demonstrated that he is presently unable to produce at rates over 25% of what a normal worker could do. Usually in these programs the client-to-staff ratio is higher to accommodate more one-to-one interactions.

The sheltered workshop is defined by the National Association of Sheltered Workshops and Homebound Programs as a nonprofit rehabilitation facility utilizing individual goals, wages, supportive services, and a controlled work environment to help vocationally handicapped persons achieve or maintain maximum potential as workers. Sheltered workshops have been criticized by some as not fulfilling their responsibilities for providing a good work environment (Gold, 1973; Greenleigh Associates, 1975; Levy, 1980). The work tasks, when available, are usually highly simplified and repetitive, frequently failing to maintain worker interest. The shop atmosphere is usually not conducive to encouraging high levels of productivity. A message frequently conveyed to the worker by the staff is that there is little need to produce at high rates. Finally, professional staff are usually not trained or knowledgeable in industrial methodology, which contributes to the situation (Levy, 1980; Levy et al., 1977; Pomerantz & Marholin, 1977). The result of all these factors is that insufficient work task and production training occurs, appropriate work behavior is not encouraged, there is infrequent opportunity to earn a sufficient wage, and few individuals move from the sheltered setting to competitive jobs.

If the sheltered setting is the major vocational alternative available to most autistic people, then the above description would paint a bleak picture for their future. In reality there are some grounds for optimism. More and more professionals and parents are beginning to recognize the problems that exist in sheltered workshops. These problems are deeply entrenched in a long-ongoing bureaucratic system and the solutions are highly complex, but are ones that can be addressed and resolved. It will take vision and commitment on the part of those who attempt to find and implement solutions, but appropriate workplaces for autistic people must be provided.

Competitive Employment

There have been several attempts to expand the vocational options of handicapped people through the development of competitive job placement models (Adams, Strain, Salzberg, & Levy, 1980; Larson & Edwards, 1980; Levy, 1978; Rusch & Mithaug, 1980; Wehman, 1980). The models have demonstrated that competitive jobs might be feasible and appropriate for some severely impaired people. All of those models adhere to the basic tenents that:

1. All people have the right to participate in all facets of society.
2. Many handicapped people have the potential to function successfully in competitive jobs.
3. Current functioning level is not indicative of potential performance.
4. Training is frequently most effective in an actual job site rather than in a simulated or artificial setting.
5. Heavy initial professional support is critical to success.

The reported success of these models in placing and maintaining low-functioning handicapped people in competitive employment clearly creates a desirable option for many and greater optimism for the more mildly handicapped. So far the demonstrations have indicated that some handicapped people might be more limited by their available opportunities than by their disabilities. Since competitive placement of severely impaired people has been at a demonstration level with selected individuals, the feasibility of this option with larger groups of handicapped people is yet to be determined.

Further attempts to place handicapped workers, including autistic people, on competitive jobs should obtain information about the types of behaviors and skills that are required to make them successful employees. Although our present training technology is highly advanced, turning handicapped people into normal individuals is not feasible. It is probable that some of their behaviors will be tolerated in competitive job settings and some will not. That information will be obtained through careful and systematic analysis of the job sites. Observations of interactions between co-workers as well as their interactions with supervisors will need to be recorded and analyzed. Determining which behaviors are necessary for successful placement will dictate training for those who do not possess them.

The reality of the present situation is that until our technology for assessing and training behavior improves, and our philosophy and economy changes to accommodate all people into the workforce, the sheltered work setting will continue to remain the primary work alternative for most impaired people.

COMPONENTS OF A HABILIATION PROGRAM

The vocational preparation of autistic people is an ongoing developmental process. Building the skills necessary for maximum participation in an appropriate vocational setting must start very early in the person's life. Starting vocational preparation in their mid or late teens may result in some unnecessary limitations. The same rationale that applies to self-help, social skill, and academic training should apply to vocational education. The rationale is that as soon as an individual is developmentally ready to learn, the training should begin. The earlier you start an educational intervention, the better chance that person will have to maximally develop skills.

To prepare an individual to fulfill his/her vocational potential, four basic areas of instruction must be addressed. They are:

1. The development of work concepts and values
2. The acquisition of general and specific task skills
3. The performance of the task skills over time and at acceptable rates
4. The development of appropriate social and work responsibility behaviors

Work Concepts and Values

To engage in work activities successfully it is imperative that an individual understand what the activities of work entail, and the value of work to individuals and society. Most normal members of society develop an understanding and a value system for work through some direct instruction from parents and schools, but primarily through observation of and participation in work situations. They are exposed to and observe the work activities of significant people in their lives. Most teachers attempt systematic instruction about work and workers very early in elementary school programs. In addition most children are given work responsibilities in early childhood which increase in scope and content as they get older. They are asked to do chores around the home or school, and in some circumstances are allowed to help a family member at his or her job. As they get older they engage in jobs for pay—delivering papers, mowing lawns, babysitting, etc. All these experiences result in the development of work concepts and values.

Most handicapped people are not given the opportunities to participate in those activities and to gain the experiences necessary for developing work concepts. Even when they are exposed to some of the experiences, they do not pick up as much information incidentally as normal children do.

It is critical that in a systematic way vocational instruction and experiences be incorporated in each child's educational plan. To accomplish this the child must be given opportunities to have work responsibilities both at home and at school. He or she must be encouraged and reinforced for appropriate participation in these activities. Field trips both at school and outside school should be conducted to expose the child to as many different work situations as possible, always directing his/her attention purposefully to key work elements. Rules and procedures that instill work values can be employed in the school and the home. In a recent article Gillet (1980) suggests specific activities that teachers and parents could use to instill those concepts. She suggests infusing career education into the school curriculum through such activities as relating classroom jobs to future jobs, using job or work situations for an experience chart story, and structuring academic activities around vocational and career concepts.

In school programs with which the author has been involved, a specific area apart from the students' other activities is used exclusively for prevocational/vocational activities. A rule that is enforced is simply, when you enter the vocational room, you work. The student is either engaged in learning a work skill or producing a work task. Inactivity is not tolerated in that room and all non-work-related activities are done elsewhere. Experience has shown that the rule is learned quickly by students at all functioning levels, and inappropriate behavior rarely occurs in that setting.

The Acquisition of General and Specific Task Skills

Most low-skilled and semiskilled competitive jobs as well as sheltered work tasks require certain levels of discriminatory and manipulative ability. In addition, skill in the appropriate use of hand tools enhances an individual's employability. These skills are obtained through systematic training and perfected with practice. Training for work skills should follow a developmental sequence, with individuals increasing the number of task skills as well as levels of complexity as they progress through a vocational education program.

Young children can be taught simple discriminations using such training techniques as easy-to-hard sequencing and match-to-sample (Gold & Scott, 1971; Zeaman & House, 1963). Industrial parts such as nuts, bolts, screws, washers, electronic components, etc., allow for discrimination training on numerous dimensions such as form, size, length, and color. In using the easy-to-hard sequencing technique the child is first asked to discriminate between objects that vary widely on a specific dimension. For example, if length is the relative dimension on a bolt-sorting task, then the first problem the child is asked to solve might be between bolts that are either 2 inches or ½ inch in length. All other dimensions are held constant. Once the discrimination is learned, the next problem is presented which reduces the dimensional difference to 2 inches and 1 inch. After the child solves that problem, subsequent problems further reduce the length differences to require finer and finer discrimination.

The match-to-sample technique is also used for teaching individuals to learn discriminations. The student is presented with a problem that requires discrimination and is provided with a sample to refer to in solving the problem. An example problem might be to pick out large washers from an assortment of parts. The child is provided with a sample washer to refer to and compare when solving the problem. This technique was used very effectively in teaching handicapped people to assemble electronic printed circuit boards (Levy, 1975; Merwin, 1973). The difficulty of the discriminations can increase by extending the number and the types of parts as well as decreasing the dimensional differences to require finer and finer levels of discriminations.

Another area for training would be to develop manipulative skills. How things fit together, attach, screw onto another part, tighten, loosen, are all skills that are acquired through training and practice. Although some people describe themselves as mechanically incompetent, which they frequently attribute to an inherent defects, it is likely that they grew up in an environment that did not provide opporuntunities for acquiring those skills. If there are few or no tools in a home and all repairs are contracted out, there is a high probability that children in such a home will not learn the skills for making repairs. If opportunities are provided for handicapped people to acquire those skills there is a good chance that they will. If that training starts early in their education, then hopefully after years of experience and practice they will be adept in performing manipulative tasks. Having a young student start with learning a simple nut-and-bolt assembly, and then gradually increasing the complexity of the subsequent tasks, should ultimately permit the individual to perform sophisticated manipulative tasks.

Using tools is a skill that is important for people to know. It is not only important vocationally but will allow an individual greater independence in home situations by being able to do simple home repairs. How to properly use a hammer, saw, screwdriver, pliers, and even some power tools are important skills to possess. A concern that parents and teachers frequently have is that the handicapped child might be injured while using tools. If students are properly trained the risk of injury from the tools is minimal. A possibility of injury should not be used as justification for not training in those skills.

Training does not have to be limited to mechanical bench assembly tasks. For some individuals other activities such as kitchen work or maintenance, and for higher functioning individuals clerical, secretarial, and academic activities, could be a part of their vocational program.

The intent of this objective is to start general and specific task skill acquisition early and gradually expand the student's repertoire to include wider varieties of skills as well as greater complexity.

Productivity

To be successful vocationally one must go beyond just possessing a skill—one must be able to repeat that skill consistently at an acceptable quality and rate. Developing acceptable and consistent rates for some autistic people has been difficult. The interest and motivation to stay on the designated task are lacking for many of these individuals. Unless these students can be taught to stay on task and produce, their vocational options will be extremely limited. This has proven to be the most challenging objective to accomplish. A few autistic individuals are motivated by the task and produce at very acceptable rates, but the majority do not. Through the use of different types of reinforcement contingencies productivity has been increased for some individuals (Levy & Kaplan, Note 1). It is important that the opportunities to develop production behavior be provided.

A suggested procedure for developing production skills is as follows. As soon as a student learns his first task, he is then asked to produce it. That is, if the student learns to discriminate between a nut and a bolt, then the production activity becomes to sort a number of the nuts and bolts. This occurs on a daily basis with positive reinforcement for satisfactory performance. Some individuals may initially need continuous prompts to sustain performance, but the prompts are gradually faded out over time. During the time the student is in production on the first task he is also being trained on a new, more advanced task. When the criterion on the new task is met, then the individual goes into production on that task and into learning acquisition on the next higher level task. In essence the student is always learning something new and given opportunities to produce.

Finding what is motivating to an autistic student is always interesting and challenging. One hopes that after an individual has acquired production experience, motivation through task performance will be realized. Levy and Kaplan (Note 1), in an unpublished study conducted at the Rimland School in Evanston, Illinois, looked at the effects of task difficulty and novelty on the production rates of autistic workers in a sheltered workshop. Two profoundly autistic men were studied under three conditions: (1) baseline, which consisted of production on a simple rubber hose and clamp assembly task (this task had been used periodically by a sheltered workshop over a 3-year time span to fill in time when contract work was scarce); (2) task change, which entailed the production of three simple tasks (the hose/clamp assembly; a bolt, washer, and nut sort; and an envelope stuff), on alternating days; and (3) the difficult versus simple task. The difficult task consisted of a nine-part bolt, washer, and nut sort. Conditions 2 and 3 were both preceded and succeeded by the baseline condition.

The results showed a low production rate (5.3%) and high error ratio (37.0%) during the initial baseline period. The change condition evidenced an increase in production and a decrease in error rate on both the bolt, washer, and nut sort, and on the envelope stuff. The difficult task condition showed increased production and lower error rates for the first 5 days and then a sudden decrease in production and increase in errors.

The authors concluded that a loss of interest due to the repetition of the job could have influenced performance on the hose assembly and eventually on the difficult task. It is possible that the nine-piece sort task was not perceived as difficult by the subjects. It does appear that when autistic workers are required to produce highly simplified tasks, periodic changes increase productivity. The effects of a more difficult task on handicapped workers' production needs to be investigated.

The Development of Appropriate Social and work Responsibility Behaviors

Another area to prepare autistic students vocationally is in appropriate social and work responsibility behavior. As previously described, social skills is the area in which autistic people show the greatest deficit and one that is probably the most critical vocationally. Training in this area is difficult since no one is quite sure exactly what behaviors and characteristics good workers possess that are directly related to their success. In addition, once the critical social behaviors are identified, the problem remains of how to teach them effectively. Investigations have recently been conducted with other handicapped populations to determine how to train social skills effectively. Some success has been reported with chronic schizophrenics (Hersen & Bellack, 1976), with psychiatric outpatients (Gutride, Goldstein, & Hunter, 1973), and with mentally retarded adults in institutions (Stacy, Doleys, & Malcolm, 1979).

It is anticipated that some of these procedures and techniques being developed to train handicapped individuals in social skills might appropriately be applied to training autistic people. Most current findings indicate that such behavioral approaches as modeling and shaping are the most effective. One program in Nashville, Tennessee, is looking at the effects that role-playing, videotapes, and self-monitoring procedures have on training appropriate work behavior with behavior-disordered adolescents. In role-playing, students rehearse social skills in simulated situations and receive feedback on appropriate and inappropriate performance. The videotapes allow the students to see their own performance in situations and evaluate its appropriateness. Self-monitoring is a procedure to help students gain self-control by assessing their own behavior. Initial results indicate that these techniques are effective with that population (Warrenfeltz, Kelly, Salzberg, Beegle, Levy, Adams, and Crouse, Note 2). The usefulness of the techniques with autistic people has yet to be tested, but could hold promise.

Work responsibilities may not be as difficult to teach as social skills. Some behaviors critical to job success can easily be identified. Using a time clock, when to use the restrooms, using work breaks appropriately, and knowing how to stop a task before completion when requested by a supervisor are some examples. Systematic instruction to develop those skills must be incorporated into a prevocational/vocational school program.

TECHNOLOGY FOR IMPLEMENTATION

An appropriate type of vocational alternative for many autistic people, especially the more mildly impaired, is competitive employment. The opportunities for normalized work activities and interactions will always be greater in real job settings than in sheltered facilities. Although it is hoped that in the future the move for sheltered settings will be toward a more realistic environment, there will always be a theraputic component that will prohibit the attainment of comparable conditions. The opportunities to engage in interesting and lucrative work, access to normal peer models, productive atmosphere, and opportunities for advancement will always be greater in competitive business and industry.

In order to maximize successful job placement and retention of the autistic worker in competitive settings an intense support system must be provided. The traditional procedure for job placement of handicapped people has been for a social service professional to help them locate and secure a job and then leave them with the employer to work out the training and adjustment considerations for the job. Sufficient support and follow-up are seldom provided. It is likely that many workers fail on the job because employers do not have the knowledge, training, and time to work with the handicapped person, and are not able to resolve simple or difficult problems as they occur.

To achieve success, intense professional involvement is required in the initial stage of job placement. Recently several educational researchers have developed methods and techniques to accomplish successful competitive job placement for many handicapped people (Levy, 1978; Rusch & Mithaug, 1980; Wehman, 1980). Similar techniques have been employed by each of these researchers. Levy (1978) developed the trainer-advocate (T-A) model to place moderately retarded sheltered workshop clients in competitive industrial jobs. The subjects in this study had been classified by the professional staff as individuals who did not possess the skills or behaviors to be successful in a competitive job market. It was further suggested by the professional evaluators that the clients did not have the potential to develop the necessary skills or behaviors.

Through the use of the T-A model the clients became successful industrial employees. One individual was trained for an assembly-line job which required quick and accurate movements as well as the use of a power tool. He quickly learned the job (in approximately 4 hours of training time) and reached 100% productivity within 2 weeks on the job. His production rate at the workshop had seldom surpassed 32% and his earnings averaged $18 per week. His salary at the factory was $140 a week, and after four years on the job he is currently earning considerably more. Presently the model is being further developed through a federal handicapped children's model program grant with moderately and severely behavior-disordered adolescents (Adams et al., 1980).

The T-A Model

Basically the model calls for providing a handicapped person with as much technical on-the-job training and emotional support as is necessary for job success. The T-A is a professionally trained individual who is responsible for the handicapped worker's complete adjustment to the job. In this procedure the T-A's involvement and assistance is faded out as the worker becomes more competent at the job and management and fellow employees become more comfortable with the handicapped worker.

The following steps are part of the placement procedure:

1. The T-A finds and secures an appropriate competitive job placement for the handicapped worker, ideally a job which matches the individual's abilities and interests. Unfortunately, with the reality of the current labor market some compromises may have to be made. With the most unskilled or semiskilled jobs the working atmosphere is probably more critical than the actual job tasks.

2. The T-A thoroughly learns the job and its requirements. In some situations this could be accomplished by systematically observing the regular workers at the job. In most cases it is desirable to actually work the job to learn the intricacies and subtleties that most jobs contain. For most low-skilled or semiskilled jobs 2–5 days are sufficient. By this time the T-A will also know the acceptability of the job for the handicapped person.

3. The T-A develops a complete task analysis of the job including the actual task(s) and the routines involved. The training procedures to be used are clearly defined and stated.

4. At this point the handicapped person is introduced to the job, the supervisors, and fellow employees. It was suggested by some professionals that the handicapped person should be involved in the initial contact interview and participate in the decision about job acceptability (Larson & Edwards, 1980). It is the author's contention that most handicapped adolescents and adults have insufficient work experience to effectively evaluate job acceptability. The T-A knows the individual's interests and capability, and can make a reasonably valid decision. Unless an initial interview is specifically requested by the employer, it is best to wait until this point to introduce everyone.

5. Training the person to the actual job tasks begins. The person remains in one-to-one training until a specified criterion for learning is achieved. The amount of time spent per training session will vary with specific individuals and situations.

6. Once the person reaches the criterion on learning the specific task components of the job, then job routine is taught. Job routine would consist of when and where to clock in and out, where to go and what to do at coffee breaks and lunch, where to go when help is needed, etc. The T-A also assists in the social aspects of the job, such as how to approach fellow employees at coffee breaks. This is primarily done by example. The T-A and handicapped worker approach a group of fellow employees

at coffee break and the T-A makes the necessary introductions and starts conversations, assuring that the handicapped worker is integrated into the activities. It is the author's experience that, once the T-A is no longer present, social interactions between the handicapped worker and fellow employees tends to fade. Co-workers are pleasant but find it difficult to maintain conversations with the handicapped employee. In many cases if the handicapped person is merely allowed to sit within a group it might be satisfying to him and acceptable to the co-workers. One individual the author worked with rejected all attempts by the T-A and fellow workers to interact on a social level. He went off by himself during breaks and lunch, and indicated to anyone who interrupted his solitude that he preferred to be alone. After a while people continued to be pleasant to him but respected his preference to be alone.

7. The worker begins the production phase of the job. At this point the worker begins to assume more and more responsibility for independently fulfilling the job requirements. If the individual cannot maintain the production demands of the job, then help is provided. However, the assistance is faded out as the individual becomes more proficient.

8. The T-A continues to fade his/her involvement and increases that of supervisors and co-workers. At this point the T-A only intervenes when it is absolutely necessary, letting the worker, co-workers, and the supervisors work things out. Judgment should be used in determining the types of problems that would require the T-A's intervention.

9. Once the worker is independently functioning on the job, the T-A should check on a daily basis with the immediate supervisor and employee about surfacing and potential problems. Daily checks are reduced to every other day, to weekly, biweekly, monthly, etc. If a problem occurs that cannot be resolved between the worker and supervisor, then the T-A attempts to resolve it.

10. If it is agreeable to both management and the worker, then a permanent employment arrangement is finalized.

This model has been criticized by some in-the-field professionals as being too costly to be practical. Their concerns are related to the intense one-to-one initial involvement. The argument is a faulty one. Through this one-to-one intervention an individual can attain a high level of self-sufficiency, be self-supporting, and pay taxes. The alternatives of institutionalization or of supplementing people in a sheltered setting would require a greater, long-term investment by society. Therefore the initial investment in a T-A's services could ultimately be the most economical form of treatment available. In addition the personal psychological benefits of more normalized alternatives to individuals and their families cannot be measured.

CONCLUSION

Presently there are few vocational programs available to autistic individuals. A reason for this is probably the low expectations society has for their potential to engage in vocational activities. Those programs that are currently available are not adequately fulfilling the needs of the handicapped people who are placed in sheltered workshops. The workshops have been criticized for not providing proper evaluation, training, and supervision, resulting in clients' not being habilitated (Levy, 1980). Some autistic people, particularly the higher functioning, could be successfully placed in competitive jobs, but because of economic considerations and negative societal attitudes toward them this is not being realized. It would appear from this description that the vocational future of autistic people is dismal. Actually, there are grounds for optimism.

Recent developments in behavioral technology have clearly demonstrated the competency of autistic people in performing vocational activities. The potential for further development of their skills and abilities is great. To realize the potential several things must occur. First, it will be necessary to find acceptable vocational sites and train autistic people for successful placement in them. This will be accomplished through the use of job and site analysis to identify the critical aspects of employment. Once the critical aspects are identified, systematic training of autistic individuals who display those skill deficits can take place. The T-A model described in this chapter could be an effective strategy for implementation. Second, the present technology for training must be disseminated and implemented by those working with autistic people at all ages and levels of functioning. This could be accomplished through professional in-services, through consultations, and through college course offerings in vocational education. Finally, the technology must be further developed for use with autistic people. This will entail not only the adaptation of research conducted with other handicapped populations but specific research conducted with autistic people. So far vocational research with autistic people has been minimal. These suggestions are not definitive, but are offered as a starting point for improving the vocational lives of autistic people.

At one time it was believed that all that was necessary in order to open employment opportunities for handicapped people was to demonstrate that they are competent workers. Judging by the continual high rate of unemployment and underemployment among handicapped people it appears that this approach has met with only limited success. Creating employment opportunities for autistic people will require determined effort by their advocates. The task is not only to open up existing opportunities, but to improve existing programs and create new, more appropriate ones. All the effort spent in training will be wasted if there are no places for them to perform their skills. The undertaking may be gigantic, but it is possible. It is clear that autistic people have the right and potential to participate productively in the labor force, and that they must be given the opportunities to do so.

REFERENCES

Adams, T., Strain, P., Salzberg, C., & Levy, S. A model program for prevocational/vocational education with moderately and severely handicapped adolescents. *Journal of Special Education Technology,* 1980, *3* (1), 36–42.

Bellamy, G. T., Peterson, L., & Close, D. Habilitation of the severely and profoundly retarded: Illustrations of competence. *Education and Training of the Mentally Retarded,* 1975, *10,* 174–186.

Gillet, P. Career education in the special elementary education program. *Teaching Exceptional Children,* Fall 1980, pp. 17–21.

Gold, M. W. Research on the vocational habilitation of the retarded: The present, the future. In *International review of research in mental retardation,* (N. R. Ellis, ed.), New York: Academic Press, 1973.

Gold, M. W., & Scott, K. G. Discrimination learning. In *Training the developmentally young* (W. B. Stephens, ed.), New York: John Day, 1971.

Greenleigh Associates. *The role of the sheltered workshop in the rehabilitation of severely handicapped.* Washington, D.C.: Department of Health, Education and Welfare, Rehabilitation Services Administration, 1975.

Gutride, M. E., Goldstein, A. P., & Hunter, G. F. The use of modeling and role-playing to increase social interactions among social psychiatric patients. *Journal of Counsulting and Clinical Psychology,* 1973, *40,* 408–415.

Hersen, M., & Bellack, A. S. A multiple baseline analysis of social skills training in chronic schizophrenics. *Journal of Applied Behavioral Analysis,* 1976, *9,* 239–245.

Kauffman, J. M. *Characteristics of children's behavior disorders.* Columbus, Ohio: Charles E. Merrill, 1977.

Larson, K. H., & Edwards, J. P. Community-based vocational training and placement for the severely handicapped. In *Expanding opportunities: Vocational education for the handicapped* (C. Hansen and N. Haring, eds.), Seattle: University of Washington, 1980.

Levy, S. M. The development of work skill training procedures for the assembly of printed circuit boards by the severely handicapped. *AAESPH Review,* 1975, *1* (1), 1–10.

Levy, S. M. *The measurement of retarded and normal workers' job performance through the use of naturalistic observation in sheltered and industrial work environments.* Unpublished doctoral dissertation, University of Illinois, 1978.

Levy, S. M. The debilitating effects of the habilitation process. In *Expanding opportunities: Vocational education for the handicapped* (C. Hansen and N. Haring, eds.), Seattle: University of Washington, 1980.

Levy, S. M., Pomerantz, D. J., & Gold, M. W. Work skill development. In *Teaching the severely handicapped,* Vol. 2 (N. G. Haring and L. J. Brown, eds.), New York: Grune & Stratton, 1977.

Merwin, M. R. *The use of match-to-sample techniques to train retarded adolescents and adults to assemple electronic circuit boards.* Unpublished master's thesis, University of Illinois, 1973.

Pomerantz, D. J., & Marholin, D. Vocational habilitation: A time for change in existing service delivery systems. In *Educational programming for the severely handicapped* (E. Sontag, N. Certo, & J. Smith, eds.), Reston, Va.: Council for Exceptional Children, Division of Mental Retardation, 1977.

Rusch, F. R., & Mithaug, D. E. *Vocational training for mentally retarded adults: A behavior analytic approach.* Champaign, Ill.: Research Press, 1980.

Stacy, D., Doleys, D. S., & Malcolm, B. Effects of social skills training in the community-based program. *American Journal of Mental Deficiency,* 1979, *84,* 152–158.

Stanfield, J. S. Graduation: What happens to the retarded child when he grows up? *Exceptional Children,* 1973, *39,* 548–552.

Wehman, P. Towards competitive employment. In *Expanding opportunities: Vocational education for the handicapped* (C. Hansen and N. Haring, eds.), Seattle: University of Washington, 1980.

Zeaman, D., & House, B. J. The role of attention in retardate discrimination learning. In *Handbook of mental deficiency* (N. R. Ellis, ed.), New York: McGraw-Hill, 1963.

REFERENCE NOTES

1. Levy, S. M., & Kaplan, E. *The effects of task change and complexity on the work productivity of autistic young men.* Manuscript in preparation.
2. Warrenfeltz, R. B., Kelly, W. J., Salzberg, C. L., Beegle, G. P., Levy, S. M., Adams, T. A., & Crouse, T. R. *Social skills training of behavior-disordered adolescents with self-monitoring to promote generalization to a vocational setting. Behavioral Disorders,* 1981, *7*(1), 18–27.

8

Medical Needs of the Autistic Adolescent

JOANNA S. DALLDORF

Adolescent health care is a relatively new medical subspecialty (Shearin, 1977) in the United States. The first adolescent medicine program was established in Boston by Dr. Roswell Gallagher in 1951. The Society for Adolescent Medicine was formed in 1968, and the American Academy of Pediatrics only recently created a section on adolescent medicine. Publications on adolescent medicine have dramatically increased in recent years, and there has been growing federal recognition (Hutchins, 1980).

Although the term "puberty" is often used interchangeably with the term "adolescence," puberty will be used in this chapter to refer to sexual maturation while adolescence will refer to all the physical and psychological changes associated with the transition period from childhood to adulthood. The growing emphasis on adolescent health care and programming mainly derives from the increased duration of adolescence due to earlier sexual maturation and activity, and the longer period of preparation required before adult independent living.

The autistic adolescent has many of the same health care needs of all adolescents, but he also has superimposed problems related to the biomedical and behavioral factors associated with the autistic syndrome. His medical care is likely to be even more fragmented because of several sources of medical consultation; he may be known to a pediatrician, a family physician, a psychiatrist, and a neurologist. It is possible that no single medical facility has assumed the role of coordinating his medical

JOANNA S. DALLDORF ● Biological Sciences Research Center, University of North Carolina School of Medicine, Chapel Hill, North Carolina   27514.

care or advocating for him. The difficulties encountered by physicians in managing the diverse and puzzling problems of the autistic child may also lead to some parental dissatisfaction with health professionals and a tendency to avoid medical consultations except in crisis situations.

The remainder of this chapter will deal with the major issues involved in the medical management of the autistic adolescent. The reader will soon become aware that the practice of preventive medicine and the availability of the past medical history play significant roles in the provision of satisfactory health care.

MEDICAL ASSESSMENT

When and if an autistic adolescent is seen by a physician, the traditional approach is often impossible. Gathering historical data may be difficult because of the fragmented care and the increased possibility that a caretaker other than the biologic parent may be the informant. The autistic adolescent, with reduced and atypical communication skills, may be unable to shed much light on the past or present medical history. Past records may be unavailable since it is likely that an adolescent would have moved several times. Since accurate medical diagnosis and proper treatment *frequently* depend more on history than examination, it would be extremely beneficial if all adolescents, particularly autistic adolescents, possessed ongoing medical record folders. The folders should include information regarding previous diagnostic studies (especially neuroradiographic, metabolic, and hematologic tests), relevant family histories, immunizations, results of screening tests, allergies, use of anticonvulsants and psychopharmacologic agents. It is a disservice to both the autistic adolescent and the physician to attempt the delivery of medical care without adequate background information. An awareness of past laboratory data could prevent costly and unnecessary repetition of studies. Adverse drug reactions might be avoided if past experiences with medications were known.

The physical examination of an autistic adolescent can present a significant challenge. It may be impossible to explain the examination procedure or to anticipate reactions. It can be most helpful to have the assistance of a parent or therapist who has a better awareness of the adolescent's behavior patterns and means of communication. Some autistic adolescents are resistant and may even react violently to the usual examination efforts. If clear-cut verbal and gestural explanations of the examination procedures do not result in cooperation, a degree of physical restraint may be necessary. However, this may become self-defeating because of the autistic adolescent's size and weight. The physician will need to determine how much physical examination is actually essential rather than doggedly following the standard examination protocol.

Laboratory studies, often essential if the autistic adolescent is on anticonvulsants or psychopharmacologic agents, can also meet with technical obstacles. The physician will again need to distinguish between necessary and routine before embarking on laboratory studies.

It should be emphasized that the dilemmas associated with the physical examination and laboratory procedures could be significantly lessened if the autistic adolescent were accompanied by accurate medical information and a parent or guardian acquainted with his current symptomatology.

PREVENTIVE MEDICAL CARE

Preventive medicine practices, which include immunizations, blood pressure checks, vision and hearing screening, are often overlooked in adolescence. Preventive medical care is often avoided during adolescence unless a physical examination is required for placement in a camp or school. The autistic adolescent may have particularly deficient health maintenance because of other concerns of higher priority or because of the variety of health care facilities and guardians involved. The medical folder recommended earlier in this chapter should therefore include information on the results of and recommended times for immunizations and screening tests. Appropriate record forms can be obtained from most health departments, medical offices, and the American Academy of Pediatrics (P. O. Box 1034, Evanston, Illinois   60204).

Immunizations may be neglected in the autistic child because of concerns that a neurologically impaired child is at slightly higher risk for adverse side effects from routine immunization procedures. Although there will be some exceptions, the American Academy of Pediatrics (1977) generally recommends that children with static neurologic disorders, which would characterize most forms of the autistic syndrome, be immunized. Because measles, mumps, and rubella, particularly measles, can have neurologic sequelae, the autistic adolescent could benefit from protection. A diphtheria-tetanus booster is usually required in adolescence and then every 10 years thereafter.

PREVENTIVE DENTAL CARE

Preventive dental practices are less likely to be followed in the adolescent period although the erratic eating habits of adolescents and their propensity for "junk foods" place them at an increased risk for dental caries. The autistic adolescent is also susceptible to dental disease because of the frequent tendency toward abnormal eating habits and food preferences, combined with difficulties in establishing good and consistent oral hygiene practices. The incidence of congenital dental deformities, known to be greater in the mentally retarded population, is probably also greater in the autistic population and further increases the tendency for dental decay. If the autistic adolescent also grinds his teeth, has other abnormal oral habits (such as biting or mouthing objects), or takes diphenylhydantoin, he is at even higher risk for dental and gum disease.

Dental care may take lower priority than other health care problems of the autistic adolescent, but periodic dental examinations are recommended since rampant dental and periodontal disease can produce significant discomfort and secondary behavioral and nutritional problems. Dental evaluation and treatment may be even more difficult than a routine physical examination and could require sedation, restraint, or even hospitalization (Kopel, 1977).

Unpleasant confrontations with the dentist could be reduced if preventive dental practices, including avoidance of sweets, routine oral hygiene, and use of fluoridated water, were employed. If the autistic adolescent cannot be taught to use a regular toothbrush, an electric toothbrush and the Water Pik might be considered. If food is used as a behavior reinforcer, it would be advisable to avoid exclusive reliance on simple carbohydrates.

Sources of Information. Dentists with special training in working with handicapped children can be located through the following organizations: American Academy of Pedodontics, the American Society of Dentistry for Children, and the Journal of Dentistry for Children, 211 East Chicago Avenue, Chicago, Illinois   60611; National Foundation of Dentistry for the Handicapped, 1739 Broadway, Suite 312, Boulder, Colorado   80302; and Academy of Dentistry for the Handicapped, 1240 East Main Street, Springfield, Ohio   45503.

DEVIATIONS IN GROWTH PATTERNS AND SEXUAL MATURATION

Differential growth patterns and rates of sexual development constitute a common cause of concern for adolescents and their parents (Root, 1980). The onset of pubertal changes and the length of time required before sexual maturity and final height are reached vary because of genetic factors, nutritional status, and associated disease processes. The physical changes accompanying adolescence include acceleration and then deceleration of skeletal growth, the development of the reproductive organs and secondary sexual characteristics, alterations in development of muscle tissue and deposition of fat, and alterations in the neuroendocrine system. Physicians are now trained to estimate stages of pubertal development, based on the degree of breast and pubic hair development in the female and genital size and pubic hair growth in the male adolescent. As can be seen in Figures 1 and 2, the growth spurt is correlated with development of secondary sexual characteristics, and the timing is variable, particularly in the male.

Delayed Adolescence. Delayed onset of puberty and associated short stature is a common situation, particuarly in boys. It is of little consolation that later onset of sexual development might result in a longer period of skeletal growth and a final height greater than that of their earlier developing peers. Although delayed adolescence is usually not a disease state, it can be secondary to central nervous system disorders, abnormalities of gonadal formation or function, and poor nutrition. A recent study (Harper & Collins, 1979) revealed delayed sexual development in a sample of autistic girls. It would not be surprising if some autistic children demonstrated delayed onset of puberty in view of the central nervous system

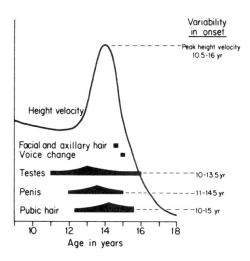

Figure 1. Diagram of sequence of events at adolescence in boys. (Reprinted with permission from Smith, D., Bierman, E., & Robsinson, N., *The Biologic Ages of Man*. Philadelphia: W. B. Saunders Co., 1978, p. 172.)

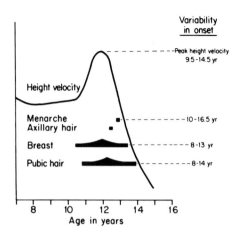

Figure 2. Diagram of sequence of events at adolescence in females. (Reprinted with permission from Smith, D., Bierman, E., & Robinson, N., *The Biologic Ages of Man.* Philadelphia: W. B. Saunders Co., 1978, p. 173.)

pathology in autism, the occasional associated nutritional problems, and the frequent use of phenothiazines, which can alter neuroendocrine function.

However, delayed sexual maturation is rarely related to an active pathologic process, suggesting that referrals for medical evaluations should be conservative. The appraisal of an autistic child with delayed adolescence would require availability of accurate records of previous heights as well as a family history of growth and sexual maturation patterns. Diagnostic studies might then include a physical examination, skeletal radiographic studies to determine the degree of bone maturation, neuroradiographic studies, and a buccal smear (a screening study for sex chromosome disorders).

Therapy for delayed adolescence is rarely indicated, but hormone replacement is occasionally necessary.

Precocious Puberty. Precocious sexual development is defined as onset of sexual development before age 8 in the female or age 9 in the male. It is of more concern than delayed adolescence because of the potential psychological consequences and the greater probability of a related disease process, particularly in males. Advanced sexual development will result in an earlier growth spurt, earlier cessation of growth, and final height frequently below adult norms. This condition is twice as common in girls, and of unknown origin in 85% of girls as compared with 50% of boys. In boys for whom the cause is unknown, a family history of precocious puberty may exist.

Etiologic factors include the aftermath of central nervous system infections (e.g., encephalitis, meningitis), brain tumors, and neurodegenerative conditions (e.g., tuberous sclerosis). Considering the central nervous system pathology in the autistic syndrome and the frequent association of autism with tuberous sclerosis, precocious puberty might prove to be an occasional complicating factor in autism.

The evaluation would again require availability of accurate growth records as well as a direct physical examination. Neuroradiographic procedures and laboratory tests to evaluate certain hormone levels might also be required.

Hormonal therapy to suppress gonadotrophic secretion and/or neurosurgical intervention may occasionally be necessary depending on the cause, the degree of precocity, and the emotional effects on the child. However, medical intervention is rather infrequent, making it an unlikely factor in the care of the autistic child/adolescent.

Short Stature. Short stature is a frequent source of concern for the adolescent and his parents, although perhaps of less import for the parents of an autistic adolescent. Short stature usually relates to familial factors or delayed adolescence. Accurate family history, growth records, and a physical examination are usually sufficient for evaluating short stature; medical intervention is rarely indicated.

Gynecomastia. Breast development in the adolescent male is not uncommon, occurring in about 40% of boys between the ages of 10 and 16 and usually associated with the period of peak growth rate. Gynecomastia rarely indicates a disease process but may cause concerns regarding abnormal sexual development. The incidence of gynecomastia may be increased in autistic boys because of their frequent use of phenothiazine medications, which can produce breast engorgement, breast discharge, and breast development. Excessive weight, also often associated with phenothiazine usage, can produce the false appearance of breast development.

DISORDERS AND PROBLEMS ASSOCIATED WITH REPRODUCTIVE FUNCTION

Irregular Menstrual Cycles. Irregular menses are common in early adolescence because of the absence of ovulation. Absence of menstrual periods, irregular cycles, or excessive menstrual bleeding may result; the latter could cause extreme anxiety for an autistic adolescent girl. Repeated episodes of heavy bleeding could also result in anemia with its associated effects on behavior, including irritability and lassitude. If menstrual irregularities persist, a medical evaluation and hormone therapy may be indicated. It should be noted that phenothiazines, frequently taken by autistic adolescents, can increase menstrual irregularities.

Dysmenorrhea. Painful menstrual periods also occur in adolescents but only after ovulatory cycles have been established. The autistic adolescent girl, like any other adolescent female, may experience severe lower abdominal pain, low back pain, pain in the anterior thighs, and gastrointestinal signs and symptoms (nausea, vomiting). Dysmenorrhea generally occurs during the earlier part of the menstrual flow and could exaggerate the behavioral difficulties of the autistic adolescent. Dysmenorrhea is no longer thought to be a psychosomatic disorder since evidence is accumulating to indicate a physiologic basis. Medications which reduce prostaglandin secretion, such as acetylsalicylic acid (aspirin) and naproxen (Naprosyn), can be most helpful, particularly if taken *before* the menstrual flow has begun. In the severest forms of dysmenorrhea, hormonal therapy aimed at blocking ovulation may be employed.

Masturbation. Masturbation is a common behavior in adolescents, particularly in boys. It may be no more common in mentally retarded or autistic adolescents, but they are less likely to be aware of the social taboos regarding masturbating in public. Masturbation is a normal behavior, which may be accentuated in some autistic adolescents because of the lack of other outlets for sexual tension and a predisposition for self-stimulating behaviors. Tight or irritating underpants and bladder infections should not be overlooked as possible contributing factors. Phenothiazines are known to inhibit ejaculation, but it is uncertain how this may affect masturbation practices.

Contraception. Birth control may become an issue for the autistic adolescent, particularly since sterilization procedures are becoming less acceptable. None of the available contraceptive methods (intrauterine devices, the diaphragm, the condom, or oral contraceptives) is totally satisfactory, although the use of oral contraceptives is generally the most manageable. The injection of long-acting medroxyprogesterone acetate (Depo-Provera) every 3 months appears to be an effective alternative for contraception in the female, but this method has not been approved by the FDA. The American Academy of Pediatrics Committee on Drugs (1980) recommended that the use of Depo-Provera be considered for approval for certain patient populations, including intellectually impaired adolescents who cannot use other contraceptive methods. It is hoped that further attention will be given to this recommendation.

NUTRITION

Adolescence is a period of rapid growth associated with an increased need for calories and specific nutrients (protein, calcium, iron, zinc, vitamins) (Marino & King, 1980). Although adolescents usually increase their food intake dramatically, they often do not eat the proper foods because of irregular eating habits and snacking behaviors. The autistic adolescent may have a less erratic eating schedule due to his more sheltered environment, but he is more likely to have specific food preferences and atypical eating styles.

Iron Deficiency Anemia. The adolescent is at risk for iron deficiency anemia because of the increased demands for iron associated with expanding blood volume and muscle mass and the loss of iron with menstrual flow. Iron deficiency anemia is rarely severe during adolescence, but even a mild anemia can produce behavioral changes and deterioration in academic performance. The adolescent should therefore be encouraged to eat such iron-rich foods as red meats, iron-fortified cereals, and leafy green vegetables.

Vitamin Deficiencies. Vitamin deficiencies are extremely rare in the adolescent in the United States unless he has a chronic digestive or malabsorption problem or participates in certain fad diets, such as pure vegetarianism. Even if an autistic adolescent accepts a very limited variety of foods, a vitamin deficiency is unlikely to result since so many prepared foods are fortified with vitamins. The autistic adolescent who is on diphenylhydantoin for seizure control might need vitamin D supplementation to counteract the adverse effects of diphenylhydantoin on calcium metabolism, but even this situation does not apply to all diphenylhydantoin users.

Proponents of orthomolecular psychiatry (Pauling, 1968), who suggest that more subtle vitamin deficiencies exist in a number of neurologic and behavior disorders, recommend a megavitamin therapeutic approach. This regimen initially referred to the administration of large doses of nicotinamide, but now other vitamins, including ascorbic acid, folic acid, pyridoxine, and vitamin B_{12}, have been added. In spite of some reports of favorable responses (Rimland, 1973; Rimland, Calloway, & Dreyfus, 1978), there are presently limited objective studies supporting the value of megavitamin therapy for autistic adolescents.

It is understandable that megavitamin therapy would have an appeal and that vitamins, even in higher dosages, would seem more "natural" than some other therapeutic approaches. However, high doses of vitamin C may interfere with vitamin B_{12} metabolism, and niacin may cause vascular flushing and skin hyperpigmentation. Excessive vitamin A may cause radiographic changes in the long bones and increased intracranial pressure. Excessive vitamin D usage has led to soft tissue calcium deposits. Those interested in the administration of large doses of vitamins must therefore recognize that there can be adverse consequences of excessive vitamin intake (American Psychiatric Association, 1973).

Obesity. Approximately 20% of United States teenagers are overweight, and the incidence is undoubtedly higher in autistic adolescents because of their tendency for less active lives and their frequent treatment with phenothiazines, which often produce significant weight gains. Obesity is a health hazard and could exaggerate the rejection already experienced by the autistic adolescent.

The use of foods for reinforcement of behaviors may be necessary, but low-calorie foods (e.g., raw vegetables and fruits) should be offered whenever possible. Regular activities, other than eating and other sedentary pursuits, should also be available. Parents should be discouraged from allowing unlimited food intake because of sympathy with the autistic adolescent's plight.

Information on appropriate diets for adolescents can be obtained from health departments and the U.S. Department of Agriculture.

Anorexia Nervosa. Anorexia nervosa, a condition characterized by marked weight loss due to voluntary food restriction, is seen most commonly in adolescent females. Although it is more likely to be noted in adolescents with hysterical, obsessional, or schizoid characteristics, it has been reported (Stiver & Dobbins, 1980) in an autistic girl in early adolescence. Anorexia nervosa is a life-threatening condition because of the physiological consequences of near starvation. Although behavior-modification therapy may help, hospitalization may also be required and particularly difficult to implement for the autistic adolescent.

INFECTIONS

Infectious mononucleosis, viral hepatitis, and respiratory infections due to mycoplasma are common in adolescents but more difficult to evaluate and manage in the autistic patient because of problems in obtaining information or performing physical examinations and diagnostic laboratory tests. In addition some of the drug therapy used by the autistic adolescent could confuse the diagnosis; diphenylhydantoin can cause enlarged lymph nodes and might mimic the findings associated with infectious processes. Major tranquilizers may cause a form of jaundice which could be initially confused with the laboratory and clinical findings in infectious mononucleosis and viral hepatitis.

The management of the adolescent with infectious mononucleosis and hepatitis primarily involves restriction of activity, which might be difficult to enforce in the autistic adolescent. Fortunately the malaise associated with these conditions will result in some self-limitation of activity.

ALLERGIES

Allergic diseases are common in adolescents and often go untreated. Allergic rhinitis ("hay fever") occurs in about 15% of teenagers and the autistic adolescent would not be spared. Allergic rhinitis causes nasal obstruction and discharge, sneezing, and itching in the eyes. These symtoms can also be associated with fatigue and irritability, thus exaggerating the behavioral problems of the average autistic adolescent. Recurrent allergic episodes can also predispose the patient to middle ear and sinus infections, again adding to the handicaps of the autistic adolescent.

Therapies include medication, elimination of the allergens (the agents provoking the allergic reaction), and desensitization programs. The major medications are antihistamines, which would decrease the symptoms but might also cause excessive drowsiness. The elimination of offending agents is a logical approach, and far simpler if an adequate history has suggested whether seasonal or perennial inhalants are involved. Some common precautions, equally appropriate for a private home or a group home, include removal of household pets, elimination of feather pillows, use of mattress covers, use of covers for hot-air vents, and elimination of other dust "collectors" (heavy rugs, drapes, stuffed animals). When antihistamine preparations and environmental alterations are insufficient, a desensitization program, which involves injections over a 3- to 5-year period, could be considered but would rarely be feasible or appropriate in autistic adolescents.

Although aggressive therapy of allergic symptomatology may not take high priority in the autistic adolescent, the behavioral effects of allergies, the behavioral effects of the medications, and the long-range complications of allergies should not be overlooked.

DERMATOLOGIC DISORDERS: ACNE

Acne, a potentially disfiguring disease, is the major dermatologic problem of adolescence, which may increase the interpersonal problems of the autistic adolescent. Acne is caused by faulty functioning of the pilosebaceous canal, the structure which surrounds the fine hairs on the face, chest, and back. The earlier phases of acne are characterized by obstruction of the pilosebaceous canal; in more severe acne there is superimposed inflammation, infection, and resultant scarring. Genetic, hormonal, and anatomical factors are involved. Dietary factors, such as ingestion of chocolate, have *not* been implicated.

Treatment depends on the severity of the acne. In mild cases, skin cleansers containing sulfur and salicylic acid, such as Fostex cream, are used. If some inflammation (redness) is present, an agent with cleansing as well as antibacterial activity, such as benzoyl peroxide, is recommended. If there is evidence of infection, an oral antibiotic, usually tetracycline or erythromycin, may be prescribed. Minor surgical procedures may also be employed.

Proper therapy of acne requires medical supervision, and the guardian of the autistic adolescent should avoid home remedies and over-the-counter preparations, some of which may be contraindicated.

TREATMENT WITH PSYCHOPHARMACOLOGIC AGENTS

Adolescence is an emotionally tumultuous time due to physiologic, physical, and environmental factors. The physiologic factors, such as changing hormonal levels and fluid retention at the beginning of the menstrual period, are less important than physical and environmental changes, particularly in the autistic adolescent. The autistic adolescent's near-adult size makes his unacceptable behaviors more obvious, possibly more frightening or harmful, and less manageable by physical means. Changes in living arrangements (e.g., group homes, respite care programs) and often reduced opportunities for a therapeutic educational program may adversely affect previously satisfactory behavioral management programs. Pharmacologic intervention in the treatment of the autistic adolescent is an acceptable approach which should be avoided until efforts have been made to achieve appropriate environmental alterations and behavioral management plans.

Sleep disturbances, aggressive behaviors, agitated behaviors, self-injurious behaviors, and withdrawn states are the more common behaviors leading to requests for drug management during the adolescent period. No drug produces dramatic or totally predictable results, and all drugs have potentially undesirable or harmful side effects. The diversity of underlying biomedical factors producing the autistic syndrome enhances the variability of drug response and the difficulties in choosing a drug. Drugs effective at a younger age may no longer produce the desired response in the autistic adolescent. The evaluation of drug effects is extremely difficult because of the fluctuating behaviors of the autistic adolescent and the impreciseness of behavior measurements, although more adequate experimental designs are being developed (Cohen, Anderson, & Campbell, 1978).

If a psychopharmacologic approach is necessary, a variety of drugs is available and can be grouped into several major categories: sedative-hypnotics, minor tranquilizers, major tranquilizers, stimulants, antidepressants, antimanic drugs (lithium). Table 1 describes these drugs in more detail.

Diphenhydramine and chloral hydrate can be helpful for nighttime sedation and in preparation for necessary examinations or laboratory procedures. Diazepam has occasional value in the anxious or agitated autistic adolescent, but its efficacy is not dramatic and physical dependence, although not necessarily severe, can occur. Stimulants may be considered for the distractible hyperactive autistic adolescent, having proven helpful in the treatment of hyperactive children with attentional deficits. However, the origin of hyperactivity in the autistic adolescent is probably different, and the stimulants may even worsen the target behaviors. The phenothiazines and haloperidol have proven useful, although not predictable, in reducing aggressive, agitated, and withdrawn behaviors. Haloperidol was observed in two studies (Campbell, Anderson, Meier, Cohen, Small, Samit, & Sachar, 1978; Cohen, Campbell, Posner, Small, Triebel, & Anderson, 1980) to decrease withdrawal and stereotypic mannerisms in young autistic children, but no similar studies have been done with adolescents. These major tranquilizers have a wide range of safety between therapeutic and toxic dosages, but they are subject to overuse because of their relative safety and effectiveness. Antidepressants have been tried in autistic adolescents who appeared to be withdrawn and/or depressed, but experience with this form of therapy is limited and generally unfavorable. Lithium, so often helpful in manic-depressive patients, has also been employed in the treatment of autistic adolescents. It has generally not been very effective, but symptoms of aggressiveness, emotional lability, and explosive outbursts have been noted to decrease. Lithium should probably be considered in those autistic adolescents for whom all other therapies have failed and where there is a cyclical behavior pattern and/or family history of cyclical affective illnesses. The indications for lithium therapy are still being evaluated (Campbell, Schulman, & Rapoport, 1978), but even the occasional positive responder will be difficult to monitor. Regular laboratory determinations of lithium blood levels must

Table 1

Classification and Effects of Major Behavior-Modifying Drugs

Drugs	Therapeutic effects	Side effects	Comments
Sedative-hypnotics Chloral hydrate (Noctec) Paraldehyde Diphenhydramine (Benadryl) Promethazine (Phenergan)	Sedation	"Hangover"	Helpful for rapid sedation of the autistic adolescent; tolerance may develop
Minor tranquilizers Diazepam (Valium) Hydroxyzine (Atarax) Diphenhydramine (Benadryl)	Sedation, reduced anxiety level	Excessive drowsiness and dizziness; diazepam has anticonvulsant and muscle-relaxant effects	Occasionally helpful for reduction of anxiety and agitation in the autistic; diazepam associated with physical dependence
Major tranquilizers Phenothiazines Chlorpromazine (Thorazine) Thioridazine (Mellaril) Trifluoperazine (Stelazine) Butyrophenones Haloperidol (Haldol)	Reduced agitation and psychotic behaviors; decreased activity; stimulation (with trifluoperazine).	Sedation; decreased cognitive functioning; weight gain; dry mouth; nasal stuffiness; constipation; urinary retention; acute dystonic reactions; pseudo-Parkinsonism, tardive dyskinesia; neuroendocrine effects.	Moderately helpful to the autistic person but many side effects of both short- and long-term significance; may reduce threshold for seizures and cause eye damage

Stimulants Methylphenidate (Ritalin) Dextroamphetamine (Dexedrine) Pemoline (Cylert)	Increased attention span, decreased distractibility and impulsivity; reduced activity level	Nervousness, irritability, depression, insomnia, tics, decreased appetite; mild neuroendocrine and cardiovascular effects	Rarely helpful for autistic people; may worsen behavior problems.
Antidepressants Imipramine (Tofranil) Amitryptiline (Elavil)	Mood elevation; ? improved attention span; reduced enuresis.	Sedation, dizziness, blurred vision, dry mouth; cardiac arrhythmias in higher doses	Rarely helpful for autistic people; may be considered if withdrawal/depressive symptoms occur; may reduce seizure threshold
Antimanics Lithium	Decreased cyclical behavior; ? decreased aggressive behavior	Muscle weakness, tremor, blurred vision, drowsiness, thirst, polyuria; possible thyroid dysfunction after prolonged use	Rarely helpful for autistic people; might be considered if cyclical behavior pattern and all other therapies unsuccessful; has reduced self-injurious and stereotypic behavior; difficult to monitor

Source: Campbell, 1978; Fish, 1976; White, 1977.

be obtained because of the narrow range between therapeutic and toxic dosages.

When medication is indicated, the prescribing physician will need to know the medical history of the adolescent, particularly regarding seizures, previous use of and response to psychopharmacologic agents, and current medications (including doses). The phenothiazines may lower the threshold for seizures, and drugs can interact either to potentiate or to diminish their individual effectiveness. Drugs should not be prescribed unless the autistic adolescent has readily available medical care. Objective means of evaluating the effectiveness of the medication should be attempted; it would be helpful if daily diaries or behavior checklists were kept and if several observers were involved. Holidays from medication are essential.

This author's hesitancy regarding a psychopharmacologic approach derives from an awareness of the potential risks of giving drugs for which the mechanisms of action in the human being are not fully understood. Drugs are essentially administered when clinical opinion suggests that the positive behavioral effects may outweigh the potential side effects.

The side effects are listed in Table 1. The sedative effects of the minor and major tranquilizers could enhance the communication and cognitive impairments of the autistic adolescent. The weight gain so often associated with the major tranquilizers could exaggerate problems with behavior management and nutrition. The neurologic problems, particularly associated with the major tranquilizers, can be severe and even irreversible. Withdrawal of a major tranquilizer may initially lead to worsening of behavior and movement disorders; several weeks off the major tranquilizers are necessary before determining whether the autistic adolescent's symptoms and signs off the medication represent withdrawal effects, more permanent neurologic consequences of prolonged drug use, or the autistic adolescent's natural behavior and motor status. The side effects described in Table 1 only represent those directly related to the pharmacologic action of the drugs. In addition the psychopharmacologic agents may produce unexpected side effects, such as allergic reactions and hematologic disorders.

The use of psychopharmacologic agents in the autistic adolescent escalates because the behavior-management techniques of earlier childhood may be less usable, and the use of any form of restraint, even to prevent self-mutilation, generates concerns about violating human rights. Although there are valid reasons for objecting to lengthy physical restraint or certain aversive procedures, the extended use of potent psychopharmacologic agents should also be considered as a form of restraint with its own harmful effects.

SEIZURES

Adolescence is a time of changing seizure patterns and greater difficulty with seizure management, but the onset of a seizure disorder in adolescence is infrequent. In contrast, the development of seizures in autistic adolescents and adults is a relatively common occurrence, having been reported for about one-quarter of cases studied (Deykin & Mac-Mahon, 1979; Rutter, 1970).

These seizures can be of several types, most commonly grand mal seizures (generalized motor) and psychomotor seizures (sudden episodes associated with specific behavioral abnormalities and possible associated motor activity). It may be difficult to diagnose psychomotor seizures in the autistic adolescent because of his already-disturbed behaviors. A seizure disorder would be suggested by suddenness of onset, associated facial or other involuntary motor movements, or alterations in level of consciousness after the suspected seizure. An electroencephalogram would help to make a diagnosis, but the interpretation of the EEG needs to be conservative. A careful description of the suspected seizures is equally important. It should be noted that phenothiazines may lower the threshold for seizures.

If anticonvulsant therapy is recommended, the effects of these drugs on the behavioral and neurologic status of the autistic adolescent must also be kept in mind in evaluating his progress. Most of the anticonvulsants have the potential for causing sedation or irritability. Personality changes are fairly common with primidone therapy. More information can be obtained from Table 2.

GENETIC COUNSELING AND STERILIZATION

Information about the risks of the autistic adolescent producing an autistic child may be requested by the adolescent's family. If a specific etiologic factor cannot be determined or if the cause appears to relate to infection or trauma, the chances of producing an abnormal child would be small. If, however, the adolescent has a neuroectodermal disorder (e.g., tuberous sclerosis), the risk is 50% for producing a child with the same biologic disorder.

It is unlikely that most autistic adolescents would be capable of rearing children (Eisenberg, 1956; Rutter, Greenfeld, & Lockyer, 1967). The employment of contraception will depend on the adolescent's potential for sexual activity. Sterilization will need to be considered in some instances in spite of the present trend away from this procedure because

Table 2
Major Behavioral/Neurologic Side Effects of Anticonvulsants

Anticonvulsant	Side effects
Barbiturates	
phenobarbital	drowsiness, hyperactivity, irritability
primidone (Mysoline)	drowsiness, dizziness, irriability, personality change
Hydantoins	
diphenylhydantoin (Dilantin)	drowsiness, personality change, ataxia, nystagmus, peripheral neuropathy, "encephalopathy"
Carbamazepine (Tegretol)	drowsiness, dizziness, ataxia, nystagmus, diplopia, ? psychotropic effect
Succinimides	
ethosuximide (Zarontin)	drowsiness, dizziness, headache, mood changes
Benzodiazepine	
diazepam (Valium)	drowsiness, irritability, behavior
clonazepam (Clonopin)	change, ataxia, reduction of anxiety
Sodium valproate (Depakene)	sedation, ? alerting effect, tremor

of previous abuses. Sterilization can enhance the opportunities for normalization of autistic and retarded adolescents.

Tubal ligation and vasectomy procedures necessitate limited risks and hospitalization time. Sterilization by abdominal hysterectomy would require more extensive surgery and hospitalization, and should only be considered for the more severely handicapped autistic girls who have difficulties with menstrual hygiene as well. A retrospective follow-up study (Wheeless, 1975) of the effects of abdominal hysterectomy for surgical sterilization in the mentally retarded yielded very favorable results.

The rights of the unborn child, the rights of the autistic adolescent's parents, and the rights of the autistic adolescent should all be considered when the issue of sterilization arises (DeMyer, 1979).

CONCLUSION

The medical care of the autistic adolescent is complicated because of the lack of understanding of the etiology of the autistic syndrome, the difficulties in obtaining medical information and performing physical and laboratory examinations, the variety of caretaking and educational programs with less opportunity for a structured predictable environment, and the increased incidence of emotional and behavioral problems. The maintenance of medical records by the autistic adolescent's family, the continuation of preventive medical and dental care, and the continued employment of appropriate behavior-management techniques would help to reduce the autistic adolescent's need for more extensive medical intervention.

REFERENCES

American Academy of Pediatrics. *Report of the Committee on Infectious Diseases.* Evanston, Ill.: AAP, 1977.

American Academy of Pediatrics Committee on Drugs. Medroxyprogesterone acetate (Depo-Provera). *Pediatrics,* 1980, *65,* 648.

American Psychiatric Association. Megavitamins and orthomolecular therapy in psychiatry. *American Psychiatric Association Task Force Report, Number 7.* Washington, D.C.: APA, 1973.

Campbell, M. Pharmacotherapy. In *Autism: A reappraisal of concepts and treatment* (M. Rutter & E. Schopler, eds.), New York: Plenum Press, 1978.

Campbell, M., Anderson, L. T., Meier, M., Cohen, I., Small, A. M., Samit, C., & Sachar, E. J. A comparison of haloperidol and behavior therapy and their interaction in autistic children. *Journal of Child Psychiatry,* 1978, *17,* 640–655.

Campbell, M., Schulman, D., & Rapoport, J. The current status of lithium therapy in child and adolescent psychiatry. *Journal of Child Psychiatry,* 1978, *17,* 717–720.

Cohen, I., Anderson, L. T., & Campbell, M. Measurement of drug effects in autistic children. *Psychopharmacology Bulletin,* 1978, *14,* 68–70.

Cohen, I., Campbell, M., Posner, D., Small, A., Triebel, B., & Anderson, L. T. Behavioral effects of haloperidol in young autistic children. *Journal of Child Psychiatry,* 1980, *19,* 665–677.

DeMyer, M. K. Adolescence. In *Parents and Children in Autism.* (M. K. DeMyer) Washington, D.C.: Winston, 1979.

Deykin, E. Y., & MacMahon, B. The incidence of seizures among children with autistic symptoms. *American Journal of Psychiatry,* 1979, *136,* 1310–1312.

Eisenberg, L. The autistic child in adolescence. *American Journal of Psychiatry,* 1956, *112,* 607–612.

Fish, B. Pharmacotherapy for autistic and schizophrenic children. In *Autism: Diagnosis, current research and management* (E. Ritvo, B. Freeman, E. Ornitz, & P. Tanguey, eds.), New York: Spectrum, 1976.

Harper, J. F., & Collins, J. K. Physical growth and development in a sample of autistic girls from New South Wales. *Australian Paediatric Journal,* 1979, *15,* 110–112.

Hutchins, V. L. Federal concerns in adolescent health care. *Journal of Current Adolescent Medicine,* 1980, *2,* 38–42.

Kopel, H. M. The autistic child in dental practice. *Journal of Dentistry for Children,* 1977, *44,* 302–309.

Marino, D. D., & King, J. C. Nutritional concerns during adolescence. *Pediatric Clinics of North America,* 1980, *27,* 125–139.

Pauling, L. Orthomolecular psychiatry. *Science*, 1968, *160*, 265–271.

Rimland, B. High dosage levels of certain vitamins in the treatment of children with severe mental disorders. In *Orthomolecular psychiatry: Treatment of schizophrenia* (D. Hawkins & L. Pauling, eds.), San Francisco: W. H. Freeman, 1973.

Rimland, B., Calloway, E., & Dreyfus, P. Effects of high doses of vitamin B_6 on autistic children: A double blind crossover study. *American Journal of Psychiatry*, 1978, *135*, 472–475.

Root, A. W. Hormonal changes in puberty. *Pediatric Annals*, 1980, *9*, 365–375.

Rutter, M. Autistic children: Infancy to adulthood. *Seminars in Psychiatry*, 1970, *2*, 435–450.

Rutter, M., Greenfield, D., & Lockyer, L. Study of infantile psychosis. II. Social and behavioral outcome. *British Journal of Psychiatry*, 1967, *113*, 1183–1199.

Shearin, R. B. Adolescent medicine in the U.S.—past, present, and future. *Pediatric Digest*, 1977, *19*, 13–17.

Stiver, R., & Dobbins, J. P. Treatment of atypical anorexia nervosa in the public school: An autistic girl. *Journal of Autism and Developmental Disorders*, 1980, *10*, 67–73.

Wheeless, C. R. Abdominal hysterectomy for surgical sterilization in the mentally retarded: A review of parental opinion. *American Journal of Obstetrics and Gynecology*, 1975, *122*, 872–875.

White, J. H. *Pediatric psychopharmacology.* Baltimore: Williams and Wilkins, 1977.

9

Sex Education at Benhaven

MARY B. MELONE and AMY L. LETTICK

PROBLEMS IN HANDLING EMERGING SEX DRIVES IN AUTISTIC ADOLESCENTS

Several of Benhaven's students entered adolescence in 1975–1976, and the staff felt a need for some action on sex education.* We were aware that a few of our students were almost the same age as our youngest teaching aides and showed signs of sexual interest in them. We needed to establish policies to guide our own behavior as well as theirs.

At the time we were not providing the students with sex education. Their lack of contact with other normal adolescents precluded their picking up information or attitudes (appropriate or not) on their own, and their parents had fewer ideas than we did about what and how to teach.

There are several problems in teaching autistic people that must be considered before developing a program. Most of Benhaven's population exhibits extreme distractibility and in some cases a lack of self-control. Although they are able to learn specific concepts during lessons, they have difficulty in generalizing the given information. They may, for instance, be able to verbalize consistently that it is necessary to look both ways before crossing the street, but in actuality they may not follow that

---

*This history of Benhaven's early attempts is based on the description in *Benhaven Then and Now* by Amy L. Lettick (1979).

MARY B. MELONE and AMY L. LETTICK ● Benhaven, New Haven, Connecticut 06511.

advice when in that situation. They display poor judgment regarding appropriate and inappropriate behavior.

Another problem area is language. The vocabulary of the majority of our students is extremely limited. There are also difficulties in expression and reception. Some students may understand the information but are unable to verbalize it; others may be able to express the correct information by rote, but have no understanding of its meaning.

Most of the students are unable to comprehend a concept which cannot be demonstrated concretely. They also have difficulty in extracting the crucial information when given an extraneous amount of material.

Many students will perseverate on a specific topic or item. They may become preoccupied with dates or numbers, or even fixate on a loose thread or misplaced object throughout the lesson. At times they may exhibit an inability to retain information for given lengths of time. They may thoroughly understand the information being presented during the lesson and the following week have no conception of what they have previously been taught. Their learning disabilities, combined with their lack of relatedness, are key considerations in choosing a sex education program.

For a start we searched for an expert on sex education. We wanted someone to educate us on the best methods of imparting information. We knew that we would have to modify others' methods for our own use, but we wanted the experience of others as to what and how to teach; we should then do the adapting and modifying. We located a specialist in the sex education of the retarded and we invited him to observe our students and help us develop a program.

After several visits, it was agreed by both the specialist and our staff that his program would be inappropriate for our students. The retarded, while low intellectually, frequently have excellent social relatedness and good communication skills, and they can and do form warm relationships that can be normal and pleasurable. His program was based on the expectation of educating low-functioning but relating, communicating adolescents, not unrelating, noncommunicating adolescents. There was no way to adapt his program to our needs. This was no surprise, but it was disappointing.

We began developing our own program. We decided to start with body parts. We used large, simple drawings of the male and female body. After several of these classes the staff, baffled and disappointed by student apathy, realized something they had not anticipated: The students were not interested! They never asked questions and they showed no desire to continue the lessons.

This was a good example of their basic autism. Their relationship with others was either a tool to satisfy their own daily needs or else it reached only to a level of external social behavior that had no drive for intimacy or deep sharing, despite superficial resemblance to normal behavior.

So the staff decided to abandon these early plans for sex education and replace them with a program of acceptable social behavior based on our own policy decisions.

POLICIES

Our first policy concerned staff–student relationships. Students' inability to discriminate, coupled with the difficulty in unlearning behavior once acquired, led us to discourage hugging and fondling as a reward for good work. The trouble with such rewards is that if a student cannot discriminate well and cannot unlearn behavior, he may sometimes hug the first person he sees after he has completed a task for which, ever since he was a child, he received a hug for a reward. If he is now 19, this can be misunderstood and can result in his being placed temporarily in jail for molestation. Therefore we recommend that our staff reward students by a pat on the shoulder and a hearty handshake instead of a hug and a squeeze.

For those who lament that we are removing the warmth of physical contact from our students' lives, we say, "We agree. It is regrettable that our students cannot know such tenderness. We shall try to substitute warm glances, warm tones of voice, and acts which, in themselves, reflect caring without involving caresses."

Our policy is: *We must teach students behavior that will be socially acceptable and appropriate in adulthood as well as in childhood.*

Students' masturbation and how we should react was also important. The masturbation, which was almost incessant around puberty, in some cases waned over the years; in others it dropped to intermittent, but often inappropriate, incidents.

Our policy is: *There is to be no disapproval of masturbation, since it is probably the only kind of sexual satisfaction that will be available to our students during their lifetime. Students must be taught, however, that masturbation is unacceptable behavior in public, and must be informed as to where it is specifically allowable.*

With our severely handicapped population it is very unlikely that opportunities for romance or marriage will be available, or that they should be sought, encouraged, or permitted. For a normal person, becoming the romantic partner and main source of strength and support to a severely mentally impaired person is a one-way street. There can be little or none of the reciprocal support that can be achieved by couples who live with *physical* disabilities in one or both of the partners.

The autistic person's inability to understand subtleties, nuances, the give-and-take of flirtation, dating, and love will then preclude any realistic relationship with a normal partner. And the possibility of finding a non-normal partner who could cope with the severe behavioral disorder of our autistic students seems remote, even if it were advisable.

Although there probably will be no other romantic objects of affection available to our students, the staff cannot provide romance as well as education. And because our students are incapable of making judgments about what is appropriate, it is up to the staff to provide the structure and the limits.

It is because we do care deeply about our students that we do not want to create patterns of behavior that will lead to later trouble or unhappiness. The experience of physical romantic relations is another one of the aspects of normal living that are not possible for our students, and we must accept that, sadly but matter-of-factly, just as we accept the other limitations on their lives.

Our policy is: *We cannot encourage behavior that will lead to frustration and disappointment for the student. Therefore we do not encourage what in normal adolescents would be predating behavior, with staff or other students. Romance must be put aside for more realistic social encounters geared to expectations of friendly sharing of activities.*

Education about female/male relationships, we said in 1976, is to be available for future use if ever it seems that a student wants to know or can understand.

In the late 1970s student behavior made it apparent that the time had come for a structured, consistent sexuality program.

Benhaven's Human Rights Committee* spent a portion of its meeting time in 1979–1980 reviewing and refining the policy on handling the sexual needs of Benhaven students, with the following conclusions:

In any relationship between a severely autistic person and another person there is the possibility of physical abuse, since the severely autistic person, in seeking his own gratification, has little awareness of, and no desire to please, another. For a partner with normal development such

*Robert Burt, professor, Yale School of Law, chairman; Dr. Donald J. Cohen, professor, pediatrician, psychiatrist, and psychologist, Yale Child Study Center; Dr. Albert J. Solnit, psychiatrist and director, Yale Child Study Center; Dr. Robert LaCamera, pediatrician and associate professor, Yale School of Medicine; Dr. Louis Lerea, clinical psychologist and speech pathologist, Southern Connecticut State College; and Amy L. Lettick, Daniel H. Davis, Larry Wood, Linda R. Simonson, and Stephen M. Simonson of the Benhaven staff.

lack of mutual feeling makes such a relationship inadvisable; for a mentally handicapped partner the relationship is a simple using of that partner, and can lead to harm or pain. The committee therefore felt that it is not advisable for severely autistic people to experience sex with another person, since that could involve possible abuse to the partner, and we felt a strong responsibility to the student's partner, who could be abused, and to the partner's parents, who trust us to look after their child.

The majority of our enrollees show no interest in sexual contact with others. Masturbation therefore seems to be the logical sexual practice for the severely autistic person.

We have had several students who were not autistic, or who were more mildly autistic, who have made advances to staff members or to other students in a rather nondiscriminating fashion. We feared for the consequences if such advances were allowed to continue.

There are risks in the noninstitutional character of the Benhaven residences. The freedom to move around and the lack of constant direct observation, which preserve the normal character of home life, are accompanied by the possible consequences of a lack of jail-like or institutional surveillance. We recognize the risks and feel they are worth taking, but while they are minimal because of the small number of individuals to whom they would apply and the limited number of hours spent at risk, we must use all sensible ways to minimize the risks.

All committee members agreed that parenthood would be undesirable, and therefore that pregnancy was to be avoided. To ensure that pregnancy should not occur, several alternatives were examined and weighed.

Segregation or Total Surveillance. One certain way to avoid pregnancy is to keep the sexes always apart, or when they are together to police all students with uninterrupted close surveillance. We are unwilling to enforce such a totally restrictive policy, but to reduce risk without the loss of general privacy or freedom of movement for all students we have installed a sensitive, selectively applicable warning system in our new residence. It can alert staff members to the movements of any particular resident about whose possible sexual activities we are concerned, indicating when he leaves his bed or sleeping quarters.

Sterilization. Some committee members felt that this would have been the answer, and regretted that sterilization is either legally forbidden or extremely difficult to carry out in all states of the country. Others felt that the past history of inappropriate sterilization of mentally retarded people, and the possible abuses of this procedure justified such legal restrictions. In any case its use is highly restricted and generally unavailable.

Abortion. A third alternative is to wait until a pregnancy occurs and then perform an abortion. Since any intimate medical procedure is very upsetting to our students, this is not a desirable solution.

Birth Control. All agreed that, all things considered, the use of a contraceptive pill is the best option available. We are not willing, however, to give a contraceptive to an individual without first discussing it with the parents and getting permission. If we see signs of sexual awakening in a student, we regard this as a welcome sign of natural growth (and discuss it with the parents as such) not as a failure of staff to prevent a prurient or sick behavior. We also take this as a reason for greater precautions.

We were concerned that reducing the risk of physical intimacy might unduly inhibit the development of any potential for normal emotional development, even the possibility of normal sexual relationships. We did not intend to encourage physical sexual relationships, but we were aware that an excessively stringent policy of avoiding the possibility of such sexual development would restrict our program's goals of maximizing normal relationships between autistic people and others. If a student were to exhibit near-normal sexual feelings, we should question the benefits to him of his placement at Benhaven, where there would be no appropriate response. Regrettably, normalcy in one area does not automatically assure normalcy in other areas. Normal sexual development would not qualify that student for inclusion with mentally retarded people, for example, because of the other, disparate characteristics of autism.

Were it not for possible pregnancy and the subsequent abortion that all members agreed would have to follow, there could be times when, if two people were mildly impaired and did have some warmth and awareness, physical intimacy in itself would not be a bad thing. What if two of our autistic people appeared physically attracted to and capable of satisfying each other without harm? Should relationships involving sexual intercourse be permitted?

The staff members on the committee were particularly emphatic in refusing to allow such activity. Not only did they feel unwilling and unqualified to provide the counseling which would be necessary, but they felt that Benhaven's physical quarters were not designed to provide sufficient privacy. They would move in to stop such intimacy. A majority of the committee did not disagree with the staff's position.

The defensibility of that position depends on the potential capacity of the autistic person. If it is clear that that person has no capacity for anything but an abusive relationship, then there is no question of a right to that relationship. But if he does have the capacity, then such a policy does interfere, and this could happen in borderline cases. Any blanket ruling is less than perfect.

The Human Rights Committee concluded by reiterating Benhaven's willingness to risk the noninstitutional setting, along with the policy of discouraging physical intimacy, and instead encouraging group relations of a nonromantic nature.

With the recommendations of the committee, we began our tasks of developing a comprehensive program that would enable our higher functioning autistic and neurologically impaired individuals to deal more effectively with their own sexuality.

Once more we examined other programs for one that would implement our philosophy and meet our needs. The only ones we found were geared to populations with social relatedness and good communication skills; the vocabulary was generally extensive and the concepts often abstract. Many lessons were based on discussions of feelings toward sexuality, which might be an excellent approach for a population which is able to identify feelings and express themselves, but was not appropriate for us. We needed a program that would clearly indicate the specific concepts, language, and teaching procedures to be utilized. The more concise and specific the lessons, the more information the students would retain. Finding no suitable program we decided to develop our own, and so we set about our task.

DEVELOPING THE PROGRAM

In addition to the development of behavioral and social growth in the area of sexuality, we felt required to provide the parameters necessary for comfortable adaptation to social environments. This would be accomplished by teaching the students the "when" and "where" of sexual behavior. We also wanted to establish a guide that would enable both the layman and the professional to teach moderately autistic and/or neurologically impaired individuals about their own sexuality.

There were several items to consider prior to the implementation of a course in sexuality and social awareness. First, the age of the student is important. One question frequently asked is "At what age should we begin to teach these students about topics such as menstruation, masturbation, etc.?" We have found that the age of the student alone cannot be the deciding factor as to whether he is ready for the program. There are several other factors that must be taken into consideration as well: Does the student possess the language ability necessary to understand the material? Is the student easily distracted? At what social level is the student functioning? Does the student exhibit disruptive behavior that will interfere with the lesson? Is the student emotionally mature enough to deal effectively with the material? Once again, as with all the other programs at Benhaven, each student must be evaluated on an individual basis.

The program was designed for a small group of verbal, moderately autistic, and neurologically impaired students aged 14–21. Although it contains basic concepts that could apply to any handicapped population, it does not include material that should be taught to individuals who exhibit high social development. This is not a program for individuals who can engage in intimate sexual relationships.

Individuals who exhibit low social development, who are unable to relate to others, are not included in this program. For these individuals, who often exhibit severe language impairment or demonstrate extreme behavior disorders, the principles of the program would be applicable but the teaching procedures would have to be adapted accordingly.

The program was called "Sexuality and Social Awareness: A Curriculum for Moderately Autistic and/or Neurologically Impaired Individuals" (see Lieberman & Melone, 1980). Program content selected was based on the needs of 13 students attending Benhaven who met the criteria. The major topics taught are: identification of body parts, menstruation, masturbation, physical examinations, personal hygiene, and social behavior. We omitted topics that we felt were beyond the scope of our students, such as dating, marriage, birth control, and childbirth.

We found it necessary to limit the terminology presented. Specific biological terms were chosen to replace the slang or baby words that the students were using.

Program content and terminology utilized were reviewed and approved by our school pediatrician, who is a member of Benhaven's Medical Advisory Committee and member of the Yale–New Haven Medical Center staff.

SEX EDUCATION CURRICULUM

The program includes six units, each containing goals and specific behavioral objectives. Each behavioral objective has clearly outlined procedures. The units are sequential and should be followed in order.

Before beginning the program with a child a parent–teacher meeting is held to familiarize parents with the curriculum and rationale. It is important that the parents be familiar with the material so that they can reinforce the concepts and vocabulary at home. We give them a copy of "Guidelines for Parents," which lists each unit, the major goals to be covered, and the vocabulary to be used. The guide also indicates when the material will be presented to their child. During this initial meeting the parents or guardians are required to sign a parental consent form permitting their children to participate in the program.

During the meeting emphasis is placed on the simplification of the material covered in the curriculum. Parents are advised to follow these guidelines and not to give students extraneous information (i.e., why females menstruate; how babies are born). Although it is the teacher's responsibility to maintain a home/school contact, parents are informed that they may contact the teacher whenever a question or problem arises.

Prior to the onset of the program a meeting is held to familiarize the staff with the contents of the curriculum. All staff having contact with the students involved in the program are required to attend in order to maintain consistency in the use of language and vocabulary provided throughout the program.

A pre- and posttest is included in the curriculum. The entire pretest is given before the onset of the program and is used as a guide to determine what to emphasize. Because of the students' difficulty in retaining information, all objectives are reviewed, regardless of pretest scores. At the end of each unit the teacher gives each student that section of the evaluation to check on mastery of the material just taught. The posttest is given at the conclusion of the entire curriculum.

A guide sheet with specific instructions and explanations precedes each unit. This includes the type of instructor required to teach the lesson (i.e., male, female, either male or female), the recommended structure of the group (i.e., all males, all females, males and females), and the duration of each lesson. The guide also lists the specific vocabulary used and any prerequisite concepts that the students should learn prior to the introduction of each unit. Any materials required for the unit are also listed on the guide sheet.

Unit I. Identification of Body Parts

The first unit in "Sexuality and Social Awareness" is "Identification of Body Parts." The students are presented with 29 specific body parts which they must learn to identify both receptively and expressively. The teacher displays two charts (male and female). He or she then points to a body part and asks, "What is this?" The student responds with the correct answer using a complete sentence (i.e., "This is a penis"). The teacher then asks the student to name a person in the group who would have that body part (i.e., "Bob has a penis"). Internal body parts and organs have been purposely omitted because of students' difficulties with abstraction and generalization. The instructor for this unit can be either male or female. The structure of the classes can be males only, females only, or males and females together. Along with the specific teaching procedures there are several suggested supplementary activities to reinforce the unit's major goals.

Unit II. Menstruation

The next unit is "Menstruation." The classes are for females only and are taught by a female instructor. Specific objectives and clearly outlined procedures are provided so that the teacher, as well as the layperson, will be able to teach procedures effectively.

In order that the students develop a basic understanding of the menstrual cycle, several specific behavioral objectives are implemented. Along with verbalizing facts pertaining to menstruation they are taught how to symbolize graphically the menstrual cycle on a calendar.

Demonstration of the correct use of a sanitary napkin is one of the most important activities in teaching the students about menstruation. The teacher demonstrates while explaining how a sanitary napkin is used. The students are then asked to demonstrate appropriate use of the napkin using a loose pair of underpants. The students are then taken to the women's bathroom where they are given a sanitary napkin and verbally instructed to put it on. The teacher intervenes when necessary. They are then instructed to remove the napkins and demonstrate the correct method of disposal of the napkin, which they have previously simulated in the classroom.

In addition there are several lessons based on the hygiene necessary during menstruation, and various ways of relieving menstrual discomforts. The students learn that while it is important to exercise every day, exercise can be especially helpful during menstruation. The teacher has the students demonstrate various familiar exercises and then shows them some new exercises and postures that can relieve menstrual cramps. The teacher demonstrates these exercises one at a time and has the students participate.

Unit III. Masturbation

The unit on masturbation allows the students to develop a basic understanding of the act. The females are taught by a female instructor and the males are taught by a male instructor. The teacher explains what the term "masturbation" means. The group then discusses any feelings associated with masturbation. It is important that the students understand when and where it is appropriate to masturbate when they feel they want or need to. For instance, although the bathroom is an appropriate place to masturbate, they do not have to masturbate every time they go to the bathroom. The teacher explains that masturbation is very personal and should not be done in front of others. In order to reinforce this concept the students and teacher compile a list of the specific times when it is appropriate and inappropriate to masturbate. Basic hygiene associated with masturbation is also emphasized in this unit.

Unit IV. Physical Examinations

This unit, which includes a description of the gynecological examination, was chosen to alleviate any fears and answer any questions the students may have. Even though these individuals will never be encouraged to engage in sexual intercourse, routine health precautions are necessary. Although not all handicapped women need to have a gynecological examination once a year, a physical history including regularity of periods, type of flow, etc., should be taken by a physician once a year. If the handicapped woman's mother was given DES during pregnancy with that child, an internal examination should be performed yearly. This part of the curriculum would be omitted for women who do not get gynecological examinations. For those to whom this unit does apply, a basic understanding of what constitutes a gynecological examination is the major goal. The unit is taught to females only, by a female instructor. Through role-play the students are taught the steps in a gynecological examination, in order to alleviate any fears or anxieties which may precede the actual examination.

Unit V. Personal Hygiene

The next unit, "Personal Hygiene," gives the students a basic understanding of the problems associated with the genital area and teaches the personal hygiene necessary to maintain a clean and healthy body. The females are taught by a female instructor and the males by a male instructor. The students are taught that if itchiness, discharge, pain, or unusual bleeding occurs from the genital area, an adult should be notified. There is also a procedure which teaches the students the correct method of wiping themselves after urination and/or bowel movements. This is an area in which many people unjustifiably assume students' competence.

Unit VI. Social Behavior

The final unit in "Sexuality and Social Awareness" deals with social behavior as it relates to sexuality. The lessons are taught by either a male or female instructor and the classes may be coeducational.

As mentioned previously, many of the students at Benhaven have difficulties with generalization. Therefore it is necessary to teach them the specific times and places for appropriate and inappropriate behavior. One of the major goals in the unit on social behavior stresses the appropriate and inappropriate times for nude, partially dressed, and fully dressed states. The students are taught that there are certain times when it is appropriate to be nude (i.e., when taking a shower), but that, for example, it is inappropriate to come to school without any clothes on. Because they have such problems with discrimination, they must be taught the specific situations to which this rule applies. They must be taught, for example, that males and females should never be nude in front of each other, but that at certain times it is all right to be nude in front of members of their own sex (i.e., changing in the locker room, changing in the bedroom). In addition appropriate choice of clothing is emphasized. Again because of their lack of discrimination many students are unable to choose the appropriate clothing for given situations. Lessons emphasizing this concept are taught (i.e., Is it appropriate to wear pajamas to school? Can we wear only our underwear to the grocery store?).

Appropriate and inappropriate forms of touching and kissing are also emphasized. The students observe other people hugging and kissing, and think it is all right for them to do the same. It is necessary therefore to teach them the "when" and "where" of these behaviors. In order to avoid confusion the number of interactions of this type must be limited. The students are taught that a handshake, a pat on the back, or a hug are acceptable during specific situations (i.e., it is all right to shake someone's hand if he has done good work; it is nice to give a member of the family a hug when saying hello, good-bye, or good-night to them). In addition the fact that they should never touch strangers is stressed. Kissing must also be limited; without specific boundaries these students are unable to determine when, and whom, they can kiss. Appropriate social distance and sitting positions are also taught. Many of these concepts are emphasized through the use of role-play.

The students must also learn to differentiate between male and female restrooms, and understand various restroom procedures. In order for them to identify male and female restrooms, it is necessary to teach them the various symbols used on public restrooms (i.e., men/women, king/queen, males/females). Once they understand which restroom to use, there are several procedures which they must learn: they must remember to close and lock the stall door when in use, flush the toilet, leave the stall fully dressed, and wash and dry their hands before leaving the restroom. In addition the males must be able to identify and demonstrate proper use of a urinal. Finally, the students are brought to a public restroom and are instructed to carry out what they have been taught in class.

PROGRAM CONSIDERATIONS

Timeliness of Topic. Questions such as whether or not students should be taught specific topics prior to the actual experience must also be considered. During the course of our program we found with several of our students that teaching them concepts which they had not yet experienced often led to frustration and confusion.

But preparing them by teaching the prerequisite concepts is most beneficial. For example, prior to teaching the unit on menstruation there are several concepts which should be taught. Since several of the lessons focus on the use of the calendar, the students must be able to count to 31, name the days of the week and months of the year, know the number of days in each month, etc. If it is decided that prior knowledge of what actually occurs during menstruation will be beneficial to the child, the unit may be taught. Again this decision is highly individualized and must be discussed with the woman's parents or guardian.

We also felt it unnecessary to teach a woman about the gynecological examination unless we were certain that she would be visiting a gynecologist in the near future. Since it is not necessary for the majority to be given an examination annually, this extraneous information would only confuse most of the women.

Several parents were concerned about the unit on masturbation. Many parents chose not to have their child participate in this unit if their child has exhibited no interest in masturbation or displayed no signs of sexual frustration due to an inability to masturbate. They feared that focusing on masturbation might increase the possibility of their child's becoming extremely confused and/or exhibiting inappropriate discrimination regarding this behavior.

On the other hand several of the parents were concerned that their child's behavior problems were due to an inability to release sexual frustration. Even though their child never masturbated, they felt that having the knowledge and opportunity to do so would alleviate many of their child's problems. Obviously there is no right or wrong answer. Each child is unique and must be dealt with on an individualized basis. It is extremely important that the parents and teacher work cooperatively for the benefit of each child.

Staff Selection. Another important consideration is the selection of appropriate staff. Although the teaching procedures are clearly outlined, the instructor must be able to develop a rapport with the students. He or she must be comfortable with the material, and know the students well enough to focus on individualized strengths and weaknesses. Also, there are certain lessons throughout the curriculum when only a male staff member will be able to teach (e.g., masturbation for males) or a female will be able to teach (e.g., menstruation or masturbation for females).

Frequency of Classes. We also found that the frequency of classtime varied with the individual student. For some of the students a 1-hour class once a week was sufficient. Other schedules allowed some of the students to have 1-hour classes twice a week. Those students who were more distractible were generally taught in half-hour intervals twice a week. At the beginning of each unit there is a projected time allotment for each lesson. Based on this projection, if all units are covered the entire curriculum should be taught to female students in 25½ classroom hours and to males in 16 classroom hours. How long the program lasts will depend on the number of classes given per week. Once the entire program is completed and the posttest is given, there will most likely be certain areas of the curriculum that will need emphasis and review. Because these students have difficulty retaining information, the curriculum may need to be repeated several times. For some students it may be taught on a continual basis.

Physical Plant. Prior to the onset of the program it is important to have specific physical plant needs available. For instance, when teaching the unit on masturbation the participating students should be in an isolated room, both for privacy and to avoid disrupting the rest of the class. For the menstruation unit a lavatory must be available exclusively for the lesson in which the correct use of a sanitary napkin is demonstrated.

Parental Involvement. Parental involvement is extremely important throughout the entire curriculum in order to maintain consistency with the home environment. Parents should be aware at all times of which lessons their children are working on in the event that a problem or question arises. The more reinforcement the students receive, the sooner the concept will be learned. It is extremely important that there be carryover from school to home. Because many students have difficulty generalizing, they may know that it is inappropriate to masturbate in the classroom but not realize that it is also inappropriate at home in the living room. No matter how many times they must verbalize these rules in school, the true test comes when they must generalize these concepts to everyday real-life situations.

PROGRAM STRATEGIES

There are several variations of procedures and additional strategies utilized throughout the different units to assist the students with their ability to generalize the given information. Role-playing is often very beneficial. The majority of the unit explaining the gynecological examination and several of the concepts covered in the social behavior unit are taught via this technique. Having the students actually go through the physical motions while explaining the concept appears to reinforce their understanding of the material. Additionally, if the students are shown concrete examples the material is learned much more quickly. In the unit which explains the gynecological examination, for example, we found it beneficial to have the females weigh themselves, just as the doctor or nurse would during the actual visit. We also tried to get as many of the materials as possible to show the women prior to their visit. Items such as a paper nightgown, the tool which is used to prick their fingers for a blood sample, and the cup in which they urinate, are generally readily available through a local physician or health care facility.

Whenever possible we tried to supplement the lessons with varied concrete examples. Many of the slides from *Sexuality and the Handicapped* (Kempton, 1976) were extremely beneficial.* Several students were unable to understand many of the concepts through verbal instruction because of their language and/or abstraction disabilities; through the use of slides these concepts were quite clear (i.e., verbal explanation of discharge versus an actual photograph of discharge).

It is therefore necessary to implement numerous variations on an objective, depending on the learning modalities of the students. Many students grasped the information exclusively through verbal instruction; for others the slides were beneficial. Having the students read and/or write the major vocabulary or concepts also helped reinforce the information. Several teacher-made games were developed to supplement the curriculum. For instance, there are several strategies used to teach the unit on the identification of body parts: the students may identify body parts on themselves, on others, from a picture, from a slide, or on a model; they can play the game "Simon Says" in a group; the teacher can implement blackboard activities to reinforce the objectives (i.e., erasing body parts, circling body parts, adding body parts); worksheets can be used (i.e., coloring in body parts, filling in missing body parts); some

---

*For those individuals who are on a higher social level, there are several existing curricula available. In our research, we discovered *Sexuality and the Handicapped* by Winifred Kempton (1976), produced and distributed by Stanfield House, Santa Monica, Calif. This curriculum and slide presentation includes material on sexual and social behavior which goes beyond the scope of individuals such as those at Benhaven.

students may enjoy categorizing body parts using word cards. The use of puzzles may also be a welcome additional activity. Tracing each other's bodies on large sheets of paper and coloring in the parts is fun for many students, and helps reinforce the objectives. There are several strategies and modalities which should be utilized to make the lessons as exciting and innovative as possible for the students.

EVALUATION AND ASSESSMENT

Evaluation and assessment of progress are based on the pre- and posttest scores and behavioral observation. It is important that a continuous record of the student's behavior be kept throughout each lesson. We found that a standardized checksheet was extremely beneficial when working with small groups of students. Prior to the use of the checksheet, random behaviors were recorded in a log. This procedure was often time-consuming and many important aspects were overlooked. The checksheet we developed includes such items as the date of the lesson, the instructor, the student–teacher ratio, the time the lesson began, the time the lesson was completed, the title of the unit, and the specific goal and objectives being taught. The general attention level of the student is recorded (i.e., was the student distracted during the entire lesson, on-task for part of the lesson, or attentive during the entire lesson?); whether the student's general behavior was moody and irritable, fair or excellent is also noted. Additionally it is helpful to have a record of the student's basic problem areas (i.e., was the student able to answer the instructor's questions when given specific verbal cues, but unable to grasp the information? does the student know the information, but cannot express it verbally? was there difficulty understanding the instructor's questions? when the question was reworded several times did the student grasp the information?). Along with the student's general grasp of the lesson, the specific concepts and problem areas are recorded. The instructor may also note what audio-visual aides were utilized and how they affected the lesson. Any other pertinent information such as additional comments or suggestions is also recorded.

THE INITIAL RESULTS

In general it appears that "Sexuality and Social Awareness" has been extremely successful with those students who have participated in the program. All the major initial goals established have been met. According to the students' pre- and posttest scores, and through behavioral observation, it is evident that all students have demonstrated a degree of behavioral and social growth in the area of sexuality. They are now able to deal more effectively with their own sexuality in many areas. For instance, they now realize that it is all right to masturbate when they feel they want or need to, as long as it is in an appropriate place, at an appropriate time. Many of the students were simply unaware of the parameters required for comfortable adaptation to social environments. They now know the "when and where" of sexual behavior. In addition we were successful in developing a guide that enables the layman as well as the professional to teach moderately autistic and/or neurologically impaired individuals about sexuality.

Although the curriculum has been extremely successful, there are certain areas which need improvement. The pre- and posttests need more flexibility in accommodating to the language competence of each student. Although the relatively good language skills of the particular group did not initially seem to require highly structured and simplified language, we found that the language disabilities did underlie the superficial performance, interfering with reception and comprehension. We had to modify and simplify the language to the individual levels of each student.

For example, during the first administration of the posttest one female student was asked "How often should you check your napkin to see if it needs to be changed?" Her response was "Every day." The instructor revised the question: "When should you check your napkin to see if it should be changed?" Answer: "In a week." Again the question was reworded: "When you have your period, you should check your napkin four times a day. . . . You should check before. . . ." The student responded, "Check napkin before breakfast, before lunch, before dinner, and before bedtime."

So we want to develop varying levels in the language component of the program, to be applied at whatever level is appropriate for each student.

Another area of weakness with the program is follow-through. Although the student mentioned above was able to verbalize the four times when she should check her napkin, whether or not she would actually do so when she had her period was uncertain. It would be beneficial if more effective methods of evaluation in various situations could be established. At this point the only available method for evaluating the carry-over of the curriculum topics to specific situations is random behavioral observation. Some form of structured checksheet that could be implemented during various situations would be a useful device in evaluating the students' generalization of the material. It would be extremely beneficial for such a tool to be utilized as a carry-over between the home and school environments.

In addition the students should be given increased opportunities to demonstrate the knowledge they have acquired. One student who was participating in the program was extremely proficient when it came to verbalizing the proper restroom procedures. He was also able to demonstrate the entire sequence correctly in the school lavatory. When taken to a public restroom to demonstrate the procedure, however, the student panicked. He would not enter the restroom; he was afraid of the "uneven tiles" on the lavatory floor. This was one thing we had not anticipated. Although the student was able to verbalize and demonstrate the proper restroom procedures, his phobia prevented him from generalizing the appropriate behavior.

CONCLUSION

Although there is still room for revision and improvement, we feel that our pilot program has been extremely successful. At last this population has a guide that enables them to have a better understanding of their own sexuality. Teachers and parents can work cooperatively and consistently to ensure autistic and neurologically impaired individuals' comfortable adaptation to their social environment. At this point our plans are to continue the current program, with continuous repetition until each student is fully aware of its major principles. We realize that it will be necessary to revise and modify the current program continually to meet the changing needs of the students, and we are prepared to do this. We hope that our contributions to sexuality education for the handicapped will stimulate others to investigate an area long in need of program research and development.

REFERENCES

Kempton, W. *Sexuality and the handicapped*. Santa Monica, Calif.: Stanfield House, 1976. (Includes a slide presentation.)
Lieberman, D. A. & Melone, M. B. *Sexuality and social awareness*. New Haven: Benhaven Press, 1980.
Lettick, A. L. *Benhaven then and now*. New Haven: Benhaven Press, 1979.

10

The Management of Aggressive Behavior

JUDITH E. FAVELL

Physical and verbal aggression is a widespread problem, one not unique to autistic adolescents (Buss, 1961; Ulrich & Favell, 1970). Nevertheless aggression can have very serious consequences for autistic individuals who engage in it. Aggression, particularly frequent or intense aggression, can severely disrupt autistic individuals' lives, as well as the lives of those with whom they live.

Aggression often interferes directly with an individual's participation in recreational, educational, and vocational programs. At the least aggression consumes valuable client and caretaker time. The behavior also evokes fear and distaste in others, and thus increases the likelihood that the aggressive individual will be avoided or treated in an undesirable or even abusive manner. Very often recreational, educational, and vocational opportunities are withdrawn entirely if an individual displays disruptive or dangerous behavior. Indeed individuals who display highly aggressive behavior often become prime candidates for more restrictive placement, or placement with individuals who are not suitable peers, i.e., those who perform below the individual in cognitive, social, or other areas of functioning. Such exclusion is usually not as arbitrary or unfair as it may appear, for aggressive behavior directly infringes on the rights and jeopardizes the safety of others. Thus treating aggression generally receives the highest clinical priority, to enable the individual to participate fully in humane, habilitative activities while ensuring others' rights to engage safely in those same activities.

JUDITH E. FAVELL ● Western Carolina Center, Morganton, North Carolina 28655.

Considering the importance of the problem, this chapter will focus on the major issues related to aggression and its treatment. These issues include: factors maintaining aggression, treatment goals, an overall treatment strategy including methods of developing appropriate alternative behavior and methods of suppressing aggression, the use of psychotropic drugs, dealing with collateral changes in behavior, and methods of generalizing and maintaining durable improvement.

DESCRIBING THE SEVERITY OF AGGRESSION

Although as a broad class of behavior aggression is considered salient and important, its clinical significance depends on its particular characteristics in a specific individual's case. The treatment priority the behavior receives, as well as the type of treatment employed, depends on several characteristics of the behavior.

First, some *forms* or *topographies* of aggression are viewed as more severe than others. Pinching others is one thing, but poking eyes or throwing furniture is quite another. The *frequency* of the behavior also varies widely. Aggression which occurs several times a day or hour is generally considered a more serious problem than that which occurs once or twice a week. *Intensity* of aggression is also a crucial dimension of the behavior. Intensity usually refers to the force used in performing the behavior or its harmful effects. Light slaps, pinches, or pokes tend to be viewed as milder intensities; similar forms which produce physical damage such as bruises or lacerations are considered more intense and severe. These dimensions of aggression *interact,* i.e., combine, to determine the seriousness of the problem. For example, an individual's aggression may be a benign form and mild intensity, but may occur so frequently that it is considered a major problem. Alternatively, aggression may erupt very rarely but be so intense and harmful when it does occur that it is given highest priority for treatment. Indeed it is the capability of adolescents to truly harm others that most often makes their aggression so disturbing, and treatment so necessary. A slap from a small child may hurt, but the same force applied by a strapping adolescent is surely more memorable.

When the characteristics of an individual's aggression are viewed as serious by virtue of either its form, frequency, or intensity, its treatment should be given highest priority. This chapter describes the most common behavioral approaches to managing aggressive behavior. It is predicated on two major assumptions: First, that aggression is most frequently maintained by the individual's environment. The behavior often occurs as a response to identifiable environmental conditions, and is sustained by its environmental effects. Second, successful treatment of aggression involves comprehensive rearrangements of the individual's natural environment, to remove the conditions and contingencies which inadvertently support the problem, and to improve support for more desirable behavior.

FACTORS MAINTAINING AGGRESSION

Most children display at least transient aggression. Sometimes a chronically aggressive child seems to "outgrow" the problem. Unfortunately more often they do not. To the contrary, there is often a disturbing increase in intensity and severity as the child's size and skill increases (Patterson, Reid, Jones, & Conger, 1975; Robins, 1966).

Several factors are commonly identified as responsible for maintaining chronic aggression in a variety of populations, including autistic individuals.

Organic Conditions

Aggression may be associated with a variety of congenital organic conditions, including tuberous sclerosis or autism itself. It may also be associated with acute medical conditions such as injuries, colds, flu, or menstruation. Clearly such conditions should be diagnosed and where possible treated. However, if no organic disorder can be identified, or if treatment is not possible or is not sufficient in reducing aggression, then behavioral treatment should be instituted. A similar recommendation can be made with regard to cyclical aggression. In some instances aggression improves and worsens rhythmically in the apparent absence of environmental changes which might account for the behavioral rhythm. Research is needed on possible biological bases of such rhythmic fluctuations in behavior. However, in the absence of such information the immediate recommendation is to attempt to identify biological and environmental conditions which are regularly correlated with regression and improvement in aggression, and to incorporate that information into a behavioral treatment program in ways described in the following pages.

Positive Reinforcement

Aggression frequently results in positive rewards or reinforcement from peers and caretakers (Patterson, Littman, & Bricker, 1967). Victims often cry, cower, or hand over their possessions; caretakers frequently scold, wrestle with, or attempt to distract or calm the aggressor by providing him or her with preferred and attractive activities. Such events may be powerful positive reinforcers for the individual, and may strengthen and maintain the aggression that produces them. The assumption is that more appropriate behavior is not as effective as aggression in obtaining these reinforcers for the individual. Appropriate forms of communication, social interactions, or other behavior are not in the individual's impoverished repertoire or do not receive the same amount, type, or certainty of reinforcement that aggression produces. In such cases treatment involves developing and strengthening alternative, appropriate means of obtaining the positive reinforcers that the individual was previously only able to receive by aggressing.

Negative Reinforcement

Aggression may also function as an escape or avoidance response, i.e., terminating or delaying unpleasant situations. For example, aggression commonly occurs when demands are placed on an autistic individual (Carr, Newsom, & Binkoff, 1980) or in other "frustrating" situations such as during periods in which positive reinforcement is withheld or delayed (Dollard, Doob, Miller, Mowrer, & Sears, 1939; Kelly & Hake, 1970; Ulrich & Favell, 1970). Similarly aggression may be observed in response to other unpleasant situations such as changes of routine, being touched, or being prevented from engaging in preferred behaviors such as stereotypies or ritualisms. These situations too may be so unpleasant or "aversive" to the individual that behavior—including aggression—which terminates or delays them may be negatively reinforced, i.e., increased in strength. The possibility that aggression may be negatively reinforced is clear when observing its common effects. Hitting, kicking, and biting often result in removal of demands, release from class, withdrawal of physical contact, or being allowed to resume a preferred activity such as self-stimulation. The aggression is thus reinforced, i.e., becomes more and more likely to occur in such situations in the future. The assumption again is that more appropriate behavior is not as effective as aggression in terminating or delaying unpleasant situations; treatment must therefore include differentially strengthening more appropriate means of obtaining reinforcers, including the opportunity to escape unpleasant situations. In addition a crucial component of treatment in cases in which aggression is motivated by escape or avoidance involves eliminating or altering the aversive properties of situations which motivate escape or avoidance in the first place.

In general, while organic factors which are correlated with aggression should be diagnosed and if possible treated, frequently the behavior appears to be a method of controlling the individual's environment, either producing positive reinforcers such as attention and/or escape or avoidance of unpleasant situations. Since aggression is often the only means of such control available to the individual, a major focus of treatment involves providing the individual with the skills to obtain similar types, amounts, and certainty of reinforcement for more appropriate behavior, and providing relatively less reinforcement for the aggression itself.

THE GOAL OF TREATMENT

The goal of treatment is to reduce the strength of aggression to an acceptable level. Strength is commonly measured by the frequency of the behavior (how often it occurs) or its intensity (the force that is used or the harm it produces). Thus after treatment aggression should rarely or never occur, or its occurrences should be judged as very mild and benign. The objective is not to interrupt aggression temporarily once it erupts. As indicated, some methods of placating, distracting, and "giving in" to an individual who is aggressing may interrupt that episode of aggression, but will increase the likelihood of its recurrence in the future. Similarly the strength of behavior is not reduced by physically or chemically preventing its occurrence. Chronic isolation, physical restraint, or amounts of medication which render the individual stuporous may indeed prevent aggression but do not reduce the strength of the behavior. In short, these do not teach individuals not to be aggressive, or teach them alternative ways of receiving the things they want and need.

TREATMENT OF AGGRESSION

Although the clinical research literature tends to be organized by individual treatment techniques, in actual practice aggression can and should be treated by a comprehensive composite of these procedures. To optimize the chances of successfully producing meaningful, durable changes in the individual's behavior, treatment should always consist of *each* of the following dimensions:

1. A careful analysis of biological and environmental conditions and consequences which might be maintaining the individual's aggression
2. Environmental rearrangements which ensure a safe, structured and responsive environment

3. Systematic strengthening of appropriate alternative behavior
4. Reduction of reinforcement for aggression
5. Rearrangement of environmental conditions differentially associated with aggression
6. In some cases, the inclusion of punishment for aggression itself

Analysis of Maintaining Conditions

Since it is assumed that aggression is most often maintained by identifiable biological and environmental conditions, the first step in planning treatment involves observing the individual under a variety of conditions and describing his or her behavior in relation to those conditions.

Both direct observations and caretaker reports can be used to collect pertinent information in several areas. First, it is important to measure the topography, frequency, and intensity of the aggression itself. These measurement dimensions were described previously, and constitute the common practice of collecting baseline, or pretreatment, levels of the behavior. However, often these data are combined across an entire day or even longer, and obscure an equally vital type of information: the *specific situations* in which aggression is more frequent or intense and the situations in which it is less prevalent. Aggression is usually "situation specific"; thus it is crucial to identify those situations which are differentially correlated with the behavior. To do this it is essential to observe the individual in a variety of situations, cataloging times, places, people, and activities during which aggression is more frequent or intense, and similarly listing conditions under which serious aggression rarely occurs. In addition it is important to record the *consequences of aggression*— what happens when the behavior occurs. For example, one might note that the individual is released from class, physically separated from his victim, sent to his room to "cool off," or obtains his victim's snack. Finally, it is equally important to inventory the individual's *appropriate behavior* and carefully note *its consequences*. Does the individual display even rudimentary communication skills? Does he work or play constructively even for brief periods? Is he affectionate or gentle with certain individuals? And when such desirable behavior occurs, what environmental response does it produce? Information about appropriate behavior and its consequences is sometimes as difficult to obtain about individuals who are labeled "aggressive" as it is important in devising their treatment.

Thus the first step in designing treatment involves observing the individual in a variety of situations to obtain information on the topography, frequency, and intensity of aggression, situations in which it is frequent or intense, situations in which it is less a problem, the consequences of aggression, and appropriate behavior and its consequences. Although such a step clearly derives from the generally held assumption that the problem is maintained by its environment, and may seem obvious as a basis of devising treatment, in actual practice it is commonly ignored. Treatments are too often arbitrarily "conceived in a vacuum," without collecting adequate information on possible factors maintaining the problem, without identifying promising rearrangements of natural conditions and contingencies that might have powerful therapeutic effects, or if not incorporated into treatment, may have powerful deleterious results. A careful analysis of an individual's behavior in relation to the environment in which it occurs enables treatment that effectively incorporates removal of the pathogenic conditions maintaining aggression, and skillful, sensitive rearrangement of natural conditions to better support improved patterns of behavior.

Environmental Arrangements

A crucial, and sometimes ignored, step in treatment of aggression involves arranging an overall safe, structured, and responsive environment. It is not uncommon to observe caretakers attempting to conduct sophisticated and arduous treatment procedures in environments which are unsafe, disorganized, and do not provide for the rudiments of humane, enriched living. Thus it is recommended that if possible prior to embarking on a rigorous program targeted at an individual's aggression, several generic features of the environment be checked, and if necessary, corrected.

Is the Situation Safe? An attempt should be made temporarily to eliminate physical features of the environmental which present danger. Every furnishing, decoration, recreational and educational material should be evaluated as to its harmful potential. The temporary removal or alteration of furnishings and materials may infringe less on the sensibilities and rights of others than does the use of those objects as an instrument of aggression against them. Subsequently, as aggression is brought under control and the individual is taught to use property appropriately the environment may gradually be restored to normal.

Similarly, in group-care situations ensuring safety usually involves arranging specific and rigorously enforced schedules of supervision. Caretakers should rotate the responsibility of monitoring the individual and intervening as appropriate. Assuming that everyone is responsible too often leaves no one responsible.

Finally, safety may involve temporarily separating an individual from his or her preferred victim. When an individual targets aggression against a single other person, it may be viewed as most expeditious to arrange that they be in separate rooms, classes, or programs. Of course in some instances such a change would be impossible or undesirable; this recommendation must be tempered with common sense and consideration of all its ramifications. Further, it should not serve as the basis for secluding the aggressor or placing him or her with individuals who are not otherwise appropriate peers.

Is the Situation Structured and Organized? Neither autistic clients nor caretakers function well in environments that are unpredictable and disorganized. Schedules of routines and activities should be planned in advance, effectively communicated to all, and proceed smoothly and reliably within and across days. Clients and caretakers should know what they are to do, when, and with whom. Careful contingency plans should be laid for emergencies, unavoidable alterations in schedules, staff shortages, and other common disruptions to continuity and consistency. Though not easy to effect, such order and organization is crucial to humane living for all and effective habilitation for aggressive individuals.

Are There Ample and Appropriate Things To Do? A setting may provide exemplary structure and organization but nevertheless be highly impoverished and unresponsive to individuals' needs. In short a crucial feature of an environment is whether it provides opportunities for constructive activity. An "enriched environment" features ample recreational and educational materials and activities. These activities and materials should be varied, and should include frequent opportunities for physical exercise and a wide variety of sensory experiences, as well as the standard use of table-tasks. Where possible there should be choices, i.e., more than one activity scheduled at a time, so that individuals may select a preferred, rather than imposed, activity (LeLaurin & Risley, 1972). An enriched environment provides for regular evaluation of what individuals actually prefer doing and provision of those preferred activities and materials (Favell & Cannon, 1977). An enriched environment provides for these activities consistently, without excessive periods during which individuals wait and have nothing to do. An enriched environment features regular reinforcement and social contact of a type the individual prefers. Caretakers should distribute their attention and reinforcement, ensuring that they regularly contact all clients, not just those who are misbehaving. These and other features of an enriched environment should be provided all day, every day, not just in "program times." The intent is not to implode individuals with frenzied overactivity, but merely to consistently provide them with constructive things to do.

Environmental arrangements that provide a safe, structured, and enriched environment serve several crucial purposes. First, it is simply humane. Second, it may effectively treat some behavior problems, including some cases of aggression. In some instances behavior problems improve when an individual is well supervised, busy with a variety of activities, and receiving regular reinforcement and contact for appropriate behavior (Horner, 1980). In cases where such arrangements are not sufficient, i.e., where the problem continues despite such changes, they are nevertheless the foundation on which other treatment procedures are built. For example, the use of time-out as a consequence for aggression depends on an enriched, structured environment in order to be maximally effective (Solnick, Rincover, & Peterson, 1977). Finally, a setting's ability to make such rearrangements is predictive of whether treatment can be conducted and conducted properly. If the setting is impoverished and chaotic, if caretakers are totally absorbed in responding to crises, they cannot effectively conduct systematic programs to treat aggression and develop alternative skills in their children and clients.

Strengthening Appropriate Alternative Behavior

In addition to overall environmental rearrangements a major focus of treatment for aggression involves developing more appropriate alternative behavior. The objective is to replace aggression with more appropriate means of controlling the environment, e.g., teaching appropriate communication, social, recreational, and other skills that will enable individuals to obtain the things they want and need. Such desirable behavior is strengthened by consistently rewarding it, i.e., following it with positive reinforcers. Thus a first step in strengthening any behavior of an autistic individual must be to identify positive reinforcers that the individual is truly motivated to work for. However, a major problem with autistic individuals is their lack of response to conventional reinforcers, particularly "acquired" reinforcers such as toy play and especially social approval (Ferster, 1961; Lovaas & Newsom, 1976). Thus a major goal of treatment is to establish physical and social contact as a reinforcer, by pairing it with already-effective reinforcers such as food (Lovaas, Freitag, Kinder, Rubenstein, Schaeffer, & Simmons, 1966). These social reinforcers can then be used to increase and maintain behaviors such as communication skills and playing with others which are commonly maintained socially. However, during the gradual process of establishing social reinforcers one must look elsewhere for other powerful reinforcers to use in strengthening appropriate behavior.

Identifying Reinforcers

In addition to the standard use of food as a reinforcer, several other possibilities may have particular applicability with autistic individuals. One is the use of high-rate behavior as positive reinforcement. The use of high-probability behavior as reinforcement for low-probability behavior is known as the Premack Principle (Premack, 1959). The concept is commonly exemplified by allowing normal students to play with toys (a high-probability behavior) contingent upon completion of school tasks (a low-probability behavior) (e.g., Wasik, 1970). Thus allowing an autistic individual access to preferred activities such as watching TV, drawing, bike riding, playing ball, or listening to music as a reinforcer for engaging in appropriate behavior is clearly a promising strategy. However, the line is typically drawn if the preferred activities themselves are undesirable. When undesirable behavior appears to be dominant in the hierarchy of preferred behavior by an autistic individual, the Premack concept of reinforcement does not seem relevant or acceptable to use. Allowing an individual to engage in rocking, finger flicking, screaming, hyperactive displays, or masturbation as a reinforcer for correct or appropriate behavior offends sensibilities and appears to be countertherapeutic for the client. It appears to sanction—indeed encourage—the practice of the very behaviors which are often the targets of treatment. The view endorsed here is that if more conventional reinforcers such as food or toy play can be identified, they should certainly be used in reinforcing appropriate behavior. However, if conventional positive reinforcers cannot be identified, and if the individual demonstrates strong preferences for nondestructive, though aberrant positive reinforcers, these should be used as positive reinforcers for appropriate, desirable behavior. Thus when an individual sits in a chair, imitates correctly, follows instructions, displays affection, and refrains from aggression, he or she may be allowed to engage for a brief time in rocking, finger flicking, or running and screaming outside. As the individual's appropriate behavior develops and increases in strength, the amount of desirable behavior required for positive reinforcement may be gradually increased and the period allowed for engaging in the aberrant positive reinforcer may be successively decreased. In this way the relative amount of time spent engaging in appropriate behavior may be steadily extended, with less and less time spent in aberrant responding.

In some cases rather than phasing out the aberrant reinforcer it may be possible to convert it into a more appropriate form. For example, if individuals enjoy hitting things and wrestling, they may be provided with punching bags, Bobo dolls, and opportunities to engage in controlled wrestling as a positive reinforcer for appropriate behavior. Transforming an aberrant reinforcing behavior into a less pathological form may be particularly relevant with stereotyped behavior. Since stereotyped responding appears to be maintained by sensory reinforcement in the form of, for example, lights or sounds, it may be possible to provide the individual with more appropriate means of obtaining those sensory events that are reinforcing to him or her (Rincover, Cook, Peoples, & Packard, 1979). If, for example, an individual engages in high rates of visual self-stimulation, it may be possible to use lights and toys with striking visual properties as a reinforcer for correct and appropriate behavior. Such visual stimulation may be an equally reinforcing, but more appropriate alternative to finger flicking and may naturally maintain behaviors such as toy play which are commonly maintained by the sensory, rather than social reinforcement that they produce. Thus, in general, when a behavior such as stereotypies is strongly preferred, it may be possible to provide the individual with a more appropriate form of it and then use that form as a positive reinforcer for other appropriate behavior.

The need for using potent positive reinforcers, including aberrant ones, may be relevant in a variety of cases where the individual's behavioral repertoire and range of positive reinforcement is impoverished. It is *particularly crucial* in cases in which the individual engages in severe and dangerous behavior problems such as aggression or self-injury, where more appropriate, alternative responses must be developed quickly and decisively as part of the treatment for these severe disorders. For example, using the opportunity to engage in stereotypies as a positive reinforcer for appropriate behavioral alternatives to aggression may indeed be a small price to pay for a reduction in aggression.

Another alternative in the search for reinforcers with autistic individuals may involve the identification of consequences for aggression and the use of those consequences, but now for more desirable behavior. If, for example, it is noted that an individual is wrestled to the floor when she is aggressive, if an individual is released from demands when he becomes agitated and assaultive, or if another is provided with distracting activities when she pushes or hits, it may be possible to use similar consequences but now contingent on more desirable behavior. The assumption is that if these events reliably follow aggression, they may be reinforcers for it; and if they are positive reinforcers for misbehavior they may be used to develop and sustain more desirable responding. Thus in the examples above some benign form of physical jostling, release from demands, or distraction may be effective as a consequence for social, communicative, or on-task behavior. At the same time their use following aggression must be greatly minimized. There are clear practical and ethical limits to the transfer of consequences for aggression to more appropriate behavior. The major advantage of such a strategy is that it provides the individual with alternative, appropriate means of gaining the specific reinforcers that previously only aggression could produce. Aggression is maintained because it more reliably and efficiently produces certain reinforcers for the individual than does more desirable behavior. It is very unlikely to expect aggression to decrease if one does not systematically provide alternative means of obtaining those same or similar reinforcers. Within that logic, one can neither simply disallow the existence of those positive reinforcers in the life of that individual nor substitute some arbitrary positive reinforcer for more desirable behavior.

Differential Reinforcement

After identifying promising reinforcers, the next step in treating aggression involves the use of these reinforcers in strengthening alternative, appropriate behavior. Several techniques employed in the treatment of aggression rest on the principle of "differential reinforcement." This concept involves providing relatively more reinforcement for appropriate, nonaggressive behavior in order to strengthen it, and less (ideally no) reinforcement for aggression in an attempt to weaken it. As stressed, the objective is to displace aggression, i.e., to establish more desirable behavior as the predominant means of obtaining reinforcement. In one specific form of differential reinforcement termed Differential Reinforcement of Other Behavior (DRO), reinforcement is provided following periods of time in which no aggression occurs. In short the individual is reinforced for refraining from aggression. At the same time occurrences of aggression typically delay reinforcement (Repp & Deitz, 1974; Sewell, McCoy, & Sewell, 1973). In a second procedure, termed Differential Reinforcement of Incompatable Behavior (DRI), reinforcement is provided for specific appropriate behavior and is withheld or delayed following aggression. Behavior which is targeted for reinforcement should not only be appropriate but also incompatable with aggression. Two behaviors are demonstrated to be incompatable if strengthening one results in a decrease in the other. Thus, for example, if reinforcing appropriate social behavior results in a decrease in aggression then these two behaviors are demonstrated to be functionally incompatable. If social behavior increases in frequency but aggression does not decline, the two are not incompatable. Though it is not possible to predict in advance what appropriate behavior may be incompatable with aggression in an individual case, there are several general types of behavior which are promising alternatives to aggression.

Social Skills. Teaching an individual alternative and appropriate ways of interacting with others may reduce aggressive modes of interaction. For example, an individual may be reinforced for sharing, playing cooperatively, and communicating with peers and caretakers. Effective "social skills training" has included several components: modeling of appropriate social behavior, verbal instructions such as "John, when you want the bike, say 'Please give me the bike,'" behavior rehearsal or practice in a variety of representative role-playing situations, and feedback and reinforcement for cooperation with training and correct social behavior (Bornstein, Bellack, & Hersen, 1980; Frederiksen, Jenkins, Foy, & Eisler, 1976; Elder, Edelstein, & Narick, 1979). Although such procedures have primarily been used with verbal clients, modifications with lower functioning individuals should also be possible. For example, it may be possible to substitute manual prompting for modeling, or shaping of behavior which more and more closely resembles appropriate social behavior for extensive verbal instructions.

Cooperation and Compliance. Frequently aggression occurs when an individual is required to cooperate or comply with a rule or routine. In some cases reinforcing cooperation and compliance may be associated with a reduction in aggression. Typically the individual initially is given repeated opportunities to practice compliance with very easy requests and is heavily reinforced for doing so. As behavior improves, the number and difficulty of demands is gradually increased. (A later section describes additional information on modifying demanding situations which evoke aggression.)

Leisure Skills. Strengthening appropriate play may reduce aggression. Though teaching and reinforcing *social* play may be one option, research also indicates that strengthening appropriate *solitary* play may be more effective in reducing aggression in some cases (Wahler & Fox, 1980). Thus with an individual who chronically demands attention and entertainment, sometimes by coercion and aggression, one strategy may be to increase independent play, i.e., entertaining oneself.

Relaxation and Alternative Physical Expression. Aggression frequently occurs as part of an overall agitated state. In such cases reinforcing either relaxation or alternative physical expression may be effective in decreasing aggression. Relaxation training typically includes prompting and reinforcing progressively relaxed states. Even nonverbal clients can be reinforced for deep-breathing, lying down, and other methods of relaxing under simulated and actual situations which tend to produce agitation. As an alternative, individuals may be taught such physical expressions as hitting a punching toy, running a track, or exercising. Though the reinforcers used to teach both relaxation or alternative physical activity may be entirely positive, it may be necessary to impose an avoidance contingency. That is, if the individual engages in these alternatives when agitated, and particularly refrains from aggression while doing so, he or she may avoid caretaker-imposed restraint or punishment.

Communication. Appropriate communication skills represent a crucial alternative to aggression for many autistic individuals. The teaching of communication may be viewed as central to providing individuals with skills to better control their environments and better regulate their own behavior (Lovaas & Newsom, 1976). Teaching communication in part involves the development of receptive language. Following verbal directions and otherwise understanding what people are saying are central to habilitation and adjustment. The common mistaken diagnosis of deafness speaks to the crucial deficit of receptive language in autistic individuals. Teaching communication also involves expressive language, ranging from manual signing to verbal expression. Autistic individuals, including those who are aggressive, must be provided with mechanisms for telling others what they need and how they feel. The procedures for training in language are well known (Lovaas, 1969, 1976). During such a training process it may be useful to provide the aggressive individual directly with one or more means of communication that serves as an immediate alternative to aggressive expression. For example, one might start with a single manual sign or a word such as "want" which is already in the individual's repertoire and may serve a generalized function. That is, when the individual signs or verbalizes, caretakers could then determine the individual's need at that time. For example, in one instance "want" might signal the individual's need for a break from demands, in another the need for a preferred toy, and in another an interest in a hug. From a single "word" vocabulary, different signs could then be developed for different needs. Alternatively, from the outset specialized responses might be developed for specialized needs. However training is approached, the major point is to directly teach and reinforce expressive alternatives to aggression (or other severe problems), to provide the individual with functional ways of controlling his or her environment which in the past only aggression was able to do.

In summary, teaching and reinforcement efforts should be directed at developing appropriate alternatives to aggression. Such behavior often includes social skills, cooperation and compliance, leisure skills, relaxation and alternative physical expression, and communication. In teaching and reinforcing such behavior several guidelines and considerations should be kept in mind:

1. The specific alternative behaviors strengthened should not only

be appropriate for the individual, but useful in producing reinforcers which are similar to those which aggression previously produced.

2. Reinforcement for appropriate behavior should be powerful, similar in strength (and perhaps form) to those maintaining aggression.

3. Reinforcement should initially be bountiful, presented after very brief periods of no aggression (DRO) and very frequently after a wide variety of appropriate behavior (DRI). In very severe cases where aggression occurs very frequently, reinforcement may initially need to be nearly continuous so long as aggression does not occur (Vukelich & Hake, 1971).

4. As behavior improves, i.e., as aggression decreases and appropriate behavior occurs more frequently, the time between reinforcement and the amount of appropriate behavior required for reinforcement may be gradually extended. If extended too far, i.e., if reinforcement for desirable behavior becomes too "lean," behavior will worsen and regress.

5. The individual should have many opportunities to practice appropriate skills. Desirable behavior should be prompted regularly throughout each day, and the individual reinforced for practicing it. Practice should particularly occur under simulated and actual conditions which typically evoke aggression.

6. Although training in alternative behavior should be intensive, it should not constitute an increase in unpleasant demands. Such training may be so aversive that it increases the likelihood that the individual will aggress to escape the demands. Graduating the difficulty of demands and using powerful and plentiful reinforcement both optimize the effectiveness of training and increase an individual's willingness to cooperate with it.

7. Effective differential reinforcement is often more art than science. Training, experience, and sensitivity are needed to modify these procedures to the individual case and to conduct them properly. With DRO for example, other inappropriate behaviors such as self-injury or self-stimulation may inadvertently be reinforced if they are occurring when reinforcement is delivered on the basis of nonaggression alone. Similarly, improvements in aggression may be lost if periods between reinforcements are extended too rapidly and in too large steps. With DRI, skillful prompting and shaping is necessary to effectively train behaviors incompatible with aggression. In short these procedures are not as easy to conduct properly as some seem to claim (Favell, 1977).

8. Treatment of aggression, including differential reinforcement, may consume a great deal of caretaker time. Caretakers' responsibilities must be arranged and organized so that they *can* differentially reinforce appropriate, nonaggressive behavior. Too often resources are organized and added only when punitive, "restrictive" procedures are used. In some cases if those same resources had been applied to enable the proper

conduct of differential reinforcement, more restrictive procedures may not have been necessary.

9. Finally, the effects of differential reinforcement rest not only on increasing reinforcement for appropriate nonaggressive behavior, but also on reducing reinforcement for aggression itself. Though desirable behavior may be consistently reinforced, if aggression continues to result in relatively *more* reinforcement, it will continue to occur. A pat on the head every 15 minutes will hardly compete with the massive social reaction which aggression may produce.

Reduction of Reinforcement for Aggression

As indicated, differential reinforcement involves not only the skillful teaching and reinforcement of appropriate, nonaggressive behavior, but the reduction in reinforcement for aggression itself. "Extinction" is the behavioral term for decreasing behavior by removal of its reinforcement.

Extinction involves withholding previously given reinforcement following aggression. If that reinforcement consists of attention, the extinction technique requires ignoring episodes of the behavior (Davison, 1964). If, on the other hand, an individual's aggression is reinforced by the opportunity to escape or avoid unpleasant situations, the extinction procedure would involve preventing escape for the behavior (Carr et al., 1980). In general when *any* event is regularly observed following aggression and the behavior is continuing or becoming worse, that consequence may be a reinforcer maintaining the problem and should be stopped. *Any* event can be a reinforcer: some individuals like to be scolded, others like to be placed in a room alone, and still others like to be physically restrained (Favell, McGimsey, & Jones, 1978; Favell, McGimsey, Jones & Cannon, 1981). Thus in order to reduce reinforcement for aggression effectively, the consequences of an individual's aggression must be carefully observed and steps taken to discontinue any possible reinforcers.

Reducing reinforcement for aggression is associated with a variety of practical problems: the problem often becomes *worse,* i.e., more frequent or intense, before better; it is very difficult to ensure that aggression is *consistently* not reinforced; *inconsistency* usually makes the problem worse; many forms of adolescent aggression cannot be totally disregarded without seriously jeopardizing *safety*; and withholding reinforcement may *itself evoke* aggression (Kelly & Hake, 1970). Because of these problems, the clinical question often becomes: "*Can* we use extinction?" The implication of such a question is that either the procedure is used or it is not. Contrary to this notion, effective treatment of behavior problems *necessarily* includes minimizing its reinforcement. Thus the decision is not *whether* to use extinction, but *how*. Since totally ignoring aggression is typically not possible, several steps may be taken to fit the procedure to the individual case.

First, it has been recommended that dangerous features of the environment be corrected so that caretakers do not have to *overreact* to protect others. Second, although some intervention is usually necessary to interrupt the aggressive episode and protect victims, that intervention should be as minimal as possible. If a training demand or other activity has to be interrupted until the individual ceases aggression, that interruption should be *temporary;* the individual should immediately return to the activity as soon as he or she becomes calm. Similarly, rather than the scolding, yelling, and reasoning that aggression often produces, caretakers should usually restrict their comments to a single descriptive reprimand such as "No, don't hit!" Likewise, in contrast to the wrestling match that often occurs, as few caretakers as possible should use "protective intervention" or "physical control" techniques, i.e., systematic, safe, and nonemotional means of physically intervening in an episode (Harvey & Schepers, 1977; Upchurch, Ham, Daniels, McGhee, & Burnett, 1980). In the interest of ensuring safety while minimizing the reaction to aggression, caretakers may be instructed to attend to the *victim* rather than to the aggressor (Pinkston, Reese, LeBlanc, & Baer, 1973). When aggression occurs, the episode may be interrupted by leading the victim away and attending to his or her needs. Such a procedure not only safely interrupts the episode but also gives caretakers something specific to do rather than asking them to "try to ignore" the behavior, an instruction that most assuredly leads to inconsistent and unspecified types of intervention. It may actually be unpleasant to the aggressor or clarify that he is not being reinforced. The technique is not appropriate in cases where peers provoke attack in order to receive comfort, or when the aggressor continues from one victim to the next until stopped. Third, decreasing relative reinforcement for aggression rests squarely on increasing reinforcement for desirable, nonaggressive behavior. Although individuals may receive some attention for aggression, they should receive relatively more when they behave appropriately and refrain from aggression. Similarly, though it may be necessary to temporarily stop demands or withdraw the individual from an unpleasant situation until aggression subsides, that client should receive *more* reinforcement, including the opportunity for breaks from demands, when he or she engages in more desirable behavior. In short, ensuring that desirable, nonaggressive behavior is heavily reinforced, and reinforced with events which previously only aggression produced, is the most crucial and effective method of decreasing relative reinforcement for aggression. Combined with reducing obvious dangers in environments and minimizing reactions to the aggression itself, these procedures increase the probability that the problem will receive relatively less reinforcement.

Rearranging Environmental Conditions Differentially Associated with Aggression

Although some aggression erupts unpredictably, more often it is very "situation specific," i.e., it occurs more frequently or intensely in some situations than in others. Which situations "control" high rates of aggression depends on an individual's reinforcement history: if an individual's aggression "pays off" in a particular situation it will be more likely to occur in that situation; if it is not reinforced it will be less likely to occur. To identify which situations regularly evoke aggression, the individual should be observed in a variety of situations and a list constructed of people, times, places, and activities during which aggression occurs. A similar list should be made of situations in which aggression rarely occurs and appropriate behavior is most prevalent. Treatment should then explicitly include extending situations in which aggression does not occur and rearranging situations in which aggression is frequent and intense.

When situations are identified in which aggression does not normally occur, consideration should be given to extending the individual's access to those situations. For example, extending the time an individual is allowed to lie on her bed, play outside, be with a particular caretaker, listen to music, or even engage in stereotypies may be amply justified if it results in reduced aggression. If such changes are not possible or desirable on a long-term basis, it may nevertheless be a useful first step in protecting others and bringing the individual in contact with reinforcement for appropriate, nonaggressive behavior, then gradually fading in situations which are more frequently associated with aggression.

In addition to considering whether and how situations associated with no aggression might be extended, it is also essential to rearrange situations in which aggression does occur. Although different individuals are aggressive in different situations, there are several common situations which evoke aggression.

Demands. Aggression often occurs when an individual is required to work on a task or follow an instruction (Carr et al., 1980), or perform other nonpreferred behaviors such as sitting in a chair or keeping shoes on. In such cases it may be possible to reduce the aversiveness of the situation in order to reduce the individual's motivation to escape. At the same time the individual's motivation to cooperate and behave appropriately must be increased. To do this the frequency of reinforcement for appropriate behavior must be increased. That is, the individual should, at least initially, be reinforced more often for behavior such as cooperation, task completion, compliance, nonaggression, and appropriate communication, including appropriate means of indicating that he or she needs a break from demands. The difficulty and number of demands should initially be reduced, then gradually increased as the individual is reinforced for complying with them. The "context" of the situation may also be improved, for example, by adding music, reducing distractions, and altering caretaker voice tone. Finally, reinforcement for aggression must be reduced, e.g., by requiring the individual to continue working or quickly returning to work when calm.

Delayed or Withheld Reinforcement. When an individual does not receive expected reinforcement, or reinforcement is delayed, aggression may occur (Azrin, Hutchinson, & Hake, 1966; Dollard et al., 1939; Ulrich & Favell, 1970). The approach to aggression induced by "frustration" is highly similar to that used with aggression which occurs in response to demands. In such cases reinforcement should initially be frequent, immediate, and contingent on appropriate behavior which is already in the individual's repertoire. As the individual's behavior improves, delays in reinforcement may be slowly introduced, the frequency of reinforcement gradually "thinned," and the response requirement steadily extended. However, individuals should never be subjected to lengthy periods of no reinforcement. Finally, episodes of aggression should never be immediately followed by returns to increased and more immediate reinforcement.

Changes in Routine and Environment, Interruptions in Preferred Behavior. Autistic individuals are often characterized as rigid and ritualistic, and interruptions in structure, routine, and preferred behaviors such as stereotypies and rituals sometimes evoke aggression or other misbehavior. Interruptions in preferred behavior and changes in routine should first be evaluated as to their importance and necessity. For example, stereotypies should not be interrupted unless there is an explicit alternative activity that should be performed. Similarly, transitions between activities should be as individualized as possible so that in most cases an individual can leave an activity when his or her attention "runs out" and not be forced either to terminate an activity while still attending to it or wait for others to finish before being allowed to move to the next (Doke & Risley, 1972; LeLaurin & Risley, 1972). In general arbitrary and capricious changes in routine and structure should be eliminated, and necessary changes made *gradually.* Throughout, cooperative, appropriate behavior should be heavily reinforced and aggression should not result in a return to a previous routine or resumption of a preferred behavior.

Social Contact. Socially withdrawn individuals may react to social contact with aggression principally to drive others away. Tolerance to social contact may be shaped by reinforcing closer and closer proximity and contact with others. During this process it is essential that social contact not be associated with unpleasant experiences such as teasing by peers or excessive demands by caretakers. The objective is to "desensitize" the individual to social interactions and to teach him or her that *people are important,* in part because they are the vehicle by which reinforcers can be obtained. After an individual tolerates social contact, more sophisticated forms of social behavior such as cooperative play and affection can be taught. Tangible reinforcement such as food used to shape social behavior should always be accompanied by social approval. Thus as social skills are trained, social approval is also established as a reinforcer through its association with tangible reinforcement. However, although approval may become a reinforcer, it is likely that it will need to be backed up regularly with tangibles to maintain its effectiveness.

Noise, Crowding, and Lack of Alternative Activities. Some aggression appears to occur in environments which are noisy, crowded, and confused (Boe, 1977). Although it is possible that such conditions may accompany overzealous efforts at enriching the environment and providing a variety of stimulating experiences, more often noise, crowding, and confusion result from *lack* of systematic efforts to enrich environments. Steps must be taken to disperse clients into small groups, eliminate "milling," alter the physical environment with, for example, carpeting to "dampen" noise, and ensure that there is an adequate array of appropriate activities available to clients.

"Bad days." Aggression often occurs when an individual is in a "bad mood" and in some cases it is not clear what environmental situation precipitated the problem. In such cases treatment should be directed at teaching appropriate means of handling anxiety and agitation. For example, when an individual begins excessive movement and vocalizes distress, he or she can be taken to a quiet place, perhaps to lie down, and reinforced for relaxing. Alternatively, an individual might be reinforced for "working off" agitation through physical exercise. It is crucial to intervene and initiate these activities before aggression occurs. Although positive reinforcement may be used to teach appropriate methods of handling agitation, it is also likely that an avoidance contingency may be necessary. That is, the individual can avoid physical restraint or punishment for aggression if he or she cooperates with training in handling agitation and refrains from aggression or some other misbehavior while upset. An individual should receive repeated opportunities to practice appropriate relaxation or exercise, particularly under actual or simulated conditions which normally evoke agitation. After teaching alternative means of dealing with agitation, the individual may be reinforced for independently initiating those alternative activities. In this way even severely disabled individuals may be taught a crucial self-control skill.

In general when situations are identified which regularly evoke aggression the overall strategy is to decrease the aversiveness of those situations, gradually change from situations controlling low rates of aggression (such as no demands) to ones associated with higher rates (demands), heavily reinforce appropriate behavior, and reduce reinforcement for aggression under a variety of actual and simulated conditions which have provoked aggression in the past.

Punishment for Aggression

In some cases aggression may be successfully treated solely by the components of treatment described previously: structuring, organizing, and enriching the environment; strengthening appropriate alternative behavior; reducing reinforcement for aggression; and rearranging situations differentially associated with aggression. However, in some cases it is also necessary to use punishment for aggression. Punishment is generally used when the problem is severe, i.e., poses a serious threat to the safety of others, and/or when the behavior directly interferes with habilitation efforts. Punishment is also used when the "positive" approach to treatment described previously has been applied consistently and competently and yet has not been effective in reducing aggression to acceptable levels.

Punishment involves decreasing the strength (e.g., rate or intensity) of a behavior either by the contingent application of an unpleasant or "aversive" stimulus or by the contingent removal of a positive reinforcer. If, for example, an individual is told "no" contingent upon (i.e., immediately following) each episode of aggression and aggression occurs less and less frequently, then "no" is said to be a "punisher" and the aggression has been decreased by "punishment." If the strength of aggression does not decrease (i.e., it continues to occur just as often or just as severely), then "no" is not a punisher. Similarly, if aggression is followed by removal of a positive reinforcer such as tokens and the behavior decreases in frequency or intensity, then that procedure is a punisher. In general a punisher reduces the strength of aggression; it does not merely interrupt the behavior temporarily. Although some approaches to aggression such as "giving in," distracting, or soothing the individual may temporarily interrupt an aggressive episode, these are not likely to reduce the future occurrence of the behavior, and indeed may actually strengthen aggression.

Different events are punishers for different individuals and it is not usually possible to predict in advance which event might be a punisher for an individual. A potential punisher must be used consistently and properly following aggression to determine if it will be effective in suppressing the behavior (Azrin & Holz, 1966). Although identifying punishers must be done on an individualized, empirically determined basis, there are several potential punishers which have proven effective in decreasing aggression in a variety of cases.

Verbal Reprimand. Although scolding an individual for aggression may be effective (e.g., Repp & Deitz, 1974), and is commonly used, very often it is ineffective in decreasing the behavior, and may reinforce the problem. However, a brief reprimand such as "No, don't hit!" should be paired with the use of the other possible punishers described below. Verbal disapproval which immediately follows the aggression and which signals that another punisher is forthcoming aids in "bridging" the delay between the aggression and the application of the more potent punisher. Pairing a reprimand with another punisher may also be effective in establishing that reprimand as a punisher, and may then be used by itself to maintain a decrease in aggression or possibly to treat other undesirable behaviors, with only occasional repairings with the original punisher (Henricksen & Doughty, 1967).

Corporal Punishment. While spanking and other forms of corporal punishment are common and often quite effective punishers, they are not allowed in many programs and are not a culturally normative way of dealing with the misbehavior of adolescents.

Token Fine. In programs in which appropriate behavior is reinforced by tokens (such as plastic chips) which are redeemable for preferred items and activities, removing a portion of those tokens contingent on aggression may be an effective punisher for that behavior (Burchard & Barrera, 1972; Repp & Deitz, 1974). In addition to the simple removal of tokens, the fining consequence may be used as an educational opportunity, whereby the individual earns back a portion of the fine by practicing appropriate, alternative behavior (May, Risley, Twardosz, Friedman, Bijou, & Wexler, 1976). Of course the effectiveness of token fines as a punisher depends directly on the effectiveness of the overall token economy.

Time-out from Positive Reinforcement. Time-out has been shown to be a very effective punisher for aggression and consists of removing the client from the opportunity to obtain reinforcement, contingent upon each occurrence of the misbehavior. The procedure presupposes that the individual is functioning in a "time-in" environment which is highly enriched and reinforcing, e.g., provides highly engaging recreational and educational activities and differential reinforcement for appropriate behavior (Solnick et al., 1977). When an episode of aggression occurs the individual is reprimanded and reinforcement is removed for all behavior for a period of time. The forms of "time-out" differ widely, and include: manual restraint such as holding the individual's arms down (Repp & Deitz, 1974), "contingent observation" in which the individual is removed from an activity to a chair to observe others behaving appropriately (Porterfield, Herbert-Jackson, & Risley, 1976), placement of the individual in an area or room which is not physically uncomfortable but is relatively nonreinforcing (Bostow & Bailey, 1969; Wahler & Fox, 1980), and contingent placement of the individual in physical restraint such as in a chair (Hamilton, Stephens, & Allen, 1967; Vukelich & Hake, 1971). Regardless of the form of time-out, the procedure should begin immediately following each episode of aggression and continue at least until the individual is calm (Hobbs & Forehand, 1977). The effectiveness of the procedure rests squarely on the relative reinforcement of time-in versus time-out. If being personally restrained or taken to time-out provides more attention than the individual ordinarily receives in time-in, or if time-out enables the individual to escape or avoid an unpleasant time-in situation, then the time-out procedure may directly reinforce aggression. Moreover if time-in is unpleasant or unrewarding, then in order for time-out to be *less* reinforcing it will have to be excessively severe, e.g., of an extended duration and depriving of nearly all sensory experiences. If on the other hand the individual is functioning in a truly reinforcing time-in situation, even a brief and benign time-out from those activities contingent on aggression is likely to be effective in decreasing the problem.

Overcorrection. The basic rationale underlying the complex combination of procedures subsumed under overcorrection is that individuals must not only correct, but *over*correct the effects of their misbehavior and intensively practice appropriate alternatives. There are two types of overcorrection generally applied to problems of aggression. *Restitution* typically involves requiring the individual to verbally or gesturally apologize to victims and others, and even to aid in administering medical assistance to those injured (Foxx & Azrin, 1972; Matson & Stephens, 1977; Polvinale & Lutzker, 1980). If property is disturbed or destroyed, the aggressor is also required to restore the environment to a better state than existed before aggression disrupted it. For example, the individual is required to straighten and clean the entire room intensively. In most applications restitution is usually intensive, effortful, and of an extended duration. Although manual and verbal prompts may be necessary to ensure compliance with overcorrection, reinforcement must be minimized during the overcorrection episode. The procedure is begun immediately when aggression occurs and is terminated only when the individual has completed the restitution and is cooperative. Further, the form of overcorrection is usually matched to the form of the misbehavior, e.g., if an individual destroys property but does not aggress against others, he is required only to clean and straighten but not apologize. However, there is some evidence to indicate that the extended duration, and matching of the type of overcorrection with the type of behavior problem, may not be necessary to the effectiveness of the procedure (e.g., Epstein, Doke, Sajwaj, Sorrell, & Rimmer, 1974). For example, Luce, Delquadri, and Hall (1980) demonstrated that a brief period of exercise in the form of repeated standing and sitting was effective in decreasing verbal and physical aggression.

A second form of overcorrection used in treating aggression consists of requiring the individual to *lie down and become calm* contingent upon aggression. The aggressor is manually held in bed, if necessary, until he or she begins to relax independently. The period in required relaxation has ranged from 10 minutes (Foxx, Foxx, Jones, & Kiely, 1980) to 2 hours (Webster & Azrin, 1973), but the individual is never released until calm. While highly effective in treating aggression in a variety of cases, overcorrection may not be safe or possible with large, physically resistive individuals.

Aversive Electrical Stimulation. Through this procedure has principally been used with self-injurious behavior, it has been employed in a small number of cases of serious aggression (Birnbrauer, 1958; Browning, 1971; Ludwig, Marx, Hill, & Browning, 1969). In this technique a physically harmless but painful electrical stimulus is delivered by a device to the client's limb or back for 1 or 2 seconds immediately following each occurrence of aggression (Carr & Lovaas, in press). Although it is a powerful punisher, there are limitations to the use of aversive electrical stimulation. One of the most serious of these with autistic adolescents is that their size and strength may prevent caretakers from administering the procedure at all. The procedure is also considered extremely "restrictive," i.e., subject to abuse and highly intrusive. Its use is therefore rigorously controlled (May et al., 1976).

In general punishment may be a necessary and effective addition to an overall program to treat aggression. Regardless of the specific punisher selected, several issues are crucial to the safe, effective and humane use of punishment.

1. The punisher should be preceded by a verbal reprimand, delivered *immediately* at the onset of the behavior (Walters, Parke, & Cane, 1965) and used contingent on *each* occurrence of the behavior.

2. If there are behaviors which reliably precede aggression, such as hitting furniture, jumping, having a tantrum, or yelling, consideration should be given to intervening with those behaviors rather than waiting for aggression to occur and consequating it. A more benign procedure such as brief manual restraint may be effective in decreasing these precursors and interrupting the chain of responses leading to aggression. However, if more benign techniques are not effective, the use of even severe punishers such as time-out in a locked room may be justified for behaviors that are themselves not serious but consistently lead to severe aggression.

3. The use of punishment for aggression may be associated with "side effects," i.e., changes in other, nontreated behavior. Positive side effects such as the collateral emergence of prosocial and cooperative behavior are common when aggression is suppressed by punishment. When negative side effects such as the emergence of new undesirable behaviors occur, these can in turn be treated by behavioral procedures, including punishment (see "Dealing with Collateral Changes in Behavior").

4. Punishment may itself evoke aggression. An individual who has been fined, placed in time-out, or shocked may react with severe agitation and aggression. Although sometimes it appears "uncontrollable and reflexive," the most likely explanation for punishment-evoked aggression in humans is that the aggression is effective in delaying or even canceling the punishment. A large and powerful individual can indeed delay being put in time-out by aggressing against those who are attempting to place him there. Indeed he might outlast and intimidate them to the point that they give up, either not following through with that consequence or discontinuing the program altogether. If aggression is not effective in escaping or avoiding punishment, it will be less likely to occur in response to punishment. On the other hand, with vigorous adolescents it may not be possible to ensure that punishment is delivered when the individual is upset and aggressive. In such cases treatment should focus on intervening *before* the individual becomes severely agitated or aggressive, and should systematically address the development of alternative, appropriate behavior—particularly in those situations which normally evoke aggression. Since punishment may represent just such a situation, the individual needs to learn appropriate reactions to, for example, being fined or taken to time-out. As indicated previously, such training should occur repeatedly and include instances in which the individual is not genuinely upset.

5. Most programs serving developmentally disabled clients have developed or adopted guidelines and policies governing treatment, particularly treatment which includes the use of punishment (e.g., May et al., 1976). These guidelines frequently include review and approval of treatment by: a Human Rights Committee (composed of lay individuals and consumer representatives) who review adherence to the client's rights; a Peer Review Committee (composed of experts in the treatment procedures under consideration) who review the technical adequacy and appropriateness of the proposed intervention; and the client's parent or guardian (Sheldon-Wildgen & Risley, 1981). It is recommended that these review mechanisms be in place in programs treating aggressive behavior, particularly when punishment is employed.

THE USE OF PSYCHOTROPIC DRUGS

There are a wide variety of psychotropic drugs that are used in an attempt to moderate individuals' emotional states and behavior, making them more tractable and less volatile (Conners, 1972; LaVeck & Buckley, 1961; Schroeder, Lewis, & Lipton, 1981; Werry, Sprague, Weiss, & Minde, 1970; Cohen & Sprague, Note 1). These may have a beneficial effect on aggression. Two major issues surround the use of psychotropics with problems such as aggression.

First, their effects must be objectively evaluated to assess their impact on aggression and on other aspects of the individual's behavior. Clearly the regime should be altered or discontinued if aggression remains unchanged or if undesirable side effects such as general lack of responsiveness occur. On the other hand if behavior is documented to improve under medication, then it should be used. The essential element is the objective documentation of effects and side effects. Although direct observation and quantified recording is most rigorous, arranging for standardized and regular caretaker reports, for example, through rating scales, may suffice (Favell, McGimsey, Jones, & Jarrah, Note 2). For most purposes the most crucial issue is directing caretakers' attention regularly and in a structured way to changes—or lack of changes—in behavior. Accurate perceptions are difficult to obtain when the effects of medication are reviewed infrequently and nonsystematically.

Second, although the use of psychotropics may facilitate and support treatment, it rarely replaces the need for environmental rearrangements which reduce the variables maintaining aggression, and builds in conditions and contingencies supporting more desirable behavior. In short medication does not teach an individual not to aggress or teach alternative appropriate behavior; that is accomplished through the components of behavioral treatment described previously.

DEALING WITH COLLATERAL CHANGES IN BEHAVIOR

Treating a specific target behavior such as aggression usually has multiple effects. For example, the suppression of aggression may be associated with decreases in other undesirable behavior such as tantrums or property destruction, or increases in prosocial, communicative, or other desirable behavior. Such changes may be termed "positive side effects" because they are both desirable and were not explicitly addressed by the treatment program. Treatment of aggression may also be accompanied by "negative side effects" such as the emergence of new inappropriate behavior, for example, emotional or asocial behavior, or a reduction in desirable behavior. Changes in collateral behavior, i.e., both positive and negative side effects, have been at least informally noted with nearly all treatment strategies, including those based on differential reinforcement and those based on punishment (Mulick & Schroeder, 1980; Newsom, Favell, & Rincover, in press).

Although research is needed on the relationships and co-variation between behaviors, and the probability and nature of collateral effects with specific techniques used to treat aggression, two clinical recommendations appear clear. First, since collateral effects are likely, efforts should be made to detect them as they emerge. Sensitive tracking of the multiple effects of treatment involves not only monitoring client behavior but caretaker behavior as well. Although positive and negative side effects may emerge in the absence of any detectable change in the individual's environment, often they seem to be accounted for by identifiable changes in caretaker behavior. For example, caretakers may "naturally" become more responsive to a client's appropriate behavior during treatment for aggression, and in that case positive changes in those collateral appropriate behaviors may emerge. Alternatively caretakers may inadvertently become less responsive to appropriate behavior while treating aggression and thus increase the likelihood that such negative side effects as the emergence of new forms of inappropriate behavior may occur. In general it is essential to track the multiple possible changes that may occur during the course of treatment for aggression, changes both in nontreated client behavior and in caretaker behavior that may in turn account for such side effects.

Second, a treatment program must remain flexible and ready to incorporate procedures to handle collateral changes when they occur. If, for example, a client becomes more cooperative, communicative, and social, provision should be made for systematically reinforcing such behavior. Although desirable behavior may emerge in the absence of deliberate training, it will not maintain, i.e., continue, if it is not reinforced. If, on the other hand, appropriate behavior declines during treatment for aggression, increased reinforcement for these behaviors may be necessary to reestablish them. Further, if new inappropriate behaviors develop, these may in turn be treated, perhaps by the same techniques used to suppress aggression or some other variation of the components of treatment described previously. Although treatment can be successively applied to each new undesirable behavior, it is in the interest of avoiding such "symptom substitution" that emphasis has been placed on developing appropriate behavior which provides the individual with alternative means of obtaining the reinforcers that aggression used to produce. Without such appropriate alternatives the individual is highly likely to attempt a variety of inappropriate means of receiving the reinforcers he or she needs.

GENERALIZING AND MAINTAINING IMPROVEMENT

The goal of treatment for aggression is to transfer (i.e., generalize) improvement to all situations which the individual encounters and to ensure that improvement endures (i.e., maintains) for long periods. The crucial point is that neither effect occurs spontaneously or naturally (Lovaas, Koegel, Simmons, & Long, 1973). Although generalization and maintenance are always an issue, they appear to be a particular problem with autistic individuals, whose behavior commonly comes under very narrow stimulus control (Schreibman & Koegel, 1980). That is, when a skill is taught or a problem is decreased by treatment in one situation, improvement often fails to generalize to other, even highly similar situations (Birnbrauer, 1968; Bucher & King, 1971; Rincover & Koegel, 1975; Risley, 1968). While generalization and maintenance do not occur naturally, they can be therapeutically *programmed*.

Although a variety of principles and procedures apply when attempting to generalize improvement (Stokes & Baer, 1977), probably the most fail-safe method involves employing treatment in all situations. Regardless of the treatment, the procedures must be employed by all people, at all times, and in all places and activities that the individual encounters. Certainly parents and paraprofessionals have proven themselves highly proficient in conducting treatment (Hemsley, Howlin, Berger, Hersov, Dolbrook, Rutter, & Yule, 1978; Nordquist & Wahler, 1973; Risley, 1968;

Schopler & Reichler, 1971). It is equally clear that without such cooperative efforts improvements will be highly circumscribed.

Although treatment must eventually be employed across an individual's entire living environment, there are several benefits to beginning treatment in circumscribed, well-controlled situations. For example, a therapist might initially conduct treatment for aggression in a 1-hour session each day in a natural or even contrived setting such as a clinic. Of course, though the situation should be well controlled, aggression must occur within it so that treatment can be applied and its effects evaluated. Indeed it may be optimal to schedule sessions at times and in situations when aggression is most likely. Treatment can then be tested and refined under conditions in which the procedures are conducted properly and consistently. During this period, features of treatment which will make it more realistic and effective to conduct in other "real world" situations can be built in. For example, verbal control over agitation and aggression may be established, and social reinforcers and punishers may be developed through pairing with other reinforcers and punishers. At the same time a variety of natural situations which normally evoke aggression can be gradually introduced. Then as aggression is brought under control in these more contrived situations, the treatment procedures may be successively applied to other settings, and others may be trained to employ them. In general such a model may enable the development of more effective treatment, and improve the manageability of that treatment.

In very severe cases, where aggression is extremely dangerous, it may be necessary to employ a highly restrictive form of this model. That is, the individual may be separated from others *temporarily* and his or her aggression treated in safe, well-controlled circumstances during which the full complement of necessary resources is available. As the behavior improves, the individual may be exposed to more and more naturalized, normalized situations. Such a strategy is only justified in the most dangerous cases, and then only as a temporary means to the end of safely reintegrating the individual into more normalized environments. It is not to be confused with secluding or isolating an individual without a treatment plan for lengthy periods.

In addition to programming generalization, steps must be taken to ensure maintenance of improvement over time. Many treatment programs for aggression seem to have very dramatic, but very short-lived, effects. Thus a client's aggression is treated over and over again by an awesome procession of techniques. Meanwhile the individual grows larger and more "streetwise," i.e., more intractable and confident that "this too shall pass," while caretakers grow relatively smaller and confident that their child or client is right!

Several issues must be addressed when programming to maintain durable improvement. First, it is usually necessary to continue some form of treatment indefinitely. After an individual has a history with the powerful effects that aggression can produce, it is often necessary to maintain a continued regime of treatment in order to prevent him or her from reverting to that method of control. However, it may be possible to change treatment to make it more practical to conduct and to maintain improvement under increasingly natural, realistic conditions. For example, positive reinforcement may be gradually scheduled more and more intermittently: for increasing periods of time in which aggression does not occur (DRO), and for increasing amounts of appropriate behavior (DRI). Such transitions must be done gradually and skillfully, and only to a point. In many cases appropriate nonaggressive behavior will not be maintained without some ongoing extrinsic reinforcement. If punishment has been used, however, it typically must be continued following *each* aggressive response. An attempt should also be made to substitute more natural rewards and punishers for the more arbitrary ones that may have been necessary during initial treatment. The opportunity to watch TV, listen to music, play outside, or have dessert are more natural reinforcers for completing tasks, complying with requests, and performing other skills than are tokens or bites of food. Social approval, the most naturally available consequence for many behaviors, should be established as a reinforcer and regularly repaired with other rewards to maintain its effectiveness. Similarly it may be possible to change to the use of more natural and perhaps more benign punishers, such as social disapproval or sitting in a chair, particularly if these have been paired with, and continue to be regularly backed up with, more intense punishers such as more restrictive time-out procedures or overcorrection. These and other changes to more natural procedures are only possible and justified if they prove effective in maintaining improvement; if they do not, a return to more intensive and contrived procedures is necessary.

Second, when treatment continues over time, it sometimes appears to become less effective, i.e., the client appears to adapt to it and aggression returns. Procedures can indeed become ineffective, and treatment must often be adjusted and refined during the course of therapy to maintain its effectiveness. However, in many cases the problem is not that the technique is no longer effective but that it is no longer used or used properly. Subtle, inadvertent slips and drifts in conducting a procedure can result in a dramatic deterioration in its effectiveness. Resorting to the use of less powerful but more available reinforcers, regular omissions of punishment, relaxation in schedules of activities, and slippage in reinforcing alternative, appropriate behavior are common, particularly when aggression is improved and the apparent necessity for rigorous treatment is less obvious. Thus an erosion in the use of therapeutic techniques should be one of the first possibilities checked when aggression worsens during continued treatment.

Finally, in the interests of maintaining durable improvement it is crucial to establish appropriate alternatives to aggression. Aggression is more likely to remain suppressed if individuals have, for example, learned alternative means of handling agitation, communicating, interacting socially, using leisure time, and dealing with the routines of life and the process of habilitation. These alternatives must continue to be functional in providing the clients with needed reinforcement. If they are not, aggression will once again emerge as the primary means of controlling their environments.

SUMMARY

Effective treatment of aggression consists not of the sequential application of individual techniques, but a comprehensive restructuring of an individual's environment to alter the factors maintaining aggression and to establish contingencies and conditions supporting appropriate, alternative behavior. Careful attention to all components of this strategy will substantially increase the likelihood of effecting meaningful, pervasive changes in individuals' behavior, happiness, and propsects for continued habilitation (Sloan & Schopler, 1977).

1. Obtain help from professionals who are trained and experienced in treating aggression. Have treatment plans—particularly those which include punishment—reviewed and approved by parents, Human Rights, and Peer Review Committees.
2. Obtain a medical examination, and if necessary treatment for biological disorders. The use of psychotropic drugs may be considered as part of an overall treatment effort.
3. Observe the individual's inappropriate and appropriate behavior in relation to environmental contexts in an attempt to identify factors maintaining the problem and rearrangements that might be therapeutic.
4. Examine and rearrange the environment to ensure that it is safe, structured, and responsive.
5. Strengthen appropriate alternatives to aggression such as social and communication skills, relaxation, and cooperation, by the use of powerful reinforcers.
6. Reduce relative reinforcement for aggression, e.g., by minimizing social reactions and disallowing escape.

7. Extend, where possible, the individual's access to situations in which aggression is less prevalent.
8. Eliminate or alter features of situations which evoke aggression, e.g., demands, changes in routines, or unpleasant social contact.
9. If aggression is severe or has not shown sufficient improvement with the above treatment, employ punishment, e.g., time-out or overcorrection contingent upon aggression.
10. Monitor side effects and incorporate those behavioral changes into treatment.
11. Program for generalization and maintenance of improvement, principally by arranging treatment in all situations and ensuring that treatment continues to be conducted properly.

REFERENCES

Azrin, N. H., & Holz, W. C. Punishment. In *Operant behavior: Areas of research and application* (W. K. Honig, ed.), New York: Appleton-Century-Crofts, 1966.

Azrin, N. H., Hutchinson, R. R., & Hake, D. F. Extinction-induced aggression. *Journal of the Experimental Analysis of Behavior*, 1966, *9*, 191–204.

Bandura, A. *Aggression: A social learning analysis*. Englewood Cliffs, N.J.: Prentice-Hall, 1973.

Birnbrauer, J. S. Generalization of punishment effects: A case study. *Journal of Applied Behavior Analysis*, 1968, *1*, 201–211.

Boe, R. B. Economical procedures for the reduction of aggression in a residential setting. *Mental Retardation*, 1977, *15*, 25–28.

Bornstein, M., Bellack, A. S., & Hersen, M. Social skills training for highly aggressive children: Treatment in an inpatient psychiatric setting. *Behavior Modification*, 1980, *4*, 173–186.

Bostow, D. E., & Bailey, J. B. Modification of severe disruptive and aggressive behavior using brief timeout and reinforcement procedures. *Journal of Applied Behavior Analysis*, 1969, *2*, 31–37.

Browning, R. M. Treatment effects of a total behavior modification program with five autistic children. *Behaviour Research and Therapy*, 1971, *9*, 319–327.

Bucher, B., & King, L. W. Generalization of punishment effects in the deviant behavior of a psychotic child. *Behavior Therapy*, 1971, *2*, 68–77.

Burchard, J. D., & Barrera, F. An analysis of timeout and response cost in a programmed environment. *Journal of Applied Behavior Analysis*, 1972, *5*, 271–282.

Buss, A. H. *The psychology of aggression*. New York: Wiley, 1961.

Carr, E. G., & Lovaas, O. I. Contingent electric shock as a treatment for severe behavior problems. In *Punishment: Its effects on human behavior* (S. Axelrod & J. Apsche, eds.). New York: Academic Press, 1982.

Carr, E. G., Newsom, C. D., & Binkoff, J. A. Escape as a factor in the aggressive behavior of two retarded children. *Journal of Applied Behavior Analysis*, 1980, *13*, 101–117.

Conners, C. K. Pharmacotherapy of psychopathology in children. In *Psychopathological disorders of children* (H. C. Quay & J. S. Werry, eds.), New York: Wiley, 1972.

Davison, G. C. A social learning theory programme with an autistic child. *Behaviour Research and Therapy*, 1964, *2*, 149–159.

Doke, L. A., & Risley, T. R. The organization of day care environments: Required versus optional activities. *Journal of Applied Behavior Analysis*, 1972, *5*, 405–420.

Dollard, J., Doob, L., Miller, N., Mowrer, O., & Sears, R. *Frustration and aggression.* New Haven, Conn.: Yale University Press, 1939.

Edler, J. P., Edelstein, B. A., & Narick, M. M. Adolescent psychiatric patients: Modifying aggressive behavior with social skills training. *Behavior Modification*, 1979, *3*, 161–178.

Epstein, L. H., Doke, L. A., Sajwaj, T. E., Sorrell, S., & Rimmer, B. Generality and side effects of overcorrection. *Journal of Applied Behavior Analysis*, 1974, *7*, 385–390.

Favell, J. E. *The power of positive reinforcement: A handbook of behavior modification.* Springfield, Ill.: Charles C Thomas, 1977.

Favell, J. E., & Cannon, P. R. Evaluation of entertainment materials for severely retarded persons. *American Journal of Mental Deficiency*, 1977, *81*, 357–361.

Favell, J. E., McGimsey, J. F., & Jones, M. L. The use of physical restraint in the treatment of self-injury and as a positive reinforcement. *Journal of Applied Behavior Analysis*, 1978, *11*, 225–241.

Favell, J. E., McGimsey, J. F., Jones, M. L., & Cannon, P. R. Physical restraint as positive reinforcement. *American Journal of Mental Deficiency*, 1981, *85*, 425–432.

Ferster, C. B. Positive reinforcement and behavioral deficits of autistic children. *Child Development*, 1961, *32*, 437–456.

Foxx, R. M., & Azrin, N. H. Restitution: A method of eliminating aggressive-disruptive behaviors of retardates and brain-damaged patients. *Behaviour Research and Therapy*, 1972, *10*, 15–27.

Foxx, C. L., Foxx, R. M., Jones, J. R., & Kiely, D. Twenty-four hour social isolation: A program for reducing the aggressive behavior of a psychotic-like retarded adult. *Behavior Modification*, 1980, *4*, 130–144.

Frederiksen, L. W., Jenkins, J. O., Foy, D. W., & Eisler, R. M. Social-skills training to modify abusive verbal outbursts in adults. *Journal of Applied Behavior Analysis*, 1976, *9*, 117–125.

Hamilton, J., Stephens, L., & Allen, P. Controlling aggressive and disruptive behavior in severely retarded institutionalized residents. *American Journal of Mental Deficiency*, 1967, *71*, 852–856.

Harvey, E. R., & Schepers, J. Physical control techniques and defensive holds for use with aggressive retarded adults. *Mental Retardation*, 1977, *15*, 29–31.

Hemsley, R., Howlin, P., Berger, M., Hersov, L., Dolbrook, D., Rutter, M., & Yule, W. Treating autistic children in a family context. In *Autism: A reappraisal of concepts and treatment* (M. Rutter & E. Schopler, eds.), New York: Plenum Press, 1978.

Henricksen, K., & Doughty, R. Decelerating undesired mealtime behavior in a group of profoundly retarded boys. *American Journal of Mental Deficiency*, 1967, *72*, 40–44.

Hobbs, S. A., & Forehand, R. Important parameters in the use of timeout with children: A re-examination. *Journal of Behavior Therapy and Experimental Psychiatry*, 1977, *8*, 365–370.

Horner, R. D. The effects of an environmental "enrichment" program on the behavior of institutionalized profoundly retarded children. *Journal of Applied Behavior Analysis*, 1980, *13*, 473–491.

Kelly, J. I., & Hake, D. F. An extinction induced increase in an aggressive response with humans. *Journal of the Experimental Analysis of Behavior*, 1970, *14*, 153–164.

LaVeck, G. D., & Buckley, P. The use of psychopharmacologic agents in retarded children with behavior disorders. *Journal of Chronic Disease*, 1961, *13*, 174–183.

LeLaurin, K., & Risley, T. R. The organization of day care environments: "Zone" versus "man to man" staff assignments. *Journal of Applied Behavior Analysis*, 1972, *5*, 225–232.

Lovaas, O. I. *Behavior modification: Teaching language to psychotic children*. New York: Appleton-Century-Crofts, 1969. (Film)

Lovaas, O. I. *Language acquisition programs for nonlinguistic children*. New York: Irvington, 1976.

Lovaas, O. I., Freitag, G., Kinder, M. I., Rubenstein, B. D., Schaeffer, B., Simmons, J. Q. Establishment of social reinforcers in two schizophrenic children on the basis of food. *Journal of Experimental Psychology*, 1966, *4*, 109–125.

Lovaas, O. I., Koegel, R., Simmons, J. Q., Long, J. S. Some generalization and follow-up measures on autistic children in behavior therapy. *Journal of Applied Behavior Analysis*, 1973, *6*, 131–66.

Lovaas, O. I., & Newsom, C. D. Behavior modification with psychotic children. In *Handbook of behavior modification and behavior therapy*. (H. Leitenberg, ed.), Englewood Cliffs, N.J.: Prentice-Hall, 1976.

Luce, S. C., Delquadri, J., & Hall, R. V. Contingent exercise: A mild but powerful procedure for suppressing inappropriate verbal and aggressive behavior. *Journal of Applied Behavior Analysis*, 1980, *13*, 583–594.

Ludwig, A. M., Marx, A. J., Hill, P. A., & Browning, R. M. The control of violent behavior through faradic shock. *Journal of Nervous and Mental Diseases*, 1969, *148*, 624–637.

Matson, J. L., & Stephens, R. M. Overcorrection of aggression behavior in a chronic psychiatric patient. *Behavior Modification*, 1977, *1*, 559–564.

May, J. G., Risley, T. R., Twardosz, S., Friedman, P., Bijou, S., and Wexler, D. Guidelines for the use of behavioral procedures in state programs for retarded persons. NARC Monograph, *M.R. Research*, 1976, *1*, 73 pp.

Mulick, J. A., & Schroeder, S. R. Research relating to management of antisocial behavior in mentally retarded persons. *Psychological Record*, 1980, *30*, 397–417.

Newsom, C., Favell, J. E., & Rincover, A. The side effects of punishment. In *Punishment: Its effects on human behavior*. (S. Axelrod and J. Apsche, eds.), New York: Academic Press, 1982.

Nordquist, V. M., & Wahler, R. G. Naturalistic treatment of an autistic child. *Journal of Applied Behavior Analysis*, 1973, *6*, 79–87.

Patterson, G. R., Littman, R. A., & Bricker, W. Assertive behavior in children: A step toward a theory of aggression. *Monograph of Social Research in Child Development*, 1967, *32*(5, 6).

Patterson, G. R., Reid, J. B., Jones, R. R., & Conger, R. E. *A social learning approach to family intervention* (Vol. 1), *Families with aggressive children*. Eugene, Ore.: Castalia, 1975.

Pinkston, E. M., Reese, N. M., LeBlanc, J. M., & Baer, D. M. Independent control of a preschool child's aggression and peer interaction by contingent teacher attention. *Journal of Applied Behavior Analysis*, 1973, *6*, 115–124.

Polvinale, R. A., & Lutzker, J. R. Elimination of assaultive and inappropriate sexual behavior by reinforcement and social-restitution. *Mental Retardation*, 1980, *18*, 27–30.

Porterfield, J. K., Herbert-Jackson, E., & Risley, T. R. Contingent observation: An effective and acceptable procedure for reducing disruptive behaviors of young children in group settings. *Journal of Applied Behavior Analysis*, 1976, *9*, 55–64.

Premack, D. Toward empirical behavior laws. I. Positive reinforcement. *Psychological Review*, 1959, *6*, 219–233.

Repp, A. C., & Deitz, S. M. Reducing aggressive and self-injurious behavior of institutionalized retarded children through reinforcement of other behaviors. *Journal of Applied Behavior Analysis*, 1974, *7*, 313–325.

Rincover, A., & Koegel, R. L. Setting generality and stimulus control in autistic children. *Journal of Applied Behavior Analysis*, 1975, *8*, 235–246.

Rincover, A., Cook, R., Peoples, A., & Packard, D. Sensory extinction and sensory reinforcement principles for programming multiple adaptive behavior change. *Journal of Applied Behavior Analysis*, 1979, *12*, 221–233.

Risley, T. R. The effects and side effects of punishing the autistic behaviors of a deviant child. *Journal of Applied Behavior Analysis*, 1968, *1*, 20–34.

Robins, L. N. *Deviant children grow up*. Baltimore: Williams and Wilkins, 1966.

Schopler, E., & Reichler, R. J. Parents as cotherapists in the treatment of psychotic children. *Journal of Autism and Childhood Schizophrenia*, 1971, *1*, 87–102.

Schopler, E., & Reichler, R. J. *Psychopathology and child development*. New York: Plenum Press, 1976.

Schreibman, L., & Koegel, R. L. A guideline for planning behavior modification programs for autistic children. In *Handbook of clinical behavior therapy*. (S. M. Turner, K. S. Calhourn, & H. E. Adams, eds.), New York: Wiley, 1980.

Schroeder, S. R., Lewis, M. H., & Lipton, M. A. Interactions of pharmacotherapy and behavior therapy among children with learning and behavioral disorders. In *Advances in learning and behavioral disabilities*, Vol. 2 (K. Gadow & I. Bialer, eds.), Greenwich, Conn.: JAI Press, 1981.

Sewell, E., McCoy, J. E., & Sewell, W. R. Modification of an antagonistic social behavior using positive reinforcement for other behavior. *Psychological Record*, 1973, *23*, 499–504.

Sheldon-Wildgen, J., & Risley, T. R. Balancing clients' rights: The establishment of human rights and peer review committees. In *International handbook of behavior modification*. (A. Bellack, M. Hersen, & A. Kazdin, eds.), New York: Plenum Press, 1981.

Sloan, J. L., & Schopler, E. Some thoughts about developing programs for autistic adolescents. *Journal of Pediatric Psychology*, 1977, *2*, 187–190.

Solnick, J. V., Rincover, A., & Peterson, C. R. Some determinants of the reinforcing and punishing effects of timeout. *Journal of Applied Behavior Analysis*, 1977, *10*, 415–424.

Stokes, T. F., & Baer, D. M. An implicit technology of generalization. *Journal of Applied Behavior Analysis*, 1977, *10*, 349–367.

Ulrich, R. E., & Favell, J. E. Human aggression. In *Behavior modification in clinical psychology*. (C. Neuringer & J. L. Michael, eds.), New York: Appleton-Century-Crofts, 1970.

Upchurch, T., Ham, L., Daniels, R., McGhee, R., & Burnett, M. *A better way—an illustrated guide to protective intervention techniques*. Butner, N.C.: Murdoch Center, 1980.

Vukelich, R., & Hake, D. F. Reduction of dangerously aggressive behavior in a severely retarded resident through a combination of positive reinforcement procedures. *Journal of Applied Behavior Analysis*, 1971, *4*, 215–225.

Wahler, R. G., & Fox, J. J. Solitary toy play and time out: A family treatment package for children with aggressive and oppositional behavior. *Journal of Applied Behavior Analysis*, 1980, *13*, 23–29.

Walters, R. H., Parke, R. D., & Cane, V. A. Timing of punishment and the observation of consequences to others as determinants of response inhibition. *Journal of Experimental Child Psychology*, 1965, *2*, 10–30.

Wasik, B. H. The application of Premack's generalization on reinforcement to the management of classroom behavior. *Journal of Experimental Child Psychology,* 1970, *10,* 33–43.

Webster, D. R., & Azrin, H. N. Required relaxation: A method of inhibiting agitative-disruptive behavior of retardates. *Behaviour Research and Therapy,* 1973, *11,* 67–78.

Werry, J. S., Sprague, R. L., Weiss, G., & Minde, K. Some clinical and laboratory studies of pyschotropic drugs in children: An overview. In *Symposium on higher cortical function.* (W. L. Smith, ed.), Springfield, Ill.: Charles C Thomas, 1970.

REFERENCE NOTES

1. Cohen, M. N., & Sprague, R. L. *Survey of drug usage in two midwestern institutions for the retarded.* Paper presented at the Gatlinburg Conference on Research in Mental Retardation, Gatlinburg, Tennessee, March 1977.

2. Favell, J. E., McGimsey, J. F., Jones, M. L., & Jarrah, A. S. *Improving the evaluation of psychopharmacological treatment in clinical practice.* Manuscript submitted for publication, 1982.

III

Family Perspectives

11

Family Needs of the Autistic Adolescent

MARIAN K. DeMYER and PEG GOLDBERG

The plight of autistic children has long brought forth efforts from the professional and lay communities to understand their needs and to try in some measure to provide treatment and education. It has only been in the last decade that the special needs of the families have been widely recognized. DeMyer (1979) has documented some major needs of families whose children were pre-school and school age, and vignettes of family needs in adolescence and adulthood. A literature review of research during the 1970s (DeMyer, Hingtgen, & Jackson, 1981) uncovered no systematic surveys or studies of family needs when the autistic family member reached adolescence. Reported in this chapter is a pilot survey of family needs and problems as the parents stated them. Because we wished to compare the adolescent period with other life periods, we also inquired about family needs during the autistic person's preschool, prepuberty, and adult years.

SUBJECTS

All but 4 of the 23 families surveyed lived in central Indiana and all but 3 families had been followed by one or both authors since the child's preschool years. Thus our knowledge about most of the families had some depth. No attempt was made to draw a stratified sample from all the adolescent autistic people known to us. We sought a range of chronolog-

MARIAN K. DeMYER and PEG GOLDBERG ● Institute of Psychiatric Research, Department of Psychiatry, Indiana University School of Medicine, Indianapolis, Indiana 46223.

ical ages from 12 years through the 20s to allow some insight into changing family needs as the age of the autistic person changed. The criterion for asking permission to interview a parent was that the autistic offspring be between the ages of 12 and 30 years. It so happened that two of the autistic children were below the lower age limit because preliminary information about their birth dates was incorrect. We decided to include information from these families because the parents expressed the same kinds of needs as those of the younger adolescents. Also, the 9-year-old boy was physically large for his age and the 11-year-old girl was developing breasts and pubic hair. Demographic data are summarized in Table 1. There were 48 siblings, 15 male, mean age 23 years (range 2–42 years). There were 16 autistic males and 7 females. The socioeconomic status of the heads of household as estimated by the North-Hatt rating system was 39% high, 26% high middle, 26% low middle, and 9% low.

QUESTIONNAIRE

Information was obtained using a semistructured interview format with 19 mothers and 2 fathers. In two cases the parents gave information in writing only. After inquiring about demographic features, the interviewers asked these questions:

1. What did your family need most during the following ages of the

Table 1
Demographic Features of Families

| | Parents | | | |
| | Chronological age | | Years schooling | |
	Mother	Father	Mother	Father
N	22	21	23	23
$\bar{M}$	48.91	52.76	13.09	14.39
Range	33–61	34–69	9–18	6–20

| | Autistic children | | | |
	Sibship	Position	Age	Sex
N (total)	73	23	22	F = 7
				M = 16
$\bar{M}$	3.09	2.48	17.27	
Range	1–6	1–6	9–29	

autistic family member: (a) 1–6 years; (b) 6–13 years; (c) 13–18 years: (d) adulthood, if the age had been attained?

2. What aspects of family life were affected adversely by problems in rearing and seeking help for the autistic person? Specific probes were used in the order given for 11 aspects of family life: intrafamily relationships, meeting needs of other children, family recreation, marital relationships, personal development of each family member, finances, housekeeping, relations with relatives, relations with friends and neighbors, emotional and mental health, and physical health.

3. What needs did you seek help for?

4. To whom did you go for help?

5. Was the service helpful, so-so, or did it make things worse?

Answers to these questions were recorded on a form using exact words of the parents liberally to reflect adequately their observations. Three types of severity ratings were then made of interview responses. (1) The interviewer rated how severely each of the 11 aspects of family life was affected over the whole life of the autistic offspring, assigning a weight of 3 for "severe," 2 for "moderate," 1 for "mild," and 0 for "not at all." The 11 ratings were then summed for each family for a maximum possible total of 33 (family life most severely affected) down to 0 (family life not affected adversely at all). (2) For each help resource the parents consulted the interviewer recorded whether the parents said they were helped, not helped at all, or received a combination of help and nonhelp. (3) The authors used their combined knowledge of the autistic person's behavior to rate severity of home management problems during the year preceding the interview. If the autistic family member was living in an institution, judgments were made about the period of a year before admission and also about difficulties while on home leave. We assigned a rating of 3 for maximal problems, 2 for severe, and 1 for moderate problems. No studies of rater reliability were conducted for this initial survey. In the following description of results all names are fictitious and all details which would identify families to others have been changed. The quotations likewise have been altered to protect the identities of parents, but all illustrations remain true in substance to the parents' description and circumstances.

RESULTS

The results of tabulating questionnaire responses will be discussed in two main sections. First will come a description of adverse effects on family life from living with and seeking help for the autistic family member. This description will set the stage for a better understanding of what the parents said the families needed in the way of help from the various sectors of society. These needs and the parents' evaluation of the adequacy of the help they received form Section 2 of the report. Although no questions were asked about the positives of living with an autistic person, several parents commented on some beneficial effects and these will be discussed in both sections of the report.

SECTION 1. ADVERSE EFFECTS OF LIVING WITH AN AUTISTIC FAMILY MEMBER

The topics are discussed in rank order of mean group severity ratings for each of the 11 aspects of family life about which we inquired (see Table 2.)

1. Family Recreation

The aspect of family life judged most seriously affected by the symptoms of autism was family recreation. Unfortunately in most families this problem did not appear to diminish with the passage of time, but took on new forms as the child became older and as symptoms changed intensity

Table 2
Severity of Effects on Family Life of Living with an Autistic Family Member

Rank order of mean	Mean severity rating[a]	Aspect of family life affected
1	2.26	Family recreation
2.5	2.22	Finances
2.5	2.22	Emotional and mental health of parents
4	2.09	Physical health of parents
5	1.96	Housekeeping
6	1.91	Meeting needs of brothers and sisters
7	1.78	Relations with friends and neighbors
8	1.65	Sibling relationships
9	1.59	Marital relationship
10	1.57	Personal development of each family member
11	1.52	Relations with relatives

[a]The higher the severity rating, the more severe were the effects of autism on a given aspect of family life.

and forms. By the time adolescence was reached most parents felt an accumlated fatigue and had reached the point of burn-out. The feeling of being on 24-hour call, 7 days a week, year in and year out, was one that we judged could only have been alleviated by the family's having access to regular recreation and respite throughout the autistic child's life at home. If the adolescent became calmer and more patient, as a few did, then family recreation became more frequent and enjoyable.

Those parents (13 of 21) who expressed maximal difficulty made statements such as the following: "Living with Dee Dee has been very confining. There is little we can do as a family together because he is very difficult to take anywhere. We have to split up and go as smaller groups even to the grocery, and then we pick where we go very carefully or we have a terrible time." One divorced mother whose husband left home early in the autistic child's life said flatly: "We've had no family recreation." Another said, "It's impossible to take Stuart many places. It takes a lot of planning and continuous supervision just to do very simple things." Another mother said their family had only one vacation together in 12 years. There were two cases where at least for some periods the autistic person was easy to take a variety of places. Joe, age 28, during adulthood became difficult to manage in the home and was admitted to a mental hospital. When he was a child he had enjoyed long car trips throughout the country with his family. The mother said, "My husband and I have very happy memories about those vacations."

2. Finances

Family finances (rank order severity rating 2½) were adversely affected in all but two cases. In the family whose children are normal the custom is for the mother to go to work when financial problems become burdensome. For the mother with an autistic child, a regular job is often not possible because substitute child care cannot be found. Also the occasions a mother of an autistic child must ask for time off the job are probably more frequent than for most other mothers. One mother, desperate for additional family income, said her employer "did not understand" and she was "forced to quit work." The mothers who went to work to be able to afford private residential placement spent their entire paychecks in addition to a portion of their husband's for such care. One mother of a highly destructive, runaway autistic adolescent said that a state-sponsored program cost more per week than the family's entire income. When payments could not be met, the parents had to bring him home; the family now works in shifts in order to care for him safely. One of the adult offspring now has to be at home at all times in order to protect both the autistic adolescent and the mother who is smaller physically than her autistic son.

At least five families were in a high income bracket and without exception spent large sums on the autistic child. Even those five couples feared for their future security because retirement will bring reduced incomes and loss of their child's access to private facilities. One mother, a widow since her autistic child's first year, said, "Brent needs 'special' everything, and everything for him costs more." One of the fruits of residential placement was that mothers could go to work and ease the family budget, a situation that most frequently happened during the adolescence of the autistic person.

3. Emotional and Mental Health of Parents

The parents' emotional and mental health (rank order of severity rating 2½) was judged by the parents themselves as worsened by the stress and anxieties of rearing, treating, and educating an autistic child in all but three families. Even in the cases where the parents denied such effect, it was obvious that more anxiety accrued from experiences with their autistic child than with their normal children. Some mothers said they were affected but denied its import with a joke: "There are days when I feel crazy—but I'm really O.K." Recurring depressive feelings and symptoms were common, e.g., "We all get so low at times—especially when we feel there is no help anywhere."

The families of older aggressive adolescents lived in fear that a weaker member of the family might be severely injured. One mother reported that she and her husband always had to "try to rise above our situation. . . . If you allow yourself to get bogged down in it, it will soon overwhelm you." This mother often felt depressed. Five mothers stated openly that they felt on the verge of mental breakdown if they had not achieved residential placement when they did, and one required psychiatric care in the aftermath of grief of "having to give up." With regard to family mental health, Lou's mother said, "When you sit on a merry-go-around all the time, you don't realize the rest of the world isn't dizzy too."

In a previous study DeMyer (1979) reported that 33% of the mothers of preschool autistic children had definite mild reactive depressions and that all parents felt anxious and upset because of the "nerve-wracking" behaviors of their autistic child. However, before the autistic child's birth there was no greater incidence of depression in the mothers than in a matched control group. This series of interviews indicated that mothers of adolescent autistic people living at home feel the same depression. Those who had "given up" and institutionalized their child retained a measure of sadness over seeing their child enter the "shadowy world of a mental institution." Sue had been institutionalized for 20 years, but her mother still had "difficulty in dealing with the heartache."

On the positive side of the picture some parents, especially mothers, seemed to have expanded their awareness of human suffering and found a "cause" they could fight for. Some found strength of character and resolve they had not believed possible previously in their interactions with educators, physicians, and others in the community. The mother of Jeremy, age 13, runs a volunteer service for parents whose children have recently been diagnosed as autistic and has found her emotional life enriched as a consequence. She helps these parents find additional services and schools, and introduces them to other parents of autistic children.

4. Physical Health of the Parents

Given the extra physical and psychological burdens the parents experienced, it is no surprise that all but four reported that their sense of physical well-being was lessened. Nearly every mother felt excessive fatigue which in some cases was chronic until respite came in the form of residential care. Several parents mentioned that their own increasing age brought increasing tiredness. Fathers nearing retirement age found that their later years were so encumbered. In all, 11 fathers and 9 mothers had chronic and severe illnesses such as heart disease, diabetes, cancer, blindness, asthma, vertebral malformations, fibrocystic breast disease, thyroid malfunction, Parkinson's disease, hypoglycemia, and anemia. While no parent thought the trials of dealing with autism caused these diseases, all parents felt the unremitting stress diminished their physical reserves needed to fight illness.

Unfortunately, as in other humans, physical illness tended to be most prevalent and burdensome for the parents after the autistic child had reached adolescence or adulthood, and after the aging process had taken its toll. Nearly every parent, even those not physically ill, had to think about the possibility of illness and of their own mortality, thoughts that became increasingly frequent during the autistic offspring's adolescence and adulthood. The next thoughts were about who would take care of the autistic family member. It was no small burden for the parents to realize it would most probably be an institution.

5. Housekeeping

Rearing an autistic offspring caused problems in housekeeping in most households. It takes no great imagination to appreciate the difficulties in keeping house when one family member takes every available opportunity to smash a dish or a mirror, or to lock out the parents and quickly smear all the food in the refrigerator over the kitchen. How can a mother keep a straight house if she must spend a great part of the day preventing the autistic adolescent from self-destruction, as four of the mothers did? Some mothers drove several hours a day to take the autistic person to a training facility, cutting down on their time for all other activities. Those mothers all mentioned that the housekeeping suffered also. Housekeeping burdens seemed not to vary with the age of the autistic child as much as with the nature of and severity of symptoms.

6. Meeting Needs of Brothers and Sisters

Almost all aspects of family living of necessity received reduced parental time and effort. The one responsibility that parents said they put most time to was seeing that the needs of their other children were met. Mickey's mother said, "We have made a real effort to keep this from being a problem." Despite the effort, all but five sets of parents believed they had succeeded only partially. Typically the siblings did not want to bring friends home because of embarrassment. In three cases school administrators and teachers either made tactless remarks or assigned a sibling to be responsible for some care of the autistic child. For example, "When Meg went to public school, her sister Eva was assigned by school authorities to be responsible for Meg on the school bus. Eva's friends didn't understand and stopped seeing her, and Eva was very hurt. I'm still angry over this." Parents never found any really effective way to blunt the siblings' feelings of social ostracism and hurt from tactless remarks by people in the community. Some of the effects on siblings were evaluated by the parents as "devastating." As one mother of an extremely aggressive adolescent said, "I now realize that we don't have just one handicapped child—all five of the kids have become limited to some degree because of the strains of Jerry. It's impossible for any of us to have a life of our own." One sibling who died suddenly while successfully preparing for a professional career was suspected of committing suicide, although autopsy results were equivocal. He was described by his mother as being "bitter" about his autistic sibling who continued to live at home in adulthood and take large chunks of the family's time and effort. Another mother described "admitting to myself" on hindsight that her other children were "extremely negatively" affected before the autistic adolescent was hospitalized at age 17 years. "Kay nearly killed us—literally. I would never have admitted it then because we were so determined to keep Kay at home." Sharing the responsibility of Kay's care finally let the parents perceive how much both parents and siblings needed time to themselves to develop their own personalities and social and work lives.

Along with the negatives, about one-third of the parents believed the siblings had been strengthened by the experience and that they had achieved empathy and care for all unfortunate people earlier and to a greater degree than other youngsters. One daughter told her parents, "Watching you raise Morrie has given me courage. I know I could do it myself if I have to."

7. Relations with Friends and Neighbors

Social relations with friends and neighbors were severely affected in 43% of the families, mainly in the direction of reduced contact rather than overt conflict. Parents mentioned difficulties in having friends in for social evenings and going to the homes of others because the autistic child could not be included due to irritating or destructive behavior. Also, substitute caretakers, who would allow more socializing, either would refuse to stay or parents found no one they thought could manage the problems the autistic family member posed.

A second source of difficulty in relations with friends and neighbors came from actions that the parents interpreted as criticism and in some cases rejection. During preschool years the common problem was un-asked-for advice about how to teach the autistic child to speak or socialize better, for example. Some parents were acutely sensitive to these implied criticisms, and to the frowns and stares of strangers when taking the child out in public. During the school-age period most parents' sensitivities diminished. However, the growth of secondary sex characteristics and the increase of body size to that of an adult reopened the old wounds as neighbors sometimes changed in their attitudes and behaviors. Pete's mother said, "He was always so welcome in all the neighbors' yards until he developed sexually. He never did anything that I know of, but the neighbors were afraid he might. I understood their position, but it hurt terribly."

While two mothers reported that none of the neighbors had any real understanding of their problems, there were five mothers who had high praise for the support and acceptance they received. Kay's mother said, "She has often screamed through an entire night and I know they can hear and it must bother them, but never has anyone been unkind. They have been helpful."

8. Sibling Relations

Early in the life of the autistic child there were frequent upheavals and quarrels. In the preschool years, before the nature of the problem was known and the family felt alone and bewildered, they were inclined to fight among themselves. Then as treatment and education were made available, "We knew we were not alone and learned to cope because we saw that others could cope." Another mother said, "We worked very hard to eliminate blame and learned to pull together as a family." However, at least four mothers stated that the other children in the family continued to fight and bicker extremely frequently until the autistic sibling was placed in residential care. Another mother said, "I think we were all in an extremely tense state until we finally accepted the fact that nothing we did made much of a difference in her condition and that she couldn't be helped in any major way."

9. Marital Relationships

The marital relationship likewise was probably more strained early in the life of the autistic child. DeMyer (1979) found innumerable daily tensions that parents said "put nerves on edge" and set off marital quarreling and diminished sexual interest, particularly in mothers. From interviewing this group of 23 parents during the adolescent period we can say that if the parents do not learn early in the life of their autistic child to be supportive of each other, divorce can result. There were six divorces among this group of 23 families, and 5 parents said the strain of coping with the problem of autism played a moderate to major role. As one father said, "Help came too late to save our marriage." Again the uses of residential care were illustrated when several mothers felt that placing the autistic child either "saved our marriage" or vastly improved the quality of it.

It must be noted that the incidence of divorce (26%) among this sample of couples was much less than that for the population of Indiana as a whole (40.3%). We do not know if this low divorce rate would hold true for a larger and possibly more representative sample of all parents of autistic offspring in a given population area. If the low divorce rate is representative, we can speculate that making decisions together about the difficult problems of living with an autistic child might serve to solidify the marital bond. Alternatively, divorce may present even more difficult problems financially and emotionally for the parents of autistic children than for other parents. At any rate most couples we interviewed openly stated or implied that bearing an autistic child had a profound effect on their marital relationship, in some cases building a stronger bond but in other cases driving the couples farther apart. (For a more detailed discussion of the effect of autistic children on the marital bond, see DeMyer, 1979.)

10. Personal Development of Each Family Member

While this aspect of family life was next to last in rank order of adverse effects on family life, it is clear that many family members, especially the mothers, had problems in this matter. First, only five mothers could manage to work regularly, let alone develop a career. If the autistic child were to remain at home through adolescence and adulthood, then mothers could never look forward to the freedom for self-development that mothers of normal children can. Few mothers had much time for reading or individual pursuits.

The mothers who came from families financially well-off had more success in finding substitute caretakers in order to pursue hobbies. As Mark's mother said, "My heart aches for those who do not have the financial means to endure the extra costs. We know many who can't afford even an occasional babysitter, even when one is available." One mother managed to do part-time professional work and pursue some additional education, but at great financial cost because of payments to sitters. On the other hand parents were zealous in helping their normal children realize their life goals, and most siblings finished high school and many attended college. Some of the siblings chose careers in the helping professions, and some openly stated that their experience with their autistic siblings provided much of the motivation for career choices.

11. Relations with Relatives

Parents mentioned fewer problems in their relations with relatives than in any other of the aspects of family life about which we inquired. It is our impression from our knowledge of younger autistic children that conflicts between the parents and the families of origin were more severe in preschool years than in later ages (DeMyer, 1979). Early in the life of the autistic child some grandparents tended to be critical of the mother for failure to toilet train and for the child's unsociability, for example. But by the time of adolescence these conflicts had largely died away and were almost forgotten. When problems with relatives continued, they were generally not across the board and those relatives could be avoided, although in some instances the feelings generated might be strong and felt for years. While a few families reported no active support from relatives, others described financial assistance, caretaking aid, and unusually good understanding from at least one or two relatives. In a few cases the mother reported an increased bond of mutual understanding between them and a relative, such as their own mother or a sister who became more supportive of the mother as she dealt with the puzzling problem of autism.

Summary

In summary, all aspects of family life about which we inquired were reported to be adversely affected by living with an autistic child. Questions may well be asked about the actual magnitude of these difficulties. For example, how much more of a problem is it to live with an autistic child than a normal one because normal children do pose problems and present strains to marriages? The answer cannot be given in exact numerical terms, but the results of these interviews and a preceding set by DeMyer (1979) and our years of clinical experience lead us to answer: it is more difficult to live with an autistic child. In our experience parents do not magnify the difficulties, although at times they may focus on the autistic child's problems while ignoring other difficulties in family living that also need solutions.

In nearly every case of autism the family must alter its lifestyle to accommodate the symptoms of autism and the special schooling required. If the child improves or has few disruptive symptoms by the time adolescence is reached, then the parents may derive a great sense of accomplishment from their many efforts and sacrifices. The stresses of earlier years are reduced and they feel many moments of contentment about their lives. Dean's mother said, "Last night we took Dean [age 18 years] to a concert. He was patient all through it. Afterwards, with a little prodding, he said 'Hello' to some people. We all had a wonderful sense of peace and enjoyment. He is easy to care for now and problems of the past seem to have faded away." On the other hand, if by adolescence symptoms remain difficult to manage, then parents are likely to feel depression and a lack of drive to continue the sacrifices. While few parents express resentment directly, in contrast to siblings, they do begin to look for a way out.

It is our clinical impression that before adolescence is reached most parents will tackle any problem concerning the autistic child as long as they have hope that their autistic child and their family will get a modicum of help from "the doctors," the school, and the community. Many give a large portion of their energies to getting "better" help. However, as we shall see in the following section, a watershed is reached in the adolescence of the autistic family member whose improvement is minimal, when often hope dies and support from the community and schools seems inadequate to the parents. No little part of the difficulty during adolescence is the parental knowledge, so long pushed aside, that their autistic child is probably never going to be "normal." With great sadness many parents "give up" and long for respite from the never-ending responsibilities of their autistic adolescent who will "remain forever a child in an adult's body."

SECTION 2. NEEDS OF FAMILY MEMBERS

The wide array of adverse effects on family life makes the needs that the parents reported to us seem appropriate. They reported that the families could have used additional services throughout the life span of the autistic family member. These needs can be grouped to the broad resource from which help could have come: (1) the helping professions; (2) the general community; and (3) the educational establishment. Table 3 lists the incidence of family needs during the four different age periods of the autistic person. The same group of autistic individuals, whose age range was 9–29 years, was used in getting information about the four life periods.

Table 3
Distribution of Family Needs by Age Group of Autistic Offspring

Needs source/Need	Age group[a]			
	1–5 (N = 23) (%)	6–12 (N = 23) (%)	13–17 (N = 11) (%)	Adult (18+) (N = 8) (%)
General community and relatives				
Respite/relief	61	65	60	12
Money	26	52	73	50
Other parent contact	30	17	20	25
Babysitters	26	35	20	12
Community acceptance	—	17	53	25
Relatives' support	9	9	7	—
Miscellaneous	9	9	—	—
Diagnosing/treating professionals				
Good residential treatment	9	26	100	88
Early/consistent diagnosis	70	—	—	—
Parent/sibling counseling	52	26	13	—
Better agency information/ cooperation	18	26	—	—
Knowledgeable/concerned professionals	22	17	—	38
Better management recommendations	18	31	7	—
Legal rights advocate	9	17	20	12
Education establishment				
Good day-/year-long program	48	61	53	25
Transportation	22	43	14	12
Curriculum additions	35	83	40	25
Teacher/staff attitudes	13	48	13	12
Sex management/training	—	17	80	38

[a]Group 1–5 includes those through 5 years 11 months of age, etc.

Thus, as can be seen in Table 3, we had information about early childhood and prepuberty on all 23 autistic people, about the adolescent period on 15 autistic people, and about the adult period on 8 autistic people.

Our information from this set of interviews tended to be more detailed about the family needs during the current age of the autistic person than about past ages. Parents were more caught up in the current period and they said more about it than earlier ages. Also, parental memories had dimmed about the preschool years of the adolescents and adults. A further problem was that we could not cover as well as we hoped all the topics we set out to do because the budget and the time allotted for the project allowed just one interview of about 1 hour per family. Because of these reasons and because we are concentrating on the adolescent period, our discussion of family needs will emphasize adolescence. However, when our knowledge warrants, we will discuss changing family needs during other age periods.

Needs from the Diagnosing and Treating Professionals

The Need for Residential Placement

When the autistic individual had reached adolescence, the need expressed by the greatest. number of parents (100%) was for "good" residential treatment either full time or part time for temporary family respite. This great need extended into the autistic child's adulthood, becoming even more urgent as parents grew older and more tired, and may have acquired chronic illness that brought their own mortality close to mind. During the preschool and grade-school periods of their autistic offspring few parents saw the need for residential treatment. Instead what they said they needed then from the professionals was an early and consistent diagnosis, counseling for themselves and their other children, and good practical advice on day-to-day management problems. In those early years, in fact, most parents were determined to keep their autistic children home at all costs unless they were offered a chance for a good residential treatment program with the idea of substantial improvement of the autistic child that subsequently would allow more comfortable living at home and adequate participation in public school programs for normal or near-normal children.

Unfortunately, like most cases of autism reported in follow-up studies (DeMyer, 1979), this goal was not realized for the autistic adolescents whose parents were interviewed. Despite special residential treatment and special education early in life, by the time of adolescence over half of the autistic people were in residential placement. Also, several other parents were actively looking for a suitable chronic-care institution. In view of the fact that nearly all parents wanted and worked hard to keep their children in the home, we looked at the unmet family needs which if met might have allowed continued home living for the autistic family member even in adolescence.

Factors Leading to Residential Placement

Several interacting factors led the families to take the feared step of institutionalization that earlier in the life of the autistic child they had vowed never to do. These factors were the age of the autistic person, the severity of symptoms, and the severity of the effect of autism on family life. The older the autistic person, the more likely he was to be in residential care. Of the 12 autistic persons over 14 years of age, 67% were placed while only 33% of the younger ones were out of the parental home (see Table 4). The mean age at placement was 12 years. When an autistic child was placed at 11 years of age or younger, parents mentioned two factors: an unusual family problem, or the large size of the child made destructive symptoms unmanageable for the family. For example, one mother became severely ill and the parents were divorced, leaving the care of all the children with the father who could not find a housekeeper willing or able to take care of the hyperactive, destructive autistic child

Table 4

Factors Associated with Residential Placement of the Autistic Family Member

		Living situation of autistic person	
Factor description	N	Residential placement % (by row)	Parental home % (by row)
Age of autistic offspring			
>14 years	12	67	33
<14 years	11	36	64
Effect of autism on family			
More severe[a]	12	75	25
Less severe[b]	9	27	73
Severity of autistic symptoms			
Maximal	7	86	14
Severe	9	56	44
Moderate	5	0	100

[a]Total family life severity rating >25 (maximum possible score 33).
[b]Total family life severity rating <25 (minimum possible score 0).

who was placed in chronic residential care at age 6 years. In two families the birth of a sibling precipitated placement because the autistic child (now nearly adolescent age) persistently attacked the baby and the mother could not match the autistic child's physical strength.

For those placed later than 12 years of age, persistent open masturbation, increase in destructive tendencies, and extreme parental physical and psychological weariness—the "burn-out" syndrome—were reported as reasons. From our vantage point it seems that before puberty of their autistic offspring the parents could shoulder all the burdens without giving up because they had hope that great improvement or even normality would result from their efforts. With the continuation of symptoms and increasing evidence that the autistic adolescent's mental retardation is not going to improve, parents give up hope. In addition the increased physical size makes many autistic symptoms more difficult to manage. Not only do the aggressive autistic individuals become more capable of hurting themselves and others because the mothers are not strong enough to contain them, but they become more difficult to get through the routine of the day. Many autistic people have to be physically guided to the dinner table, in and out of the car, and to go to the bathroom. The physical effort required of the mother, great as it was when the child was young, becomes an impossible burden for many mothers as the child grows to adult size.

The physical evidence of sexual maturity may also bring added problems, in some cases so persistent and severe that parents could find no effective solution. Even if the autistic adolescent did not openly masturbate, several mothers found no good way to take care of their autistic son's toileting needs in public once he passed the age of 7 or 8 years. The open masturbation was a worry and an embarrassment, and relations with neighbors and friends became strained. The masturbator was not welcome in the neighborhood and shunned by all but the staunchest relatives.

Not unexpectedly the severity of symptoms was related to residential placement. Of those autistic people whose behavior problems were maximally difficult to manage, 86% were in residential care in comparison to 56% of autistic people with "severe" ratings. On the other hand none of those people whose behavior problems were judged "moderate" to "mild" was placed outside the home (see Table 4).

The more severe the behavior problems of the autistic family member, the greater the adverse effects on family life. The mean ratings for severity of effect on family life was 20.6 (see Table 5). Two families had the maximal rating of 33 while the lowest rating was 4. In those families severely affected (>25), 75% of the autistic individuals were placed out of the home while only 24% of those whose families were less severely affected were so placed.

Table 5
Interaction Between Magnitude of Home Management Problems and Effect of
Autism on Family Life

Magnitude of home management problems of autistic symptoms	N	Effect of autism on family life	
		Severe[a]	Less severe[b]
Maximal	7	50%	10%
Severe	9	33%	56%
Moderate	5	17%	34%

[a]Total family life severity rating >25 (maximum possible score 33).
[b]Total family life severity rating <25 (minimum possible score 0).

Is it realistic to expect that if families were given regular respite that the autistic family member could remain longer in the home? We believe that only a test by providing adequate respite care and upgrading all services to the families could answer this question, but certainly the quality of life for the families would be improved. Obviously, once a parent loses the will to try any longer, or becomes physically ill or advanced in age, of necessity society will need to find a way to provide complete care for the dependent autistic person.

Changing Needs from Professional People During Autistic Adolescence

It is interesting to note that by the adolescent period not a single parent professed a need for diagnostic services or better information about autism from agencies and professional people. Also, the expressed need for parent and sibling counseling about family feelings concerning autism was down from earlier years. The parents' remarks gave no sure reason for the changing needs, but perhaps the fact that more than half the autistic adolescents were institutionalized made these needs less pressing. However, our clinical practice strongly suggests that parents of all autistic adolescents and adults do need knowledgeable and concerned professional advice at certain critical periods: namely, at sexual maturity, particularly if sexuality is expressed in a way that frightens or repels other people; at termination of school programs; if parents cannot agree on whether to institutionalize; on choosing appropriate institutions; on continued family stress because of difficult-to-manage symptoms of autism; on development of seizures. Any change for the worse in the autistic person or in availability of services can upset the balance of family life because symptomatic gains and satisfactory services have often been won through great effort by the whole family. The relatively great numbers of parents who consult us during these crises attest to the fact that knowledgeable professionals are a need in the autistic offspring's adolescence and adulthood.

Marital strife that has been absent for years can erupt with divisive bitterness if certain problems arise during the autistic child's adolescence. If the parents disagree on whether to institutionalize the marriage can disintegrate. It is our experience that during the early life of many autistic children it is the father who is more likely to push for institutional care. During adolescence it is often the mother who is worn out psychologically and physically and the father may disagree with her about chronic care. We have also been consulted by adult siblings who report that their parents' marriage is failing because of new differences in opinion about how to manage the care of the autistic now physically fully grown but still fully dependent. It may not be possible to arrange a rapprochement between the parents, but professional counseling can relieve the intense pain both parents suffer and effect some reasonable living arrangement for the autistic person.

Siblings' Needs in Adolescence

We have known families where siblings have suffered burn-out and need to move to distant cities in order to assuage their own pain. Sometimes the siblings as children have been intensely involved in the care of the autistic family member and have submerged their own needs until some urge within them in adolescence and early adulthood propels them to independent expression. These siblings may need professional help to recognize the legitimacy of their needs and to deal with the guilt arising from their emancipation proclamation. Parents need help to deal with the anger and hurt over what they perceive as a defection by a child they could previously trust to help.

Professional Services Needs of the Autistic Adolescent

Last but not least, the autistic adolescent or adult often needs professional services. We professionals have done too little in the way of systematic study or discernment of their needs or provision of the high-quality residential care that dependent autistic adults ultimately will need. Also relatively unstudied are techniques for helping high-functioning adolescents who nearly, but not quite, make it into the mainstream of normal life. Consulting me one recent week were two young men, both with more than adequate general intelligence but with problems in organizing their activities well enough to make the grade in school and in their work. Also plaguing them both was an inability to make friends despite a desperate desire to do so. While both were referred to able psychotherapists, the question remains if the young men will be able to profit from such therapy. As Mr. A (another autistic man, now in his 30s) said in anger to me, "You doctors spend all your time getting an autistic child to talk and stop screaming and wetting his pants; but you do nothing to help us in the later stages of development. We need to make friends and succeed on the job." On a happier note, Mr. A recently called to tell me he had been able to make significant progress in making friends with women by attending "a Masters–Johnson type program for single people." He was interested in my giving word of this to other patients with problems similar to his. Mr. A's success has come because he has been persistent and self-motivated to search. What can we professionals do for others less intelligent and less motivated?

Needs from the Legal Profession

An important issue for 20% of the parents during the adolescent period was the need for a legal rights advocate both for their child and for themselves. With the passage of Public Law 94–142 assuring high-quality education for all handicapped youth, parents often felt that educators were not providing the optimum education and they wished legal advisors to help them when personal confrontations with the schools did not achieve enough improvements in curriculum.

Because the burgeoning sexuality of the autistic teenagers brought so many thorny and often unsolveable problems, many parents seriously considered sterilization procedures. When they found such operations difficult to arrange, they expressed a need for a legal advocate to present their views to the public and to the courts. One couple who arranged for a sterilization procedure found themselves sued by the Legal Services Organization, which obtained a temporary injunction stopping the operation. This couple, impoverished by years of caring for their autistic child, would have been unable to afford a defense without private financial aid. The issue of whether sterilization should be denied to all handicapped persons is a controversial one, but as one mother said, "I wish those people who think all handicapped people should have the right to bear children would have to care for them [the adolescent] and protect them for just 6 months. Also they should have to feel the heartache of caring for the baby of an adolescent autistic girl or see an autistic son suddenly shunned by everyone." While it is difficult to locate cases of childbearing in autistic women, the contemplation of the possibility is a heavy burden for many parents already greatly stressed.

Parents' Evaluation of Professional Services

Every parent we interviewed expressed a need for professional services and all sought such help beginning early in the autistic child's life. Physicians (including family practitioners, pediatricians, psychiatrists, and neurologists) without special training or experience in autism were the most commonly mentioned resource. Others frequently consulted were psychologists and social workers. (Teachers and educators will be discussed in a subsequent section.) Because parents often could not remember all the professional people consulted over the years, we grouped them together and then rated the parents' perception of how helpful they were as a group. Only three parents said that all "the doctors" they consulted were uniformly helpful. Most parents gave at least a few of the doctors a "good" rating while reporting "unhelpful" experiences with "most" of them.

Professional people who had specialized in the diagnosis and treatment of autism received more "good" ratings than those who had not so specialized. To the parents, the specialists in autism seemed to understand where to find the various available resources and could at times open doors to the autistic person that had previously been closed. Their advice about management of behavior problems also seemed more realistic and useful to parents than the advice of the nonspecialists. In addition to specialized knowledge about autism, the attitudes of caring, empathy, and intelligent listening were requisites in the parents' perception of a "good doctor." Those parents whose opinions and observations were belittled or who were accused of lying felt a bitterness that never fully died away. The doctors who projected an attitude of caring and respect were remembered with good feelings. Here are some examples of parents' perceptions of their consultations with professional people:

Ken's mother: "He was 12 years old when he started attacking our baby and became very difficult to manage at school. No doctor we talked to gave us any useful advice until a neurologist recommended a state school and helped us get him in. But the other doctors didn't have the foggiest idea about how to help us."

Marie's mother: "Some doctors must think parents don't have feelings and they don't listen. Our daughter (now age 14 years) has been very self-destructive. She hits herself and digs at her skin to the point she is covered with sores. One time she injured herself to the point that we took her to _____ Hospital emergency room. Without even hearing us out the doctors thought we have been guilty of child abuse. That was very hard to take."

Donny's father: "I must say most of the doctors we talked to confused us. They used terms we didn't understand and seemed to disagree about what Donny's problem was. We appreciate those who took time to listen, but my blood still boils about the doctor who looked at him about 10 minutes and said his case was hopeless. Then he asked us what we had done to cause it. Finally we saw someone who knew what he was talking about and we got some practical help.''

Quality of Institutions

Since about half of the autistic persons whose parents we interviewed were currently in institutions, we had a fair sampling of parental perceptions of their quality. On the whole the private institutions received better ratings than the large state institutions. If the latter had a "good" staff–patient ratio and care was taken to communicate with parents regularly, then the state institution was rated as "good." As Marie's mother said, "When we first took Marie to _____ State Hospital, we talked to a social worker who had been there long enough to know what was going on and we felt comfortable about telling her things Marie needed. That social worker left and now we get a new one every few months. Some seem O.K., but they have too much to do and none of them knows what is going on. We feel very uneasy about the quality of her care now. It has deteriorated."

One main drawback to private institutions was the high cost, and at times they refused to keep patients whose behavior became "unmanageable." Several parents noted how difficult it was to get a child in the state institutions and how expensive they had become. Illustrating some difficulties these situations can bring is the following account from Chuck's mother: "Chuck [age 23 years] was in a private residential school for 6 years. Suddenly they called my husband one day at work to say Chuck was being discharged immediately because they couldn't control his masturbation. We hadn't been told before about this problem and my husband was in a state of shock. I feel the only reason I was able to arrange a transfer to _____ State Hospital was because I was tenacious and refused to take "no" for an answer. Many parents I know have thrown up their hands and then lived forever with a bad situation. I knew that if Chuck came home, our marriage in effect would have been over and I would have had to quit work. I couldn't pay that price."

Needs from the General Community and Relatives

First and foremost, families needed respite and relief, and this need did not diminish until adulthood when most of the autistic people who remained in the home were not difficult to care for. This need, of course, parallels that of the needs of the parents from the professional community, the need for respite residential care. All those autistic individuals too difficult to manage at home were in chronic-care institutions by late adolescence. Parents expressed a need for a source of trained "babysitters" who could take over on a night out for the parents or a week or two for family recreation. Lee's mother spoke for all of the parents when she said, "We really need some time off from caring for Lee; but when we have tried to arrange it, the struggle we go through is exhausting, expensive, and often doesn't get results." Families of those autistic people with acutely severe symptoms of course need the temporary respite of their offspring's emergency hospitalizations in the local community, which were very difficult to arrange. Many parents expressed a need for relatives to help out more than they did, but also realized that these relatives might need some training to perform well.

While financial needs of the families were at their height during the adolescent period, few parents had any good ideas about how to achieve substantial relief except for more agencies and schools to be publicly supported. The irony of this suggestion was that parents tended to evaluate critically the public schools and the state-supported hospitals. Several parents mentioned that they felt public moneys were wasted because agencies too often offered only a repeat of diagnostic services and too seldom provided continuing treatment and counseling services needed not only by the autistic person but by all family members.

About 20%–30% of parents, especially mothers, felt a strong need for continuing contact with other parents of autistic people. They felt that no other resource understood what the family was suffering or knew the nature of community resources quite as well as other parents. This need of course is responsible for the sturdy growth of the National Society for Autistic Children. "Other parents" and "parent groups" received mostly "good" ratings as valuable sources of help at some time during the autistic child's life. Most parents used this resource most heavily during the school-age period when hope was high that great improvement might occur and when many were still struggling to solve home management problems. As adolescence was reached, and as more children were in chronic residential placement, parents tended to lose interest in parent groups and membership in NSAC. Every time we talk to parent groups, we ask for a show of hands concerning the age group of the autistic people whose parents are attending. Invariably the school-age group (6–12 years) wins. Only a handful of parents of preschool and adolescent people attend, and often none from the adult age group.

Finally, a poignant need expressed by over half the parents of adolescents was for more community acceptance of their autistic offspring. There was a definite shift after the child developed mature body sexual characteristics and adult height and weight. Jamey's mother said, "I wish people wouldn't act afraid of him in the stores and parks. He's big, yes, and he still does some odd things with his hands, but he's not going to hurt them. This [fear of public] never happened when he was little." Parents also wanted someplace for the adolescents to go to socialize since ordinary social relationships with peers were generally not possible. Even the higher functioning autistic people needed these services.

Education Establishment and Sexuality Management

The schools assume a pivotal role in family life all through the developing years of the autistic person. If the parents perceive the education establishment as failing their autistic offspring to any serious degree, the whole balance of the family can be thrown out of kilter. It is moot whether some parents expect too much, but these 23 parents were quite outspoken with us over their needs from the schools. They wanted "good" programs that were available for 8 hours a day throughout the year. They wanted the curriculum to be varied, with opportunities for physical education. Although some parents wanted increased emphasis on reading and writing, others wished for "practical" education in living, socializing, and preparation for vocations.

Many wanted summer programs so that the mothers could spend needed time with their other children and so that the autistic child would not lose the gains made in the regular term. The parents needed continuity of good school programs. When by virtue of chronological age alone an autistic child was required to go to another program in another school, the whole energies of the parents could go into searching out and evaluating available schools. The whole family felt the anxiety of these transition periods. Those parents who had encountered demeaning and hostile attitudes in teachers and administrators wanted these persons fired from their jobs. Several parents sought legal help to effect changes they thought were absolutely necessary. The drawback to these tactics was a sense of further alienation from the teachers and school administrators.

When adolescence was reached the need for schooling did not decrease; but in the parents' estimation there was need for a shift in curriculum emphasis. The developing sexuality of the autistic adolescent took precedence in the minds of many parents. They felt "completely unprepared" for the problems it brought. Rightly or wrongly, 80% of the parents wanted the schools to take over the role of educating them how to deal with the sexual behavior of their adolescent autistic offspring. They wanted counseling concerning their own and their normal children's painful feelings in this regard. For the adolescents themselves, parents wanted the schools to offer sexuality training programs. Parents wished for help in teaching the girls how to care for menstrual needs and preventing open masturbation, for example. Some of the young men, in addition to open and frequent masturbation, rubbed their genitals against others and thus courted not only rejection but legal prosecution. Parents were particularly concerned about preventing such behaviors because once started they proved extremely hard to extinguish.

Parents' Evaluation of Schools

Public school programs tended to be less highly regarded than private schools and special agency programs. Public school administrators were sometimes viewed as "not even trying" to provide high-quality and innovative, useful programs, and as disinterested in the individual child. One parent indignantly told of an administrator who "took 3 months to fill out a simple form that held up our child's admission to a greatly needed program." The bigger the school system or class, the more the parents felt unheard and unknowing of "what was going on" in the schoolroom. One mother of a severely self-destructive child said: "The school teachers in _____ [previous large city of residence] seemed very insensitive about our other child's feelings about her autistic sister, and the school provided a very short school day. Because of this, we moved to _____ [small city in another state] where the school program is much better and occupies a whole day. We still cannot get help if an emergency arises and we are very concerned that she may get pregnant. What a catastrophe that would be! What will we be able to get for her in a few years when her schooling stops?"

One should evaluate the parents' critical comments in the light of their great expectation from the schools. Parents hope that if education can be applied with sufficient skill and persistance, then great changes for the better will result. Parents want their autistic child to have every chance to advance to as close to normal as possible. If they feel that that chance is denied, then they can be angry and push hard for changes. Educators on the other hand have a limited budget and must provide equally for all students. Nevertheless the school personnel could alleviate the burden of the family with an autistic child considerably by listening carefully to parents, sharing the education goals with them, and being careful not to respond with angry defensiveness when parents push for better programs. These parents for the most part will respond positively to an honest and forthright discussion of sincere efforts to upgrade programs.

SUMMARY

While some positive experiences accompany living with and seeking help for an autistic child, there are great stresses on the families who must alter their lifestyles in order to accommodate the symptoms of autism and find help for the afflicted child. Of 11 aspects of family life about which we inquired, parents reported that the most severe problems came in achieving family recreation. This lack, together with unavailability of respite care when symptoms or family problems were severe and the chronicity of autism, finally led a large proportion of parents to lose hope and the will to keep the autistic adolescent at home. About 67% of autistic adolescents over 14 years of age, and all of those whose symptoms were judged "severe," were in institutions. Other aspects of family life adversely affected were finances, emotional and physical health of parents, housekeeping, personal development of each family member, and relationships among family members, friends, and neighbors.

To meet the stresses of autism, parents said the families needed additional services from three broad resources:

1. *Professionals.* Parents want concerned, caring "doctors," knowledgeable about autism, who can provide useful recommendations about home management, family counseling, community resources, and "good" institutions within reach of the family budget. These institutions are needed for treatment, for respite periods during family illness, and to provide time for restorative recreation of the family unit.
2. *The General Community.* Again, the parents' highest expressed need is for aid in achieving time out from being on call for their autistic child 24 hours a day, year in and year out. In addition they need financial and legal aid, continuing contact with other parents of autistic children, and more community acceptance of the autistic person.
3. *The Educational Establishment.* Because so much is expected of schools to effect basic and substantial improvement in the autistic child, parents want all aspects of schools to be of high order. Many parents want curriculum changes, better trained and more empathic teachers, longer school days and school years. The sexual maturity of autistic adolescents stimulated parental fears and real management problems if sexuality was expressed in a way that repelled or frightened other people. Many parents wish for help from the schools in managing these problems.

Needs of the family with an autistic adolescent show some changes over earlier years, but do not diminish. The physical growth to adult size and sexual maturation bring new problems that can be overwhelming to families already stressed to their limits. Without respite care and counseling for the new and painful family feelings, the family members suffer a burn-out syndrome and the autistic adolescent must be placed in an institution. While not all cases of autism could be managed in the home if services were upgraded, certainly the quality family life could be made better. We need to develop methods to help high-functioning adolescents achieve friends and job proficiency. Society needs to develop satisfactory care for all dependent autistic people of adult age because, ultimately, old age and illness of parents forces them to give their autistic offspring to other hands.

REFERENCES

DeMyer, M. K. *Parents and children in autism*. Washington, D.C.: Winston, 1979.
DeMyer, M. K., Hingtgen, J. N., & Jackson, R. K. Infantile autism reviewed: A decade of research. *Schizophrenia Bulletin,* 1981.

12

Stress and Coping in Families of Autistic Adolescents

MARIE M. BRISTOL and ERIC SCHOPLER

Our understanding of the problems and needs of autistic adolescents and adults is still in its infancy, compared with what we know about autism in children. During the past decade some important strides have been made in the study and treatment of autistic children and their families (Paluszny, 1979; Rutter & Schopler, 1978). These have included the recognition that autism is not primarily an emotional illness but a developmental disability (Schopler, Rutter, & Chess, 1979). Autism is not caused by parental pathology; instead parents can be productively involved in their own child's treatment (Schopler & Reichler, 1971). Moreover the optimum treatment for such children is not psychotherapy, but special education made available in our public schools and implemented with the collaboration of parents (Schopler & Bristol, 1980). However, in most of our public schools special education ends when the student reaches 18 years of age. What happens to the adolescent with autism? What happens to the struggles of his parents?

MARIE M. BRISTOL ● Carolina Institute for Research on Early Education of the Handicapped, Frank Porter Graham Child Development Center, University of North Carolina, Chapel Hill, North Carolina 27514. ERIC SCHOPLER ● Division TEACCH, Department of Psychiatry, University of North Carolina Medical School, Chapel Hill, North Carolina 27514. The preparation of this chapter was supported in part by the Special Education Program of the Department of Education, Contract Number 300–77–0309. However, the opinions expressed do not necessarily reflect the position or policy of the U.S. Department of Education, and no official endorsement by the U.S. Department of Education should be inferred.

In this chapter we discuss the best answers available to us at this time based on both our research and our clinical experience with families of autistic adolescents. First, we will consider the problems of adolescence endured by families with normally developing children. This is followed by a discussion of the special family stresses of parents with handicapped children and parents of autistic youngsters. Their problems and needs change with development as do the problems and needs of their parents. However, there is a wide range in parental coping skills, the resources they bring to their handicapped offspring, and the sources of support supplied to them by their community. We will review briefly what we know about family coping in crisis situations in general and then discuss predicting and avoiding crises in families of autistic children. The contribution of child characteristics and family resources to successful coping and active coping strategies will be discussed. In addition the relationship to stress and coping of both informal social support from extended family, friends, and neighbors, and formal support from schools, churches, and related social agencies will be examined.

Our information comes primarily from three sources: (1) the research literature; (2) our clinical experience; and (3) our longitudinal research with families of autistic children. Except for the work of DeMyer (1979) and Holroyd and McArthur (1976), few systematic data are available specifically regarding the impact of autistic children on families. Accordingly we have reviewed some studies of children with other handicaps which seem particularly relevant to families with autism.

Our clinical experience is primarily based on our work with the community-based North Carolina program for the Treatment and Education of Autistic and Communications Handicapped Children (Division TEACCH). This program has been devoted to the study and treatment of such children for the past 15 years, and also includes adolescents and adults with autism. A more detailed description is provided in Chapter 19.

At Division TEACCH we are also engaged in systematic research on coping and stress in families of autistic and communication-handicapped children. From these studies we hope to be able to answer two basic questions: First, how can we best predict which families are most at risk for family crisis and most in need of assistance? Second, what are the differences between families overwhelmed by the stress of having an autistic child and those that are coping well? We are particularly concerned with coping strategies and supports used by the more "successful" families that might have implications for interventions with families that are not doing as well.

An initial cross-sectional study of stresses and supports reported by 40 mothers of autistic children aged 4–19 years (Bristol, 1979), and three separate studies on sources of help for families of autistic children served as pilot studies for a longitudinal study of coping and stress now underway.

Families of consecutive evaluations in the TEACCH program are asked to participate. Data on child characteristics and progress are collected in the course of clinical evaluations. At the time of initial evaluation, mothers complete a standardized family assessment battery in their homes and participate in a second 2-hour interview in their homes 9 months later. Much of the material in this chapter regarding North Carolina families is drawn from the pilot studies and from preliminary data from this ongoing program of research.

GENERAL PROBLEMS OF ADOLESCENCE

A mother of a nonhandicapped adolescent, on hearing the expression "I'd love kittens if only they didn't have to grow up to be cats," remarked that she'd love children more if only they didn't have to grow up to be adolescents. This mother was echoing the distress that almost all families face at some time when they are helping their children do the "two steps forward, one step back" march to adulthood.

We know, for example, that in families of nonhandicapped children one of the lowest points in marital happiness generally occurs during the children's adolescent period. Family life cycle studies show that during their children's adolescence parents report not only the lowest level of satisfaction with their children, but also one of the lowest levels of satisfaction with companionship, financial management, allocation of household tasks, and sex (Burr, 1970). Families are dealing with adolescent

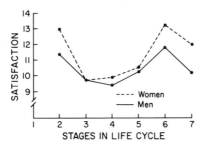

Figure 1. Satisfaction with children over the life cycle. Stages in the life cycle: 1, no children; 2, oldest child under 6; 3, oldest child 6–12; 4, oldest child 13–20; 5, oldest child 20 or one child has left home; 6, all children launched; 7, retirement. From "Satisfaction with Various Aspects of Marriage Over the Life Cycle: A Random Middle Class Sample" by W. R. Burr, *Journal of Marriage and the Family*, 1970, *32*, 29–37. Copyright 1970 by Wesley R. Burr. Reprinted by permission.

rebellion, their children's successful and unsuccessful attempts at independence, and their children's emerging sexuality. At the same time the parents themselves may be dealing with their own midlife crises. Marital discord and divorce, career shifts, sexual problems, depression, and newly awakened fears about health and mortality are common among parents of adolescent children by virtue of the developmental tasks that many parents themselves are facing (Levinson, 1978; Sheehy, 1976). Without minimizing the real and acute problems faced by parents of adolescent autistic children, it is well to keep such problems in the perspective of "normal" family development. We must also learn to recognize that some of the problems of parenting an autistic adolescent are normal and even necessary if adolescents are ultimately to be able to exist independently of their parents.

SPECIAL PROBLEMS IN FAMILIES OF HANDICAPPED CHILDREN

Mothers

To suggest that there is stress in families of nonhandicapped children is not to imply that there are no special family problems in caring for a handicapped child. Some studies in fact indicate that in families of mentally retarded children the divorce rate may be triple the national average, and the suicide rate may be twice the national average (Love, 1973). The prevalence of depression among mothers of handicapped children has also been documented (Cummings, Bayley, & Rie, 1966). A study (Cox, Rutter, Newman, & Bartak, 1975) of mothers of autistic and dysphasic children suggests that almost a third of the mothers in these families of handicapped children reported incidents of depression in response to stress associated with the birth or presence of the handicapped child in the family. DeMyer (1979) and her associates found a similar proportion of mothers of autistic children who reported depressive symptoms.

Fathers

Although most research has been conducted with mothers, reviews of research on fathers of handicapped children (Bristol & Gallagher, 1982; DeMyer, 1979; Price-Bonham & Addison, 1978) reveal that significant emotional and financial strains are experienced by fathers, who often lack outlets to deal with such stress or to contribute to the child's progress.

Siblings

Studies of siblings of handicapped children also reveal mixed outcomes. Some siblings suffer from emotional and behavioral disorders (Cohen, 1962; Farber, 1959; Gath, 1974; Schwirian, 1976). The pervasive nature of this stress is highlighted by studies which indicate that the negative effects on siblings may continue into adult life (Cleveland & Miller, 1977; Grossman, 1972) and are not merely a temporary reaction to the increased childrearing demands posed by the handicapped child. The case for stress in families of handicapped children then is rather well documented.

Successful Families

In contrast to the rather bleak picture painted above, we know from both clinical experience and research studies (Caldwell & Guze, 1960; DeMyer, 1979; Graliker, Fischler, & Koch, 1962; Grossman, 1972; Gallagher, Cross, & Scharfman, Note 2) that at least some families are able to cope successfully and may even be enriched by the presence of a handicapped child. In a recent study of marital happiness in families of children with a variety of handicaps (Krause-Eheart, Note 3) approximately half of the mothers reported that the handicapped child did not affect their marriages. The remaining half of the mothers were divided into two approximately equal groups—one felt that the children had adversely affected their marriages, the other felt that having a handicapped child had actually strengthened theirs. Our clinical experience suggests that the same may be true for families of autistic children.

STRESSES IN FAMILIES OF AUTISTIC CHILDREN

Comparison with Other Handicaps

When families of children with different types of handicaps are compared, families of autistic children report more coping problems and stress than families of children with other types of handicaps such as Down's syndrome or psychiatric disorders (Holroyd & McArther, 1976). Mothers of both Down's syndrome and autistic children reported similar problems of poor health, depressed moods, excessive time demands, and excessive reliance of their children on them, pessimism about the child's future, and limits on family opportunity (jobs, education, etc.) because of the handicapped child. Mothers of autistic children, however, reported more problems and tension in areas such as taking their children to public places and more embarrassment and disappointment than parents of Down's syndrome children. They also reported that their children were more physically dependent on them for care, had fewer activities that occupied them, and fewer services and resources in the community including poorer prospects for independent living. Autistic children were reported to be more disruptive of family integration in activities such as meals, vacations, and family outings, and had more difficult personality characteristics.

In fact there may be a characteristic profile of stress associated with parenting an autistic child. Data collected on stresses reported by 40 mothers of autistic children in North Carolina (Bristol, 1979) reveal a striking similarity to those reported for parents of autistic children in California (Holroyd & McArthur, 1976) (See Table 1).

Stresses in North Carolina Families of Autistic Children

A Developmental Progression

In our initial research (Bristol, 1979) all mothers (N = 40) reported problems or stresses in dealing with their children, although the particular problems differed with the age of the children. It is interesting to note that a similar developmental progression of stresses in families of autistic children was found by DeMyer in Indiana. Since these stresses are discussed at length by DeMyer in Chapter 11, they will only be summarized briefly here. Stresses include the negative impact of the child on the parents and family, parental concerns for the "survival" of the child and the family, and finally the survival of the child in the community. Mothers of very young autistic children focused on constant caretaking demands, lack of sleep, and concern for the physical survival of the children who might run into streets or get up and wander in the middle of the night. As children got older many of these problems abated, and management problems shifted from survival to self-help issues, difficulties with the children's behavior in public, and attempts to maintain some semblance of normal family functioning or family survival. Management problems with older children, although less frequent, took on greater importance because of the increasing physical size and strength of the children and the decreasing strength and energy of the mothers. If physical aggression became a problem in adolescence, this had the potential for acute family crisis unless parents were highly skilled or help was available. As children grew older and larger, parents also noted less community acceptance of deviant or bizarre behavior and began to worry about the child's survival in the community.

Concern about the adolescents' sexual problems such as masturbation, and, for mothers of girls, self-care in menstruation and fear of pregnancy also emerged. Other parents, however, noted that they would probably worry about a daughter's becoming pregnant even if she were not handicapped. Still others spoke of adolescent problems such as alcohol and drugs that they would never have to face with their autistic children.

Child Age and Family Stress

One of the clearest findings of this initial research was that older autistic children (9.5–19 years, N = 20) were more stressful than younger autistic children (4–9.5 years, N = 20). This was true even though families in the younger and older groups did not differ in terms of socioeconomic status, number of children in the family, hours of maternal employment, the children's mean IQ scores, or the adequacy of both formal and informal supports discussed below. Age continued to be a significant factor even when other family stresses, mother's age, and the degree of the children's dependency were taken into consideration.

A clear difference between parents of older and younger children was a greater realism and pessimism regarding the child's eventual outcome. As Marcus (1977) has pointed out, parents of young autistic children often focus on the child's lack of language and assume that when the child learns to communicate all will be well, if only the parents work long enough and hard enough. By adolescence the permanency of the child's handicap is apparent and early hopes for normalcy give way to concern about care for the child when the parent will no longer be able to provide such care. More than two-thirds of the parents reported worries about what would happen to the child when they got older. As the child approaches the upper limit of school eligibility, the immediacy of the future looms large.

Almost half the total group of parents (N = 40) felt that caring for the autistic child had limited the growth and development of some family member, usually themselves. Slightly fewer than half the mothers reported that they had to give up an education or a job because of their autistic child. These concerns were more common among parents of older children because of the greater length of time involved and the increased difficulty of finding child care for older children. Concerns about lost opportunities for employment and education are also common among parents of non-handicapped adolescent children (Sheehy, 1976).

A significant difference was found between parental perception of

Table 1

Comparison of Mean QRS Scale Scores for Mothers of Autistic, Down's Syndrome, and Psychiatric Outpatient Children in the Bristol and Holroyd & McArthur Studies

QRS scale	Child's diagnostic category			
	Autism[a]	Autism[b]	Down's syndrome[b]	Psychiatric outpatient[b]
Parent Problems				
1. Poor health/mood				
$\bar{x}$	5.5	5.2	3.5	4.4
σ	2.9	3.1	2.4	3.3
2. Excess time demands				
$\bar{x}$	6.9	5.6	4.7	5.3
σ	3.2	2.2	2.9	4.0
3. Negative attitudes toward child				
$\bar{x}$	11.4	13.0	8.6	7.8
σ	4.0	3.6	4.1	5.3
4. Overprotection/ dependency				
$\bar{x}$	6.4	7.0	5.0	5.2
σ	2.4	2.6	2.4	2.7

QRS scale	Child's diagnostic category			
	Autism[a]	Autism[b]	Down's syndrome[b]	Outpatient[b]
Family Problems				
8. Lack of family integration				
$\bar{x}$	4.5	6.1	3.1	4.5
σ	3.1	4.5	2.6	3.2
9. Limits on family opportunity				
$\bar{x}$	3.2	2.3	1.0	1.8
σ	2.6	2.2	1.7	2.4
10. Financial problems				
$\bar{x}$	4.3	4.5	5.0	5.7
σ	2.8	2.9	2.7	3.3
Child Problems				
11. Physical incapacitation				
$\bar{x}$	3.4	3.2	2.1	1.9
σ	2.2	2.2	1.8	1.7

Lack of social support and related scales

5. Lack of social support				
$\bar{x}$	3.4	4.8	4.3	3.8
σ	1.4	1.3	1.2	2.0
6. Overcommitment				
$\bar{x}$	3.8	3.5	3.4	2.6
σ	1.0	1.1	1.3	1.5
7. Pessimism				
$\bar{x}$	3.8	4.6	3.4	2.6
σ	2.1	3.3	2.2	2.5

12. Lack of activities				
$\bar{x}$	2.3	2.7	1.2	1.7
σ	1.6	1.8	1.7	1.7
13. Occupational limitations				
$\bar{x}$	4.0	3.9	3.3	1.9
σ	1.2	1.0	0.8	1.8
14. Social obtrusiveness				
$\bar{x}$	2.6	2.8	2.2	1.8
σ	1.2	1.1	1.4	1.6
15. Difficult personality				
$\bar{x}$	19.2	18.5	12.7	13.0
σ	5.6	5.9	4.7	6.8

[a]Data from Bristol (1979).
[b]Data from Holroyd & McArthur (1976).

adequacy of available services for younger and older autistic children. As in studies of other areas of the country (Sullivan, 1976) parents reported a lack of vocational training, alternative community placements, and recreational programs for adolescent autistic children.

Stresses of Adolescence vs. Lack of Services

When discussing stress related to having an adolescent autistic child, it is important that a distinction be made between problems associated with adolescence per se and problems that are caused by lack of appropriate services. The mother of a 6-foot-tall adolescent recounted how her child had suddenly become assaultive both at home and at school. Instead of assuming that the behavior was an immutable characteristic of adolescence, the mother judged that it was probably her son's response to a new school program. The mother went to school, observed the program, and helped the teacher adjust the program downward to her adolescent's level and also developed a strategy with the teacher for responding to the assaults both at school and at home. In a short time the crisis passed and the assaultive behavior ceased.

Another mother, when asked if her son masturbated in public, replied that he used to, but that "That was not allowed in our home. He had to learn to go to his bedroom or bathroom to do that." The mother had received adequate parent training to be able to work with a teacher to successfully change the problem behavior. The need here was for adequate parent training in response to what is essentially a normal adolescent behavior. Many of the behaviors attributed to adolescence in handicapped children such as high rates of repetitive behaviors may be more accurately characterized as the result of inadequate programming and lack of activities for the child, not as problems of adolescence per se.

Burn-Out

Also apparent with a limited number of mothers of older children was a sense that the parents had simply "burned out." The parents had done as much as they could for as long as they could. If the child was not continuing to make progress and good services were not available, there was a sense that the mothers felt they could no longer justify sacrificing their lives for the autistic child. If the adolescent was doing well, the mother seemed to feel that any sacrifices she had made were worthwhile. If the child was not, the sacrifices appeared to have been in vain. This group represented a distinct minority and was usually comprised of parents living in isolated areas with few high-quality services available.

Other parents had also grown weary, but had not "burned out" because they were confident that if necessary they could find a suitable group home for the child which would provide independent living skills for the child and respite for the family.

Although all families of autistic children, particularly adolescents, reported stresses, most were functioning well and had not been destroyed by the presence of the autistic child. How were these people, these families, or their environments different from those families who had been overwhelmed or "burned out" by the real, chronic stress of caring for their autistic child?

Before attempting to answer that question, it is well to consider the growing body of data which helps us to understand how any family copes with serious stress, whether that stress is the presence of a handicapped child, physical illness, the stress of military separation, or natural disasters such as tornadoes and floods (Cohen & Lazarus, 1979; Hill, 1958; McCubbin, Dahl, Lester, Benson, & Robertson, 1976).

GENERAL FAMILY COPING WITH STRESS

For some time now sociologists have been attempting to determine what factors in families precipitate family crises in the face of stress and what factors provide families with the resiliency which makes them "crisis-proof." Although many questions remain unanswered, there are some conclusions that can be drawn about family coping after more than three decades of research.

First, it is clear that not every stressor, no matter how serious, causes a family crisis. Hill (1958) has proposed a classic, interactive model of family stress:

$$A \longrightarrow B \longrightarrow C \longrightarrow X$$

stressor	family resources	family perception of the stressor	crisis

In this model the family's crisis-meeting resources and definition of the problem mediate the family's ability to prevent a stressor event from creating some crisis in the family system. Although the severity of the stressor is important (Hill, 1958; McCubbin, 1979), what is equally important are the resources the family has to deal with that stress and the subjective definition the family makes of that stress. Clearly the past tendency of professionals to blame problems in families of autistic children on parental personality defects had the effect of increasing the potential for crises, and undermining coping efforts. It is also clear that successfully functioning families do not avoid the impact of the stress, but rather that they bounce back in a "roller-coaster" form of adjustment (Hill, 1949), first dealing with a period of disorganization, a period of recovery, and then a reorganization. It is not that these families are never depressed or never feel overwhelmed, but that these families somehow have the resiliency they need to begin over and over again. It is also clear that coping successfully is not simply an achievement of mastery at one point in time, but a process that continues, and changes over time.

SUCCESSFUL COPING IN FAMILIES OF AUTISTIC CHILDREN

How do these principles of family coping apply to families of autistic children, particularly families of adolescent autistic children, and what are the resources and definitions that affect families' abilities to function in spite of the awesome burden of caring for their child? Although we do not yet have unequivocal research results that directly answer these questions, based on our clinical experience, the general literature on family coping, and some preliminary results from our ongoing research we can speculate on the differences between crisis-prone or high-risk families and those seemingly crisis-proof or "invulnerable" (Ackerley, 1975) families which are somehow coping successfully with their autistic adolescent.

Child Characteristics

Among the key elements in whether families can cope is the severity of the stressor, i.e., characteristics of the autistic children or adolescents themselves. In our initial pilot study (Bristol, 1979) with 40 mothers of autistic children it was clear that the number of coping problems reported by mothers was significantly related to both the characteristics of the autistic children themselves and the adequacy of programming available to them. For the total group the best predictors of parent and family problems were the autistic family member's difficult personality characteristics including their management problems, their degree of dependency, and their need for assistance in self-help skills; and on the other hand a lack of activities, services, and prospects for independent living. These problems cut across all social classes, did not differ for black or white families, and were not related to the mother's age or the birth order of the child. Clearly, then, families with "easier," less dependent children and adequate services will be more able to cope successfully. Fortunately the types of child characteristics identified as related to stress are those that, within limits, can be improved through intervention. Access to activities and services is also something that is within our power to change. Characteristics of the autistic family members and their service environments alone, however, do not determine whether the family will be able to cope successfully.

Family Resources and Beliefs

The resources the family can muster in their day-to-day care of their autistic adolescent are also important. These include personal resources of the parents, resources of the family system, and active coping strategies that parents use to deal with the problems they are facing.

Personal Resources

As McCubbin (1979) and others have pointed out for successful family coping in general, families with resources such as adequate finances and good physical health will be more able to deal with additional stresses. Both McCubbin and his associates (1980) and Rabkin and Streuning (1976) suggest that more intelligent and better educated parents may be able to understand stressful situations better and may have more effective general problem-solving skills. While this is generally true for parents of autistic adolescents, these same families sometimes have higher vocational aspirations for their children and may be more stressed by the discrepancy between what they had hoped or imagined for their children and the reality of what the adolescents are able to accomplish as they approach adulthood.

Other personal characteristics such as self-esteem and a sense of having some control over one's own life have also been shown to influence a family's ability to cope with stress. (McCubbin, 1979; Pearlin & Schooler, 1978). In fact with successful parents of autistic adolescents both these qualities were evident in our pilot studies.

As parents became more realistic about their children, most seemed to become more optimistic and self-confident about themselves. They had survived the sleepless nights and the temper tantrums. They were justifiably proud of the skills they had succeeded in teaching their children. With the exception of those parents whose children had physically aggressive behavior, most parents reported that their adolescents were calmer and more responsive than they had been as young children. Most attributed these changes to maturation and special services, and to their own work with the child. Many of these same parents reported that they had once been shy and nonassertive, but now knew how to take on school boards, county commissioners, or state legislatures in order to get services for their children. These people knew that they were facing difficult situations, but they also knew that they had faced and overcome difficult situations in the past. They were effective people and they knew it.

In our TEACCH training we help parents become more effective in dealing with and obtaining services for their children. We are currently investigating whether such training increases parents' perception of control over their child's future and reduces stress (Devellis, Revicki, & Bristol, 1981).

Family System Resources

These resources for preventing family crisis include a family system's vulnerability to stress, its previous history of successfully overcoming problems, and the sources of support it has to draw on to meet its needs. Families with a moderate amount of cohesion and adaptability are generally less vulnerable to stress (Hill, 1949; McCubbin et al., 1980). The successful families of autistic adolescents described themselves as "close-knit," "able to roll with the punches," and able to adjust as the child's needs changed. Most important, they seemed able to laugh and somehow maintain their sense of humor and their larger perspective on life so that all of the family's financial and emotional resources were not expended only on the autistic child. These family resources are internal sources of support and crisis prevention. Sources of support outside the family are discussed below.

Coping Strategies

When we speak of stresses and resources in these families or even when we discuss personality traits such as self-esteem that affect the family's ability to deal with their autistic adolescent, the picture that emerges often appears to be a rather passive one. The parent seems to "be" a certain type of person who "receives" emotional support, advice, or assistance from others. In fact, as McCubbin and his associates (1980) have pointed out, effective coping is a very active process which includes not only what you are or what you receive, but what you actually do to deal with a stressful situation. It is a process that continues and changes over time and from situation to situation, one that will have to be studied over time before conclusions can be drawn about the ways in which parents actively cope with the realities of having an autistic adolescent. What we do know, as Cohen and Lazarus (1979) have pointed out, is there are at least two distinct types of coping strategies—those that attempt to change the stressful situation directly (instrumental) and those that help families minimize, tolerate, or ignore the stressful situation (palliative). These latter strategies do not change the situation itself but may affect the way parents cope with having an autistic adolescent. Although at this time we cannot empirically define effective coping strategies for families of autistic children (although such studies are underway), our clinical experience leads us to speculate on possible effective and ineffective ways of dealing with having an autistic adolescent.

Instrumental Coping Strategies. These action-oriented coping strategies are aimed at reducing stress by changing either the child or his environment. They include such things as learning new information and skills to help parents deal with their autistic adolescent, actually modifying the adolescent's problem behaviors through parent interventions, advocating for services needed by the adolescent, changing the adolescent's school or vocational placement, and being certain that any prescribed treatments for the adolescent are carried out at home.

Research at Division TEACCH has demonstrated that providing information and training parents to be co-therapists for their autistic children is effective in improving parents' teaching skills, reducing children's inappropriate behaviors, increasing functional skills, and preventing unnecessary institutionalization (Marcus, Lansing, Andrews, & Schopler, 1978; Schopler, Mesibov, DeVellis, & Short, 1981; Short, 1980) (see also Chapter 19). More recently (Bristol, Note 4) it has been demonstrated that this training for active involvement in their children's program is significantly related to reduced maternal stress. Becoming actively involved in the treatment process then is clearly an effective coping mechanism. Parents without such training may struggle inappropriately, too often interpreting the child's handicap as willful opposition, and expect the autistic person to shape up with overly severe discipline. This is a form of active involvement that is not effective, and leads not only to poor prognosis for the child but guilt and frustration for the parent.

Because a particular coping strategy may be effective at one time and not at another, the actual form of involvement that a parent should have in an intervention program depends on the particular parent, the specific child, and on the age of the child. As autistic children reach adolescence, parent training should be focused on helping the child become increasingly independent of the parent, a much different focus than one takes with a 4-year-old learning to approach his parents and make contact for the first time.

To be effective, then, we must ask not "What is the best way?" but rather "What is the best way of coping with this particular child at this point in time given a specific set of circumstances?"

Palliative or Intrapsychic Strategies. These coping mechanisms include both effective and ineffective attempts to minimize, tolerate, or ignore the stress of having an autistic adolescent. They include such processes as holding certain beliefs about the cause of the autism or about its outcome, taking medication such as antidepressant drugs, or holding more general views on life such as believing that you always have things to be thankful for, or finding alternate sources of satisfaction.

Parental Beliefs. Hill (1949, 1958) has pointed out the importance to family coping of subjective definitions or beliefs about the stressful event. For example, he points out that family crisis is less likely to occur in cases where the family believes the stressful event is due not to their own inadequacy but to circumstances outside the family (as in the case of natural disasters such as tornadoes) and the belief that others are in the same circumstances as they are. Previously parents were told they were the cause of their child's autism and they had few other parents in similar situations with whom to identify.

In our ongoing research we are examining the definition that parents give to having an autistic child before they receive any intervention or training. Some parents speak of the "burden" of having an autistic child and its cost to family progress ("Our family can never achieve what I'd hoped now that we have a handicapped child"). An alternative view sees the autistic child as a punishment for something someone in the family has done or as a proof of their inadequacy as parents ("If we had been better parents, my child would not have the problems he's had"). A third definition addresses the challenge of having an autistic child and the opportunity to learn new skills ("Caring for my child gives meaning and purpose to my life"). Depending on the choice of definition, the task of coping may be easier or more difficult.

Some parents' belief in God sustains them, leading some to believe that He will give them the strength necessary to carry on and that there is a purpose for all of their suffering. For others religion offers the promise that the child will be "healed," although this belief becomes less tenable the older the child gets. In both cases the parents feel that they are "not alone" and that having an autistic child has a higher meaning and an ultimate reward.

Palliative Actions—What You Can Do to Feel Better. We spoke above of actions directed toward changing the child or improving and accessing services and of parental beliefs that make having an autistic child more or less stressful. Here we include those actions that do not change the child's situation but are successful or unsuccessful in reducing stress. These include taking medications such as antidepressants, eating or sleeping more, shopping, or jogging. An important form of coping is developing interests and activities such as hobbies or a career that provide alternative sources of satisfaction and make the stress bearable. As the child reaches adolescence parents of both handicapped and nonhandicapped children may begin to have a sense of loss of career opportunities or time for hobbies. Those parents of adolescent autistic children who have been able to have interests of their own are more apt not only to be happier themselves, but to have encouraged their adolescent to be able to be less dependent on them and more prepared to face adult life. For parents to do this, however, the family must have had access to services such as child care and the adolescent must have opportunities to be away from home participating in school or community activities.

Support in High- and Low-Stress Families

Cobb (1976) describes social support as information leading the person to believe that he is cared for and loved, esteemed and valued, and part of a network of mutual communication and obligation. Cobb believes that meeting relational needs is more important in this type of support than the exchange of goods and services. In fact there is a rather extensive literature relating informal social support to a reduction in stress and improved health outcomes for persons dealing with other kinds of stress ranging from complications of pregnancy to unemployment (Cassel, 1974, 1976; Cobb, 1976; Eaton, 1978; Finlayson, 1976; Gore, 1978; Nuckolls, Cassel, & Kaplan, 1972).

In the pilot studies done at TEACCH, perceived adequacy of social support was one of the factors that distinguished the highest and lowest stress groups. In both the older and younger groups it was clear that some parents were coping with the strains of having an autistic child very well while others were overwhelmed by the stress. To try to understand the differences in these groups, the highest and lowest stress groups were compared (top and bottom quartiles, $N = 10$ in each group). Although there was a tendency for the highest stress group to have children who were older than those of the lowest stress group, this difference did not achieve significance. Age of the children alone, then, could not be the deciding factor in successful or unsuccessful coping. The highest and lowest stress groups were also comparable in terms of mother's age, family income, number of children in the family, percent of firstborn children, percent of children who were more severely autistic, and number of mothers who were employed outside the home. The groups differed significantly in characteristics of the children, their environments and school placements, mother's satisfaction with employment status, and perceived adequacy of informal support received.

The lowest stress group had children who had fewer difficult behavioral problems, more self-help skills, more activities and services available, and consequently better prospects for independent living. From a clinical perspective it is interesting to note that the child characteristics which separated the high- and low-stress mothers were not fixed characteristics but rather those that are amenable to intervention.

Some 80% of the lowest stress group had children receiving direct TEACCH services. The majority (70%) of the children in the highest stress group were receiving services in "regular" local special education programs which generally do not provide parent support services. Another striking difference between the groups which did not differ in terms of number of mothers employed outside the home was a substantial difference in the mothers' satisfaction with their employment status. In the low-stress group 90% of the mothers reported that they would choose their present employment status (either working or not working outside the home) regardless of the handicapped child. Only 20% of the mothers in the highest stress group felt that their employment status was unaffected by the autistic child. The issue apparently was not one of working or not working outside the home, but rather the matter of having some choice or control over that decision. That choice often depended on the availability of adequate child care.

Mothers in the lowest stress group reported the same degree of social support from their own children as mothers in the highest stress group, but considerably more support from husbands, both the wife's and spouse's relatives, friends, and other parents of handicapped children (8 of 10 of the highest stress mothers had relatives who were available but not helpful, so it was not simply a matter of dealing with "mobile" families).

Informal Support and the Adolescent

Informal social supports for families of autistic adolescent children may include both the immediate and extended family, friends, neighbors, and other parents of handicapped children (who form a unique category of friends and consultants). The adolescents' advanced ages, the reality of the permanency of their handicaps, and diminished community acceptance for bizarre or deviant behavior by someone nearing adult size may all affect the kind and amount of social support available to the adolescent's family.

The Spouse. Husbands may be less supportive than previously because the child is no longer making rapid improvement. The husband's fuller realization of the permanency of the handicap may also make him reluctant to invest heavily in the child or support the wife in her efforts to do so. (In some cases, however, the reverse is true. The wife may be suffering from burn-out and the husband may have developed a deep attachment for the child and be able to support his wife in her efforts.) Tavormina (Note 5) has described four styles in which fathers may relate to their handicapped children. Each of these styles was observed among the parents of autistic children. In the first style the father emotionally divorces himself from the child and leaves the care of the child entirely to the mother, involving himself completely in outside activities. Although the child does well initially, mothers in this situation are likely candidates for burn-out by the time the child is an adolescent. In a second form of adaptation both mother and father join together in rejecting the child. Children with this type of father "support" tend to be institutionalized regardless of the severity of their handicaps. (Only one possible case of this form of adaptation was observed.) A third and common form of adaptation, especially for parents of young children, is for both parents to make the child the center of the universe and subordinate all their needs and desires to the service of the autistic child. These parents are prime candidates for burn-out. By adolescence this type of adaptation would be expected to take its toll both on the marriage and on the siblings. A fourth style, and the one that seemed most characteristic of successful coping, was when the mother and father joined in mutual support of each other and the child, but maintained some semblance of a normal life and some sense of their own identities and needs. Parents who had achieved this sort of adaptation, and for whom adequate child services were available, seemed to be weathering the storms of adolescence rather well. This form of adaptation requires adequate support services such as child care so that parents, especially the mother, can meet her needs as well as the needs of her family.

Single parents of handicapped children experience greater stress than parents with spouses (Beckman-Bell, 1980; Holroyd, 1974). Mothers alone with adult-size autistic children may be physically unable to cope with them as they reach adolescence. The lack of an adult male in the home may precipitate residential placement of a child who might otherwise be able to continue living at home.

Siblings. Siblings of adolescent autistic children may be the only persons besides the parents and teacher who can handle the management of their autistic brother or sister. This may present an enormous source of support for parents and give them precious opportunities to shop and do other things without worrying about the autistic child. On the other hand as siblings themselves enter adolescence they may be more self-conscious about having an autistic sibling and less willing to be seen in public with the family. Siblings may be dealing with fears of having handicapped children themselves. Many parents expressed concern that siblings were now at an age to leave home themselves and that soon one of the parents' best sources of support would be gone. However, some parents reported that once siblings left home and had their own families they were more sympathetic and supportive than before, and helped the parent by caring for the adolescent children overnight or by taking them on special outings.

Extended Family. Although much has been written about the demise of the extended family, modern methods of communication and transportation make it possible to stay in touch with relatives who live considerable distances away. In addition, medical advances have increased longevity so that not only three-, but four-generation families may become common. Relatives outside the immediate family, including the child's grandparents, aunts, uncles, and cousins, are at least potential sources of support for families of adolescents.

By the time the autistic child reaches adolescence the pattern of acceptance or rejection by these relatives is often well established. The extended family may be either a valuable source of support or no longer an important part of the child's life. By this point more stressful relationships have often led to an accommodation where negative relatives are avoided. Parents who have received adequate training may also have increased both their skills and their self-confidence enough that insensitive remarks made by relatives are either frankly rebutted or ignored.

In our initial work it appears that families turn first for support to parents and then brothers and sisters, with neighbors being called upon mainly for short-term emergency situations. These family members provide not only the emotional support of an understanding confidant, but also actual physical care for the child, transportation, and in a few cases financial support. In some cases the autistic adolescent's cousins are the only peers he has ever really interacted with besides his own siblings outside structured settings like schools. One problem mentioned by a number of mothers of adolescents was that the size and strength of the adolescent combined with the increasing frailty of aging parents eliminated persons such as grandma from child care and left the mother without an important source of babysitting or respite care.

Other Parents of Handicapped Children—Friends and Consultants. Some parents of autistic adolescents interviewed had well-developed networks of support from other parents of handicapped children, especially from parents who had been involved with them in efforts to develop services in their communities. Some were active members in the National Society for Autistic Children and took pride in the services they had helped obtain. Those mothers of adolescents who are not in contact with other parents of handicapped children appear to be the most highly stressed. In addition to providing general emotional support and understanding, other parents of handicapped children appear to provide needed norms that indicate to parents that keeping their child in the community is important and that all of their efforts are worthwhile.

In addition to informal social support parents need formal support and services from community organizations and service providers.

Community Resources—Formal Support

Formal support is defined as assistance that is either social, psychological, physical, or financial, and is provided through an organized group or agency or for which a fee is paid. In general these formal organizations or agencies provide services directly to the autistic adolescent, although most also directly or indirectly serve the family's needs for maintenance and growth. The adequacy of these services is an important determinant of a family's ability to cope with the stress of their autistic adolescent.

When professional services are provided, it is generally assumed that these services are supportive of parents. This is not necessarily true, and, in fact, various authors (Schopler & Loftin, 1969; Turnbull & Turnbull, 1978) have noted that some such services might even be sources of stress for parents. Simply providing formal services, then, does not guarantee that they will meet parents' needs or will be helpful to them in coping with their autistic adolescents.

Since services needed by autistic adolescents are discussed at length in other chapters of the book, only a few service needs will be highlighted briefly here. The focus will be on those thought actually to affect the family's ability to cope with their autistic adolescent.

Educational and Vocational Training. The primary purpose of educational and prevocational and vocational programs is to increase the adolescent's social interaction and skills. However, the adequacy of such services also directly affects the family's ability to cope with the stress of caring for their adolescent. The family perceives that, in addition to providing the family with some much-needed respite from the adolescent, such continuing intervention efforts are necessary to help their adolescents develop the skills required to function independently when the parents are no longer able to care for them. This concern about the adolescent's future is a real and continuous one for parents and a significant source of stress. Such stress is greatly alleviated by the knowledge that the adolescents are receiving appropriate services or are being helped to reach their full potential whether the adolescent continues to live at home or in some alternative residential placement.

Parent Training. In a study of over 200 TEACCH families (Bristol, Note 1) parents consistently rated parent training and their children's intervention programs as among the three most helpful sources of support to them as parents. (Other consistently high ratings were reported for their spouses, their other children, summer camp, the wife's relatives, parent groups, and physicians. Some of these other choices will be discussed below.)

Although direct educational/vocational services are critical for the autistic child and adolescent, they are not sufficient to enable the family to deal with their autistic adolescents' problem behaviors or to provide continuity in their skill development. One hopes that long before their child's adolescence the parents will have received training in behavior management and in stimulating and maintaining language development, social interaction, self-help, and other independent living skills in their children. It is important that professionals and paraprofessionals in school and work settings have these skills, but in order for the family to be able to continue to function the persons most directly responsible for the adolescent, their parents, must know how to prevent problems from becoming family crises.

In the TEACCH program this training is usually completed long before the child approaches adolescence, but parents may call on the parent therapists when they need additional training or consultation for particular home or school problems, or for assistance in finding community or residential services. (See Chapter 19 for a more detailed description of TEACCH services.)

Medical and Dental Care. Although some parents have had unfortunate experiences with both physicians and dentists, both groups received generally high ratings from North Carolina parents of autistic children. Experience with developmentally disabled children is gradually becoming an accepted part of some (but not all) medical and dental training. When asked in what way these groups were helpful, parents replied "He took my child." In some cases parents were simply grateful to find someone who would care for their autistic child during stressful periods of illness or dental distress. In other cases parents were grateful for the understanding shown of the special needs of their child or even for the simple recognition that a problem existed and for referral to appropriate diagnostic and programming services.

Churches and Synagogues. One of the important sources of support expected, but not listed, in the top ten was services provided by churches or synagogues. Churches were consistently ranked in the bottom third in all three studies. Although some parents spoke of the importance of their personal religious beliefs in coping with their autistic child (and even believing that the child would ultimately be "cured"), few parents rated organized religion highly. Parents commented that at least in churches or synagogues they had expected their children to be accepted. Few spoke of a place in the liturgies for their autistic children or even a tolerance for noisy or bizarre behavior. Parents often reported a gradual decrease in church attendance as the child got older and more conspicuous.

Respite Care. Some form of periodic or regular respite care may mean the difference between family crisis or residential placement of the adolescent and the continued maintenance of the child in the community. Tavormina and his associates (Tavormina, Ball, Dunn, Luscomb, & Taylor, Note 6) have demonstrated with families of other handicapped children that even a 2-week respite provided by a camping program improved mothers' mental health and made them more capable of coping with their children on their return. The less adequate available educational/vocational and recreational services are for the adolescent, the more critical respite care becomes.

Parent Groups. In the TEACCH study cited above mothers listed parent groups as one of the top ten sources of help to them. In organizations such as the National Society for Autistic Children parents exchange information and advice with other parents of autistic adolescents, find the support of a group that values their efforts on behalf of their children, and also participate in generating and maintaining high-quality services for their adolescents through advocacy and political action. The benefits to the autistic adolescents are obvious. Less obvious perhaps is the opportunity such collective action provides for the parents to overcome the feelings of helplessness that having a severely handicapped child often brings.

Alternative Living Arrangements. Unfortunately, in our zeal to prevent autistic adolescents from living in the institutional warehouses of yesteryear we may have also communicated to parents that anything other than home care is proof of lack of concern or caring. As pointed out by Lettick (Note 7) in a position paper for the National Society of Autistic Children, parents of most autistic adolescents, like parents of all adolescents, have a right to expect that their children will some day achieve a measure of independence and live apart from them. For most this will mean living in group homes or independent living arrangements in their parent's community (NSAC, Note 8). For others who do not have the luxury of appropriate community services this will mean placement in a residential setting at some distance from their homes. The important point is that parents, while continuing to advocate for appropriate community facilities, are forced to make decisions that take into consideration not only the needs of the autistic adolescent but of the entire family. Any such decision, whether to keep the adolescent at home or eventually to place him in an alternative setting, is made with thought and much pain. No one placement is appropriate for all autistic adolescents and parents must not be made to feel guilty for choosing what is for them the best of the available options. In any case, whether the adolescent or adult will continue to live at home or in an alternative setting, the development of independent living skills is necessary so that he can enjoy the maximum amount of independence possible.

Other Services. Social, legal, and public health services among others are also available for families of autistic adolescents. In the North Carolina sample, however, these services were generally seen as not available, not helpful, or too expensive for parents of autistic children. Some parents in remote areas were unaware of available benefits such as the North Carolina state tax deduction for the home care of their handicapped children or the possibility that their adolescents might receive benefits through such programs as Supplementary Security Income (SSI). The lack of coordination of different kinds of services for autistic adolescents makes it imperative that professionals stay current regarding services and benefits available in their areas. They can at least make parents aware of such services and, if possible, assist them in obtaining needed services and maintaining some continuity across service boundaries.

SUMMARY

Previous institutional programs for autistic adolescents have attempted and failed to adequately substitute for families. We need to find ways not to substitute for, but to support families in the care of their autistic adolescents in their homes and/or communities.

We need to interpret the problems of autistic adolescents in the context of the problems of normal adolescence and the life crises of the "normal" family life cicyle.

The stress of caring for an autistic child is both real and acute. Autistic children are more stressful for families than children with other types of handicaps. Older autistic children are more stressful than younger autistic children for a number of reasons, including parental realization of the permanency of the child's handicap, the lack of services for autistic adolescents, the conflict between the child's needs and the parent's own developmental needs, and the consequent risk of parental burn-out.

Whether the stress of having an autistic adolescent will result in family crisis and disintegration depends on personal and family resources, coping strategies available to the family, and both formal and informal support supplied by extended family and the community.

Coping strategies include both parental beliefs and actions which the parents can take either to change the autistic adolescent or his environment or to help them tolerate the stress involved.

The sources of parental stress which have been identified are not fixed or immutable characteristics of the child or his environment, but are characteristics amenable to intervention such as behavioral difficulties, lack of self-help skills, placement of the child in a nonsupportive classroom environment, and the lack of services leading to good prospects for independent living.

Some parents are coping well with the stress of having an autistic child. Many have gained confidence in their own ability to teach their children and to mobilize resources to provide services for them. Highest and lowest stress mothers differed on child characteristics amenable to intervention, adequacy of informal support, satisfaction with the mother's employment status, and in the child's placement in a supportive classroom environment.

There may be special problems in mobilizing support and services from spouses, siblings, and grandparents during the child's adolescent period, and community services may have to be developed to provide badly needed respite care. Other parents of handicapped children may be needed not only for emotional support, but as a norm group which communicates to the family that their efforts on behalf of their child are worthwhile.

Parents need social and emotional support, services to facilitate child growth and development, and services to enable the family itself to grow. The top ten sources of support named by parents of autistic and communication-handicapped children in our North Carolina sample were TEACCH parent training, TEACCH classroom services, spouses, the family's own children, other (non-TEACCH) special education and parent training programs, summer camp, the wife's relatives, physicians, and parent groups. Ratings of helpfulness of these sources were not related to a measure of social desirability.

Many problems which are attributed to adolescence are in fact due to failure to provide adequate services—both direct services for the child and support services for families. Autistic adolescents, like all adolescents, deserve an opportunity to grow toward independence from their parents. This requires prevocational and vocational training programs and alternative community living arrangements which are not presently available. There is no one best living arrangement for all autistic adolescents.

Parents are forced to make choices from available and less than optimal options. They need the support of professionals and other parents in learning about the options available and in obtaining the best available services for their autistic adolescent.

REFERENCES

Ackerley, M. The invulnerable parent. *Journal of Autism and Childhood Schizophrenia,* 1975, *5,* 275–281.

Beckman-Bell, P. B. *Characteristics of handicapped infants: A study of the relationship between child characteristics and stress as reported by mothers.* Unpublished doctoral dissertation, University of North Carolina, Chapel Hill, North Carolina 1980.

Bristol, M. M. *Maternal coping with autistic children: The effects of child characteristics and interpersonal supports.* Unpublished doctoral dissertation, University of North Carolina, Chapel Hill, North Carolina 1979.

Bristol, M. M.. & Gallagher, J. J. A family focus for intervention. In *Finding and educating the high risk and handicapped infant* (C. Ramey & P. Trohanis, eds.) Baltimore: University Park Press, 1982.

Burr, W. R. Satisfaction with various aspects of marriage over the life cycle: A random middle-class sample. *Journal of Marriage and the Family,* 1970, *32*(1), 29–37.

Caldwell, B. M., & Guze, S. B. A study of the adjustment of parents and siblings of institutionalized and noninstitutionalized retarded children. *American Journal of Mental Deficiency,* 1960, *64,* 845–861.

Cassel, J. C. Psychosocial processes and stresses: Theoretical formulation. *International Journal of Health Services,* 1974, *4,* 471–482.

Cassel, J. C. The contribution of the social environment to host resistance. *American Journal of Epidemiology,* 1976, *104*(2), 107–123.

Cleveland, D. W., & Miller, N. B. Attitudes and life commitments of older siblings of mentally retarded adults: An exploratory study. *Mental Retardation,* 1977, *15,* 38–41.

Cobb, S. Social support as a moderator of life stress. *Psychosomatic Medicine,* 1976, *38,* 300–314.

Cohen, F., & Lazarus, R. Coping with the stresses of illness. In *Health psychology: A handbook* (G. C. Stone, F. Cohen, & N. Adler & Associates, eds.) San Francisco: Jossey-Bass, 1979.

Cohen, P. C. The impact of the handicapped child on the family. *Social Casework,* 1962, *43,* 137–142.

Cox, A., Rutter, M., Newman, S., & Bartak, L. A comparative study of infantile autism and specific developmental receptive language disorder. II. Parental characteristics. *British Journal of Psychiatry,* 1975, *126,* 146–159.

Cummings, S. J., Bayley, H. C., & Rie, H. E. Effects of the child's deficiency on the mother: A study of mothers of mentally retarded, chronically ill and neurotic children. *American Journal of Orthopsychiatry,* 1966, *36,* 595–608.

DeMyer, M. K. Comments on "Siblings of autistic children." *Journal of Autism and Developmental Disorders,* 1979, *9,* 296–298.

Devellis, R., Revicki, D., & Bristol, M. Development of the child improvement locus of control (CILC) scales (Unpublished paper). Frank Porter Graham Child Development Center and Division TEACCH, School of Medicine, University of North Carolina at Chapel Hill, 1981.

Eaton, W. Life events, social support and psychiatric symptoms. *Journal of Health and Social Behavior*, 1978, *19*, 230–234.

Farber, B. Effects of a severely retarded child on family integration. *Monographs of the Society for Research in Child Development*, 1959, *24*, No. 71.

Finlayson, A. Social networks as coping resources: Lay help and consultation patterns used by women in husband's post-infarction career. *Social Science and Medicine*, 1976, *10*(2), 97–103.

Gath, A. Sibling reactions to mental handicap: A comparison of the brothers and sisters of mongol children. *Journal of Child Psychology and Psychiatry*, 1974, *15*, 189–198.

Gore, S. Effect of social support in moderating the health consequences of unemployment. *Journal of Health and Social Behavior*, 1978, *19*, 157–169.

Graliker, B. V., Fischler, K., & Koch, R. Teenage reaction to a mentally retarded sibling. *American Journal of Mental Deficiency*, 1962, *66*, 838–843.

Grossman, F. K. *Brothers and sisters of retarded children: An exploratory study*. Syracuse, N.Y.: Syracuse University Press, 1972.

Hill, R. L. *Families under stress: Adjustment to the crises of war separation and reunion*. New York: Harper, 1949.

Hill, R. Sociology of marriage and family behavior, 1945–1956: A trend report and bibliography. *Current Sociology*, 1958, *7* (May), 1098.

Holroyd, J. The questionnaire on resources and stress: An instrument to measure family response to a handicapped member. *Journal of Community Psychology*, 1974, *2*, 92–94.

Holroyd, J., & McArthur, D. Mental retardation and stress on the parents: A contrast between Down's syndrome and childhood autism. *American Journal of Mental Deficiency*, 1976, *80*, 431–436.

Levinson, D. J. *The seasons of a man's life*. New York: Knopf, 1978.

Love, H. *The mentally retarded child and his family*. Springfield, Ill.: Charles C Thomas, 1973.

Marcus, L. Patterns of coping in families of psychotic children. *American Journal of Orthopsychiatry*, 1977, *47*(3), 383–399.

Marcus, L., Lansing, M., Andrews, C., & Schopler, E. Improvement of teaching effectiveness in parents of autistic children. *Journal of the American Academy of Child Psychiatry*, 1978, *17*, 625–639.

McCubbin, H. Integrating coping behavior in family stress theory. *Journal of Marriage and the Family*, 1979, *41*(2), 237–244.

McCubbin, H. I., Joy, C. B., Cauble, A. E., Comeau, J. K., Patterson, J. M., & Needle, R. H. Family stress and coping: A decade review. *Journal of Marriage and the Family*, 1980, *42*(4), 855–871.

McCubbin, H., Dahl, B., Lester, G., Benson, D., & Robertson, M. Coping repertoires of families adapting to prolonged war-induced separation. *Journal of Marriage and the Family*, 1976, *38*(3), 461.

Nuckolls, C., Cassel, J., & Kaplan, B. Psycho-social assets, life crises and prognosis of pregnancy. *American Journal of Epidemiology*, 1972, *95*, 431–444.

Paluszny, M. *Autism: A practical guide for parents and professionals*. Syracuse, N.Y.: Syracuse University Press, 1979.

Pearlin, L., & Schooler, C. The structure of coping. *Journal of Health and Social Behavior*, 1978, *19*, 2–21.

Price-Bonham, S., & Addison, S. Families and mentally retarded children: Emphasis on the father. *The Family Coordinator*, 1978, *27*(3), 221–230.

Rabkin, J., & Struening, E. Life events, stress, and illness. *Science*, 1976, *194*, 1013–1020.

Rutter, M., & Schopler, E. (Eds.), *Autism: A reappraisal of concepts and treatment.* New York: Plenum Press, 1978.

Schopler, E., & Bristol, M. *Autistic children in public school,* an ERIC Exceptional Child Education Report. Reston, Va.: Council for Exceptional Children, 1980.

Schopler, E., & Loftin, J. Thought disorders in parents of psychotic children. *Archives of General Psychiatry,* 1969, *20,* 174–181.

Schopler, E., & Reichler, R. Developmental therapy by parents with their own autistic child. In *Infantile autism: Concepts, characteristics, and treatment* (M. Rutter, ed.), London: Churchill Livingstone, 1971.

Schopler, E., Rutter, M., & Chess, S. Editorial: Change of journal scope and title. *Journal of Autism and Developmental Disorders,* 1979, *9,* 1–10.

Schopler, E., Mesibov, G., DeVellis, R., & Short, A. Treatment outcomes for autistic children and their families. In *Frontiers of knowledge in mental retardation,* Vol. I (P. Mittler, ed.), Baltimore: University Park Press, 1981.

Schwirian, P. Effects of the presence of a hearing-impaired preschool in the family on behavior of older "normal" siblings. *American Annals of the Deaf,* 1976, *121,* 373–380.

Sheehy, G. *Passages: Predictable crises of adult life.* New York: E. P. Dutton, 1976.

Short, A. *Short-term treatment outcome using parents as co-therapists for their own autistic children.* Unpublished doctoral dissertation, University of North Carolina, Chapel Hill, North Carolina, 1980.

Sullivan, R. Autism: Current trends in services. In *Autism: Diagnosis, current research and management* (E. R. Ritvo, ed.), New York: Halsted Press, 1976.

Turnbull, S., & Turnbull, H. *Parents speak out: Views from the other side of the two-way mirror.* Columbus, Ohio: Charles E. Merrill, 1978.

REFERENCE NOTES

1. Bristol, M. M. *Sources of help for parents of autistic children.* Paper presented at the International Conference of the Society for Autistic Children, Boston, July 1981.

2. Gallagher, J. J., Cross, A., & Scharfman, W. *The characteristics of successful parents.* Unpublished manuscript, University of North Carolina, 1980.

3. Krause-Eheart, B. *Special needs of low-income mothers of developmentally delayed children.* Paper presented at the National Conference of the Society for Research in Child Development, Boston, May 1980.

4. Bristol, M. M. *Impact of handicapped children on mothers: Some research results.* Paper presented at the OSE Handicapped Children's Early Education Program / CEC Division for Early Childhood Conference, Washington, D.C., December 1980.

5. Tavormina, J. *Fathers and families of handicapped children.* Unpublished manuscript, University of Virginia, 1977.

6. Tavormina, J., Ball, N., Dunn, R., Luscomb, B., & Taylor, J. *Psychosocial effects of raising a physically handicapped child on parents.* Unpublished manuscript, University of Virginia, 1977.

7. Lettick, A. *On growing—up and away.* A position paper approved by the Board of Directors of the National Society for Autistic Children, Washington, D.C., 1974.

8. National Society for Autistic Children. *Community policy resolution.* A position paper approved by the Board of Directors of the National Society for Autistic Children, Washington, D.C., July 1981.

13

Growing Out of Autism

CLARA CLAIBORNE PARK

This chapter is about one autistic child, as she was and as she is today. It cannot be a case study—there is no room for that. It took nearly 300 pages to describe her first 8 years (C. C. Park, 1967). But because her earlier development has been described in more published detail than, I believe, that of any other autistic child (see also C. C. Park, 1977, 1978, 1982; D. Park, 1974; D. Park & Youderian, 1974), it should be of use at least to sketch her continuing progress as she has grown, not to young womanhood in any complete sense but into a person able to enjoy her life and to make a real contribution to her family and to society.

Progress it has been. These have been years of slow yet accelerating learning. Jessy Park—"Elly" in the published materials—unlike earlier generations of autistic children, was able to stay in school until she reached 22. The fact that the laws of her state guaranteed her that continuing education has been central to her progress. We all remember the years when special education stopped at 14 or 16, if it ever began, because people thought that children with mental disabilities had learned all they could learn by then. But Jessy was in her mid-teens before she began to learn *how* to learn, and the social and academic learning she's done since age 16, when in the old days her education would have been over, has been the most important of her life.

Psychologists talk about a "critical period"—we've heard, for instance, that a normal child learns more between birth and age 5 than in all the rest of its life. That might just be true of normal children, though I don't believe it; I'd argue with any psychologist that I learned more

CLARA CLAIBORNE PARK • Department of English, Williams College, Williamstown, Massachusetts 01267.

between 16 and 22 than I did between zero and 5. Certainly I learned far more between 37, when Jessy was 2 and I began to realize I had an autistic child, and today. For ourselves, and even more for our autistic children, the adolescent and adult years keep on being years of learning, if we can find the means to teach.

The severity of Jessy's symptoms was evident before she was 2. She was 3 when we first heard the word "autistic" from Dr. Sidney Gellis of Boston Children's Hospital. What he saw then was a classic case of infantile autism, displaying Kanner's symptoms with textbook exactitude: remoteness from persons, hyperreactivity to minute deviations in the environment, nonexistent social and verbal comprehension, lack of speech, marked retardation in general functioning. Even then she showed (though not to him) a grasp of abstract forms and systems that denied conventional retardation. She could match shapes and colors; she understood numbers unusually early; she could do a jigsaw puzzle as easily upside-down as right-side-up. Yet it was not easy to lure her to do these things, harder yet to extend them to wider or more useful competencies. The most frustrating of all her symptoms was the eerie inertia which held her from doing even the few things she could do. The core criteria of autism—abnormal responses to external stimuli, stereotyped automatic behavior (rocking, etc.), abnormal language development, abnormal affective contact—all were present, and crippling.

Today Jessy is 24, slim and shapely, but still with a child's transparency of expression. School is over for her, though learning remains a lifetime task. She has passed the state's minimum competency test, surprising us all—not only the basic mathematics, easy for her, but even (by a bare point) the reading comprehension. It was an extraordinary achievement for her and for her teachers, for when she arrived at the regional high school 9 years before, she could read only a few words, with massive resistance and doubtful comprehension, and her speech, still minimal, was intelligible only to those who knew her well. Her IQ then on the Wechsler Intelligence Scale for Children tested at 76 (66 Verbal, 92 Performance). Five years later, at 18, newly tested on the Wechsler Adult Intelligence Scale, it was recorded at 101–106 (Verbal 88–95, 119 Performance). Though the new numbers may be explained partially by the social progress which made her more accessible to testing, the increase in comprehension and the extension of reasoning capacity beyond the realm of shape and number are a clear tribute to the power of patient education.

But school is over and the IQ is only a number. Far more important than these achievements, *Jessy has a job!* With the help of vocational education, job counseling, and transitional CETA funding and employer backup (now no longer needed), she has passed the hurdle we feared so long would be too high for her. She works in the mailroom at Williams College, where in addition to sorting mail she processes the telephone billing for the entire college and even—most astonishing of all—is able to answer the phone. She handles her own growing bank account and has just received a raise. Technically this is not sheltered but ordinary employment; actually it is something in between, since her father and I teach at the college, it is within walking distance of home, and college offices tend to be staffed with friendly, understanding people who are willing to make allowances for the peculiarities of an efficient and reliable worker, especially one with a small child's simplicity and attractiveness. Nevertheless she is employed not because people are kind but because she is doing useful work, as well as anyone else could do it.

Jessy is home a good deal since her job as yet occupies her only 20 hours a week. She gets herself up in plenty of time for work, for she becomes anxious if she has to hurry; she doesn't like the sound of the alarm clock and doesn't need one. If her father or I have breakfast with her, it's for sociability, not supervision. She makes her bed, changing the sheets if needed, selects her clothes by her own accurate color sense, prepares her breakfast, and leaves the house on the dot, even if we're not there. At home she takes responsibility for much of the household routine: the laundry, the vacuuming, the garbage, making bread and yogurt, keeping the cookie jar filled. Though she leans toward desserts, she cooks entire meals too; recipes are the kind of straightforward reading she does best. She can repair a dripping faucet. She weaves on the loom she bought with her own earnings. She paints, with such vivid colors and unusual themes that she has sold many pictures.* Seeing this cheerful and useful member of our household, the long, inert years when she did nothing without inspired coaxing, and little enough with it, might almost be forgotten.

But not quite. Jessy is most at ease—and appears most normal— when there is work to be done. Painting can fill some leisure, and she can listen to her favorite radio station—although a stranger might be surprised to discover that she is listening more for the station call letters than to the music. But eventually she runs out of things to do, and if there are no companions to step in to encourage a new activity and share it, one can see that the old Jessy is still there, sitting on her bed, or rocking in a rocking chair (if we don't stop her, wildly and in the dark, often with smiles or laughter). Then the vision of what she might have been, what she might still become if the world abandons her, is made frightening real.

---

*For the poster of their 1981 international conference, the National Society for Autistic Children used a painting Jessy made when she was 13.

She wants companions now. She is even able to say that she is bored or lonely. She no longer tells people to go away, as she did in the years when she sat by the hour and sifted her "silly business," the bits of paper—often her own pictures—she had made into confetti. She says of an absent sister, "I am missing her"; when she hears a friend is delayed, "Oh no! When will Joan come back?" If autism retains its root meaning of "immured within the self," Jessy is not autistic any more. Recently we looked down from a plane and saw a small island with one house on it. We had been talking about the meaning of the word "isolated," for Jessy had become very interested in the words on her school vocabulary lists. So I said the house was isolated and that it would be lonely living there, but that it would be nice if you didn't like people. To which Jessy replied that she *did* like people.

And she does. When siblings or friends come back she is all smiles and hugs. She would hug acquaintances too, and the people who sometimes come to the house to meet her—hug them regardless of age and gender. She has had to be taught that a smile and a handshake are more appropriate. For all her progress, her comprehension of language, of gestures, of the social world is still in most ways simpler than that of a normal 7-year-old.

It improves, however. A measure of this is her steadily expanding capacity to enjoy simple films and stories, and to understand the necessary explanations. In her mid-teens she would follow a picture book of the kind one reads to 4-year-olds if the pictures were explicit and if there were no more than a sentence or two per illustration. Today she listens with attention to *Little House on the Prairie* and enjoys the matter-of-fact account of frontier life and family relationships. She neither could nor would read such a book alone. Reading is hard and reading stories harder; she does best with the literal prose and familiar subject matter of her cookbooks. But being read to is a richer educational opportunity than solitary reading—it is a social activity. We talk about the story. I read slowly, so Jessy can follow the print; eye and ear work together. Often I stop so she can read aloud the next sentence. We are both glad Laura Ingalls Wilder has written many books; the library now opens promising new avenues of learning.

Bizarre behavior, of course, has not entirely disappeared, nor has "evidence of bizarre thinking"—the phrase the psychologist used when he evaluated her 5 years ago, reporting that in 3 hours of testing he found none. That was certainly gratifying. But it was there, and still is. I expect he didn't talk to her about roads, or crickets, or about the click the refrigerator makes; he never discovered that each of the household appliances is inhabited by a "make-believe family" of "little imitation people."* Jessy still speaks haltingly and with effort; words are hard to find and sentences hard to put together. She has little ordinary conversation. But anyone who asks her about the little imitation people will get an earful. "Guess what! The oven is a make-believe family also! Noise of the oven same as the buzzer of the washing machine. This part of the family has only two children and both get married and one of them has children and the other don't. And there are four parts of the family. 'Member our family has two parts. Second part are my cousins. Stove has three sets of cousins. Some of the sisters and cousins and family are Karens [her favorite name]. There are two Karens in two different sets of cousins, and both didn't get married. Too young." Asked about the names of the other children, Jessy said, "I know one of them, but I don't want to tell you." Later, after looking at a children's book on astronomy, she extended the concept: "Every galaxy has lots of sun families. Know why I say that? Pretend the sun is the parent, and the planets are the children and the earth is me!" Then she sensed a difficulty: "But the sun is not married."

Jessy tells about the appliance families with glee. But a little imitation person can mean trouble. For years Jessy avoided saying thank you; pressed, she would swallow the words and avoid our eyes, so as not to encounter the imaginary hangman visible there, the little fellow who hangs from trees or is pinned to clotheslines (see Figures 1 and 2) or jumps lower or higher according to various formulas of conventional politeness. A "late politeness" or "double you're welcome" will no longer cause Jessy to cry as if—or rather, much more than if—she'd lost her last friend. But the word "cricket" can cause either smiles or dark mumbles, even tears, it's unpredictable which; Jessy insists she doesn't know why the value of the word changes. By extraordinary efforts, reinforced by the knowledge she cannot cry or mumble on the job, Jessy has brought the outward evidences of her bizarre thinking under control. It's many months now between the times when she shrieks like an inconsolable banshee; she does it only at home, and when she does, she gets it under control in minutes rather than hours. For our part, now that she can tell us about it, we see that the material of her "bizarre thinking" must always have been correlated to a far greater degree than we realized with her bizarre behavior.

Bizarre thinking must be controlled, even minimized. Yet to miss out on Jessy's bizarre thinking is to miss out on a good deal of her charm. Jessy smiles and laughs more a lot—more than most people her age.

---

*Compare the word "Lilliputian." Long ago we looked at the pictures in *Gulliver's Travels* together. It has been "little imitation people" ever since.

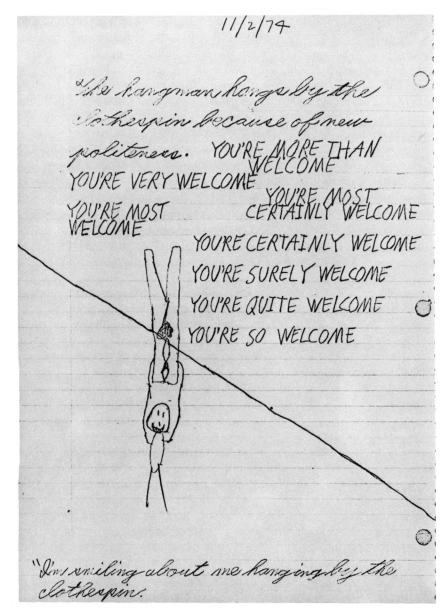

Figure 1. Drawing by Jessy Park at age 16.

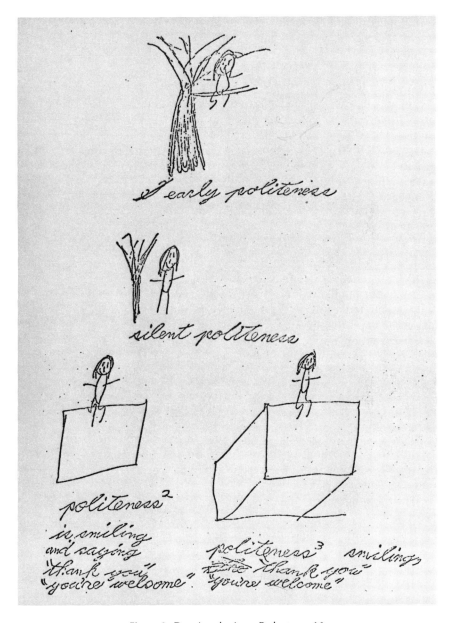

Figure 2. Drawings by Jessy Park at age 16.

Sometimes it's at "normal" pleasures. But often it's her secret, autistic smile at delights we can't understand, in realms of emotion where we can't follow. Though Jessy can at last tell us why she feels happy—or sad—the explanations don't explain. Who cares about "cricket," or the click of the refrigerator? Why, we normal people ask, should anyone feel joy at the sight of a road under construction so that the very sight of a construction project makes a hike worthwhile? "Three layers; pebbles, stones, tar! How about *four* layers?" Jessy hates what she calls " partly heard song." Why? She can explain that. "Partly heard song is just like 'I don't know'"—and she hates to hear "I don't know," though she often says it. It's absolutely logical if you accept the premises: the "un" of "unheard," says Jessy, is like "no," and "heard" is like "yes." So "partly heard" is to "unheard" and "heard" as "I don't know" is to "no" and "yes"—it's in between. That figures, and figuring is what Jessy's always been good at; she worked out the prime factors of all the numbers up to 1000 before she was 13. It figures, but it's not quite the same as making sense—our kind of sense.

I do not think anyone at work knows about the little imitation people who undoubtedly inhabit their calculators and electric typewriters, and I devoutly hope that in the unlikely event that her boss says "cricket" Jessy can keep her reactions under control. Yet we have not wished completely to bid farewell to these strange products of the imagination, especially as in their absence her conversation is flatly factual, limited, and uninteresting. One does not wish to encourage "bizarre thinking," yet to discourage it entirely is to sacrifice much of the individuality and charm which are among her greatest assets. In the adolescent years, however, it had to be discouraged since it led so often to behavior too bizarre to be tolerated in the social world she was increasingly able to enter. We were regretful but resigned to what seemed to be a necessary and permanent loss.

In the long years when speech was so limited, art had been one of our chief ways of communicating. Jessy between 8 and 14 produced literally thousands of consecutive pictures which she stapled into "books," presenting a curious, repetitive, yet attractive universe of rapid, stereotyped renditions of the adventures of herself, her family, and little imitation people among roads, dials, record players, numbers, clouds, and whatever else had mysteriously attracted to itself her emotional interest. We would spend hours together talking about them. While speech was still too much of an effort to be elicited by the commonplace events of normal life, the books could lure her to communication—but also to greater and greater elaboration of her bizarre obsessions.

At 14 Jessy arrived at the fine arts department of the regional high school, and for 9 years art was a continuing item in her Individualized Educational Plan. It proved easy for her to learn to draw from life and to execute assignments with increasing skill and refinement. Bizarre subject matter dropped entirely out of sight. She produced creditable still lifes, perspective sketches of rooms and buildings, even—on assignment—Cubist compositions. But these displayed no particular individuality beyond that conferred by her fine sense of design and color and her tendency to render her subjects from unusual visual angles (for more on her artistic development, see C. C. Park, 1967, 1978). Nor did she produce this sophisticated artwork spontaneously, as she had her "books"; it was done obediently, on demand, and in contrast to the books she had nothing in particular to say about it. Art apparently was something she could do, and do extremely well. But it did not interest her, and with regret we assumed that her naïve spontaneity of her earlier art had been sacrificed necessarily, if indeed she had not, as normal children do, simply outgrown it.

Not so. In the last 2 years the discovery that her painting can elicit substantial checks, those ultimate reinforcers, has brought an unprecedented surge of creativity. Jessy now uses her polished technique to communicate her vision of the objects which hold for her so much obscure meaning. Radio dials, railroad crossings, electric blanket controls, quartz heaters—and crickets—are now transformed into nearly abstract design elements and charged with a surreal intensity through the sense of color and form she possessed before she could speak and that she can now use to render her private preoccupations public. Jessy is a natural pop artist; in the singing colors of her acrylics the bizarre becomes both original and beautiful, and autism's stereotyped repetition becomes the artist's exploration of a theme. So we now hope that through art she can have it both ways—that she can keep in touch with the bizarre springs of her emotional life, yet without threatening her life in the normal world.

For that is the world into which, for 20 years, we've been trying to bring her. And most of her pains and pleasures now are like those of other people—less intense, certainly, than the joys and anxieties of her private universe, far less interesting to read about, yet reassuring in their ordinariness. Life for us all is full of commonplace annoyances—things break, the hot water runs out when we're in the shower. Jessy overreacts to these, but she now verbalizes instead of shrieking—progress, although the verbalization is always tending toward the ritualized and bizarre, as when she says, "Oh well about the water hang hang!" And life is full of ordinary pleasures that Jessy and we can now enjoy together—when Christmas brings friends or family home, when we or she make one of the patently untrue or impossible statements that are her idea of what's funny. ("Jokes, such as eating roads, a man has three arms, a house is upside down, and flowers are growing on a telephone, make me laugh.") Most remarkable of all to us is her pleasure when she's praised for one of her accomplishments. Once the surest way to cut short an activity was to notice it. For a long time after that she paid no attention. For the past 8 years, though, she has recognized praise and now she delights in it. "I'm proud of myself," she says, echoing a phrase we've taught her but a phrase she now thoroughly understands.

She has much to be proud of. There have been so many firsts in these years—the first time she answered a question with more than yes or no; the first time she spontaneously used speech to transmit information, putting words together to tell us something we didn't already know; the first time she greeted someone by name; the first time she used a third-person pronoun (more than 10 years ago, and she still can't do it reliably or with ease); the first time she used a past tense; the first time she answered the telephone and wrote down the message; the first time she bought groceries alone; the first time she swam the length of the pool; the first time she noticed we were out of milk and *herself* took off downtown to buy it. Only when we think what it would be like to have to learn explicitly all those activities of normal life and language that people "pick up naturally" can we understand how much she has to be proud of. Her speech is labored and telegraphic, and syllables get garbled if there are too many of them—but still, she communicates what she needs to so that even people who don't know her can understand it. She's learned to control the more bizarre manifestations of her emotions; she doesn't flap her arms any more, or rock except in rocking chairs. Though when she's frustrated or displeased she still may mumble under her breath the tags of stereotyped phrases which have long since lost whatever meaning they once had for her ("cigar three, cigar three," "we go on," "in the morning"), she's trying hard and the mumbles are audible only to the alert ear. For perhaps the most important thing she has learned is to make an effort, and to persevere. The disappearance of the inertia, the "willed weakness" that was the most frustrating and pervasive of her handicaps, was an unexpected side effect of a behavior-modification program that will be described latter in this chapter. Jessy is still gravely handicapped in language, behavior, and social comprehension. But the long years of refusal are over. "If at first you don't succeed, try, try again." What she once echoed, she now practices and understands. She no longer must be lured into action or into learning. She will do what she can.

How did she reach this point? Through the hard work of many people. Jessy has had no therapy from professionals in psychiatry or psychology, but education is therapy. At school and at home Jessy has been surrounded with teachers.

I need not describe her school program to those familiar with the materials and methods of primary and special education. It was some time, however, before Jessy had the benefit of the systematic application of those methods. Mandatory public education for the "emotionally disturbed" did not arrive in our state until Jessy was 13, and since we wanted above all to keep her at home with us, we could not bring ourselves to send her to a residential school. So for years she was in school for no more than 2½ hours a morning—for 6 terrible months in her 10th year, not even that long (C. C. Park, 1977). At last at 14 Jessy entered the regional high school where she was to remain until she was 22, in a full day program focused on spoken and written communication, comprehension, and social behavior. She was able over the years, with the help of understanding teachers, to take not only art but gym, sewing, cooking, typing, office skills, and bookkeeping with normal children.

She did not make friends among them, though some of them were very nice to her. Even now she makes few social initiatives on her own. At school it seemed to make little difference to her if she had lunch alone or with others; she could understand little of teenagers' rapid conversation and none of their concerns. Only in the last years of school—she was already 20—did she acquire a friend in the conventional sense, her first and only peer relationship, with a frail, childish, but very sociable boy from her special class. Joe comes every Sunday to play records; sometimes he takes Jessy for a walk to visit one or another of the old ladies whom he calls *his* friends. (They mumble, Jessy reports.) They giggle together; he too likes radio call letters. She looks forward to his visits.

But over the years she has had another kind of friend. Today she no longer needs a live-in companion, but for years, especially after her sisters and her brother moved on to college and left the house empty, we had an extra daughter, a young woman living with us to provide the stimulation and practice in social living that comes so much more naturally from somebody young than from increasingly middle-aged (and tired) parents. I lost count of them when the number passed 20. Jessy calls them her friends, and they are—the dearest and most devoted of friends. She doesn't call them her therapists, but they are that too—the most devoted and resourceful of therapists. In Jessy's early years her family were her primary therapists and teachers. It was her good fortune, and ours, that we found such friends to take over the work of helping Jessy so as to keep our home a place of learning even when we grew tired of teaching.

It is these young women who more than anyone else have been responsible for her continuing progress. I could not even hope to list all the things they taught her—most of the things she does today, readily and easily, she learned to do with them. It is they who taught her to buy groceries downtown, to wash up after cooking, to answer the phone; they too taught drawing and painting. They taught her to bicycle and ski, to mend her clothes—the list is endless, and built into each item has been the continuing expansion of speech and social comprehension which remains her chief, permanent task.

Companions, therapists, *friends*. For all those years Jessy was unconscious that most people do not hire friends—unconscious too that devotion and imagination like theirs was beyond what any money can buy. But a couple of years ago for the first time she asked a question about that—another measure of progress. Jessy had noticed—finally—that the college girl who has replaced the live-in companions picked up a $10 bill for the two afternoons a week she came. "Why don't *I* get paid for being Joe's friend?" she asked. We told her that it was because the friends who got paid were teachers too, and reminded her of some of the things they'd taught her and what hard work it had been sometimes when she'd shrieked or even hit them. She wasn't Joe's teacher and so she didn't get paid. That satisfied her; simple, matter-of-fact explanations usually do. Friends who teach are paid; others not; both are precious. It has been through friends who teach, both at school and at home, that the needs addressed in the earlier chapters of this book—educational needs, language needs, recreational and leisure needs, social and interpersonal needs—have been met.

What have we learned? From an experience that has changed our lives so fundamentally, the temptation is to answer "Everything." But to keep my answers practical rather than metaphysical I will try to be specific.

We have learned how useless intellectual progress is without social development. Of course we knew this. Long before Jessy was even thought of my grandmother had used to say to me (to my intense irritation), "Be good, sweet child, and let who will be clever." But we are a family of intellectuals—even my grandmother was rather more clever than good—and in the years when there was little to rejoice in it was natural to rejoice in Jessy's square roots and prime numbers. But one cannot live in a world of prime numbers. It helped put things in proportion when we met, as we sometimes did, other autistic young people who were intellectually far more advanced and fluent in speech than Jessy, but whose demeanor and behavior made it unlikely that anyone would enjoy spending much time with them. Unquestionably Jessy has intellectual capacities which have not been developed. She has learned far less mathematics than she could have. She could have gone farther in algebra. It is possible that she could have learned to work with computers; perhaps she would have if the right friend had come along. Though I regret a possibility left unpursued, I do not regret that instead of mathematics Jessy's energies, and theirs, went into the development of as attractive a human being as the circumstances allowed.

Friendliness is learned among friends and social behavior in society. Such learning is what is making it possible for Jessy to work in the mail-room today—more broadly, for her to remain in the community. And this is another thing we've learned: that ordinary members of the community will be extraordinarily helpful when they know how much they too contribute to Jessy's development. Storekeepers, bank clerks, checkout girls, no less than those in more formal positions, will be patient, smile, make allowances—if the behavior they see is not too disruptive or bewildering. They will smile out of the goodness of their hearts, and once they involve themselves they will smile because they see progress and are pleased at their part in it.

Somewhere here among the lessons learned belongs what in fact belongs everywhere: a recognition of the supreme importance of gaiety and laughter. There is no more useful a teaching tool in dealing with the autistic than a kind of rollicking high spirits. "Assume a virtue if you have it not." If you don't feel like laughing, ham it up anyway. Jessy's cheerfulness is one of her great charms. Laugh and the world laughs with you. We have learned that to add glumness to disability is to double a handicap's crippling power. There is a sense in which the most important thing Jessy ever learned was to smile and say hello.

How did did she learn to do this? Certainly a cheerful household contributed. But it was by no means enough. And this brings me to another lesson of Jessy's adolescent years less obvious than the previous ones— one which we were unprepared for. A friendly, cheerful world may have helped Jessy be cheerful and friendly (and I should note that even in babyhood she had a happy disposition within her autistic stronghold). Nevertheless, however we coaxed and encouraged, she did not in fact learn to greet another human being until she was 14 years old. She learned it not through imitation or osmosis, but through a behavior-modification program. The power of these new teaching methods, so much more flexible and more widely applicable than we had thought, is certainly one of the things we learned. But that was scarcely a discovery, except to us who had delayed so long to learn to use them. The real discovery was the shallowness of that inertia and negativism that we had thought so profound, and for so many years regarded as the core of Jessy's condition.

Jessy learned to say "Hello, Mrs. Jones" via an ordinary, scorekeeping golf counter, available at any sporting goods store. "Hello" earned her one point; eye contact, another; the proper name, a third. "Hello, Mrs. Jones" . . . and people at school began to report their astonishment. Jessy was suddenly so much more friendly. Of course they were all smiles, greeted for the first time after Jessy had so long ignored them. Social reinforcement could hardly have been stronger or more naturally delivered. It was some time before they noticed the click-click-click of Jessy's counter.

This was only one of many behaviors which could gain or lose points. Jessy kept track of them all, with autistic literalness. Autistic people don't cheat. We had stumbled onto the system by accident; Jessy had seen the counter on a visiting child, been fascinated by an instrument that combined two of her strongest interests, clicks and numbers, and decided she wanted one of her own. Only slowly did we discover how to use it, to utilize her strengths—her exactitude and thoroughness, her grasp of numbers—to address her weaknesses. Through points Jessy was actually able to begin to control the aggressive behavior which in this passive child had never before been a problem, but that had begun to surface as school put more demands on her. (Hitting carried a massive penalty—minus 100.) Through points, and the exact specifications made necessary by the weekly drawing up of the behavioral contract, such abstract concepts as "helping" began to take on a little meaning, teaching her what helping might consist of, and showing us what we should have known, that this 14-year-old girl had no idea of the content of even so obvious a social concept as this.

Clicking up 100 points earned a popsicle, but it was not until the day that Jessy racked up 167 that we realized that the system was its own reward. We watched in amazement as Jessy, via our homemade behavior-modification program (for more details, see D. Park, 1974), rapidly acquired a large repertoire of new behaviors and eliminated others we had assumed we must live with forever, spurred on by something no more concrete than a rising tally. (Years later, she was to watch with the same satisfaction the rising balance in her bank account.) It now seemed necessary to conceptualize the whole matter of Jessy's inertia and passivity differently. For all those years Jessy had done so little and refused to do so much. For example—one of thousands—she could set the table efficiently at 7, but who had the patience or the stamina to get her to do it? "Willed weakness," I had called it. Yet now that she had a reason to make an effort, she did. For a popsicle! For points on a counter! The realization, when we arrived at it, seemed ridiculously simple: Jessy had never had a reason to make an effort before.

The normal child has any number of reasons why it wants to make an effort, to grow, to perform the myriad tasks of development. They are social reasons, rooted first in relations with its family, and later, as it grows, with peers. Talking, perhaps, is biologically programmed; certainly it requires undamaged speech centers in the brain. But beyond any natural unfolding the baby has social reasons to pay attention to the sounds its mother makes, to make sounds in return, to practice and refine them, to notice what effects those sounds produce. It knows its mother and wants to talk to her. It imitates naturally, as Jessy did not. But it also has reasons to imitate; it wants to sweep just like mommy, to button its own coat the way Johnny does, to use the toilet like daddy, it wants not to be a baby anymore. It has reasons to do things and reasons to refrain. As it grows, parents and teachers exhort it not to pick its nose, not to scratch in embarrassing places. Children learn to inhibit these natural activities because they have good reason to. They know adults will scold; more important, they know that their peers will think they're gross.

> Cinderella, dressed in yellow,
> Went downtown to meet her fella.
> On the way her britches busted,
> How many people were disgusted?
> One, two, three, four . . . .

But Jessy was immune to emulation or embarrassment. Of all these natural motivations for activity and growth, not one had any meaning for her. Yet the developmental work she had to do was far harder than a normal child's: not only to acquire ordinary self-help behavior, but above all to surmount her communications handicap, to attend to speech and practice it, and to control her bizarre anxieties and the bizarre behavior that accompanied them. Why *should* she try to do these things?

We had constructed the concept of an autistic refusal of experience. Yet how deep is a refusal which can be melted with a golf counter? As we watched external reinforcers supply the motivation which had so long been lacking we learned the culminating lesson: that external rewards— and penalties—can bring about internal changes. For Jessy now enjoys praise; she would rather be active than idle; and the counter has been shut away in a drawer for 7 years.

Now that Jessy has learned to try the formal contract is no longer necessary. If a behavior which threatens social integration does not respond to ordinary approaches, money substitutes for points; the mere agreement on a possible fine is so effective that she hardly ever actually has to pay up. (She enjoys setting fines for us too, since our behavior, too, now and then leaves something to be desired.) And we continue to apply another lesson the contract first taught us: Jessy can grasp a social concept only through clear specifications.

Two years ago, for example, one of the young companions set a new goal for Jessy: "thinking of others." Together they specified a few things that might consist of, all very concrete. It has not worked a miracle; it has not given her insight into how people think or what they are feeling. You have to *tell* her you are sad, and her ritualized "I hope you will feel better" is not really very comforting. But recently she told me with pride that she was making tapioca with nutmeg instead of cinnamon because "you like that better," and she puts on classical records for me at lunchtime "because you don't like rock music." She is thinking of others in the only ways she knows how.

Does she know she's different? Does she care? Not yet, I think. She knows about physical handicaps; she talks about them freely and cheerfully, mostly to recall the rule she's been taught—that you don't talk about people's handicaps unless they mention them first. Never has she shown the slightest indication that she's made the generalization from physical to less visible handicaps, that she feels herself to have anything in common with our friend with only one arm, or the tiny, dwarfed ladies who keep the store where she sometimes buys milk. A mental handicap in fact is a perfect example of the kind of social generalization Jessy's mind has such difficulty forming. Jessy knows she has trouble talking and controlling her behavior—that it has taken her a long time to learn to do these things and that she still has to work hard at them—harder than other people. That's the way we've presented her difference to her. But the comparison with others is ours, not hers. To feel your own difference and suffer because of it you have to form a concept of what other people are like, what they expect, what they do—not what autistic people are good at, even when their IQs average out as high as Jessy's. Last year, doubtless thinking of his thick cataract glasses and frail body, Jessy remarked unexpectedly, "I think Joe is handicapped." I said that he was, and that there were all sorts of handicaps, some in the body and some in the mind, and that some people would call her own difficulty in talking and behaving a handicap. This was obviously a completely new idea; she gave it her full attention for a minute or so. It seemed to arouse surprise rather than feeling. The subject hasn't come up again; if it does, we can elaborate on the idea as seems best—perhaps even teach her a new word, "autism."

Will she ever leave home? Or will she live with us, a help and a sunny presence much (not all) of the time, and move when we are gone to the sisters and brother who say "Of course she'll always have a home with one of us"? We have never wanted that to be necessary, and as the number and quality of group homes improves it very likely won't be. But Jessy has grown into an attractive person, with a simplicity and transparency that are very winning in this complex world. Her siblings, like her friends, genuinely love her. If we live 20 more years, Jessy will be 43 and they will be moving into their 50s. It no longer seems preposterous that in their busy professional lives they could find a place in their homes for an affectionate and industrious cook-housekeeper. For so many years Jessy absorbed so much of other people's time, energy, and attention. Now she is able to give—more and more. All we can know about the future is that she will continue to change and develop, if she continues to find people who will help her. That learning need never stop is for us the most important lesson of all.

REFERENCES

Park, C. C. *The siege*. New York: Harcourt, Brace & World, 1967. (2nd ed. with epilogue and plates), New York: Atlantic-Little, Brown, 1982. Translated as: *Histoire d'Elly*, Paris: Calmann-Levy, 1972; *Eine Seele lernt leben*, Bern: Scherz, 1973; *Het Beleg*, Baarn: Bosch, 1974; *Belägringen*, Stockholm: Aldus, 1975; "Isolated Elly," Tokyo: Kawade Shobo, 1976; *Et Barn bag faestnings mure*, Denmark: Gyldendal, 1977, *Beleiringen*, Oslo: Gyldendal, 1978; *Ciudadela Sitiada*, México: Fondo de Cultura Económica, 1980.)

Park, C. C. Elly and the right to education. *Phi Theta Kappan*, 1977, *4*, 534–537. (Reprinted in R. E. Schmid, J. Moneypenny, & R. Johnston, [Eds.], *Contemporary issues in special education*. New York: McGraw-Hill, 1977.)

Park, C. C. Review of *Nadia: A case of extraordinary drawing ability in an autistic child* by L. Selfe. *Journal of Autism and Childhood Schizophrenia*, 1978, *8*, 457–472.

Park, D. Operant conditioning of a speaking autistic child. *Journal of Autism and Childhood Schizophrenia*, 1974, *4*, 189–191.

Park, D., & Youderian, P. Light and number: Ordering principles in the world of an autistic child. *Journal of Autism and Childhood Schizophrenia*, 1974, *4*, 313–323.

14

Parental Perspective of Needs

MARGARET AVERY DEWEY

In moments of strength, when they are not so overwhelmed that they crave only sympathy, parents of autistic adolescents realize that what they want is understanding and help. Whose understanding? Everyone's—the teachers', the neighbors', the corner policeman's, and the therapists'. What kind of help? Practical help that meets the unique needs of their autistic son or daughter.

From the perspective of a parent of a 33-year-old autistic man, this is how I now view the needs of an adolescent with autism. Basically, he* has the needs of every human being. The difference for an autistic person is in ease of attainment. These basic needs are: a place to live, bodily nurture, joy in living, self-esteem and acceptance, and freedom from suffering and abuse.

Adolescence is a tortuous pathway at best. Most of us manage to follow it to independence with a little guidance, but autistic individuals need more than a little help. Unexpected impediments, like great boulders, seem to crash in their way. If, after tremendous effort, they succeed in climbing over one block, they are next likely to stumble into a hole because they were watching for rocks, so to speak. Lessons learned in one crisis are seldom adapted to a different situation.

When our autistic son Jack was a teenager we were absorbed in helping him get along in school and at home. We assumed he would learn

---

*I will use the masculine pronoun for ease of style. This suits the gender of my primary example, and the fact that there is a 3:1 preponderance of males over females with the disorder of autism.

MARGARET AVERY DEWEY ● Special Education Materials author, 2301 Woodside Road, Ann Arbor, Michigan 48104.

what to do in different settings as our other children learned, by a sort of social osmosis. Watch, listen, imitate, consult, experiment, adapt, and refine. Now I realize that the malfunction of autism seriously impedes social learning, just as it delayed the acquisition of Jack's speech to age 4½. Furthermore the quality of an autistic person's social behavior is often eccentric. This too is true of their speech. Jack was echolalic in the beginning, and now his contributions to conversation are likely to be pedantic monologues.

I use Jack as an example because I know him, not because he is a typical autistic person. The fact that he was able to remain in a public school system until he graduated from high school puts him in the "high-functioning" group. Yet it was not an easy trip for him, for us, or for his teachers. Readers who like to compare IQ scores can puzzle over this. Generally, Jack tested to have an IQ of about 83. The year he was 10, however, it jumped by 28 points. When I asked him whether the test had been easier than usual, he replied that it was the same test he had had the year before. He had remembered the questions and pondered them during the year. On a fresh test he was again near 80.

I now believe that autism, like retardation and cerebral palsy, comes in degrees of severity. In addition, each individual afflicted with autism has a unique personality. What is misleading is that a disability is likely to evoke similar reactions in different people. We do not assume that blind people are all alike because they all make use of touch and sound to compensate for lack of vision. Aside from their reaction to blindness, they are different.

Observing Jack and other autistic adolescents during the past 10 years has helped me make recommendations which can be applied, with modifications, to autistic people who are more or less severely handicapped than our son. Methods of guidance which worked for him would not be effective for every autistic person. Yet I was much helped by contact with parents who showed me that certain attainments were possible within the framework of autism. It remained for us to test by trial and error how far our son could go. Thanks to the example of Fran Eberhardy (1967) we had the courage to support Jack's desire to learn piano tuning. He now makes his living tuning pianos.

Returning to the basic needs I listed earlier, let me list some questions we should have asked long before we did so of necessity. These questions apply to an autistic person of Jack's level of competence. Autistic adults who live in a sheltered environment will have some assistance in achieving the first two needs. For their parents, however, finding a suitable placement is a major obstacle. There are not enough places to begin to meet the need for good residential care.

A Place to Live. If he wants to move away from home, will he know how to go about it? Can he locate safe, affordable quarters? Can he maintain his place, keep it marginally clean and free of incapacitating clutter? (Comparable questions parents of a less able child might ask: Where will he live as an adult? Is he learning skills which will make him an asset in a group living situation? Is he being rewarded for good control of antisocial impulses?)

Bodily Nurture. Does he know how to shop wisely for food? Can he prepare it for eating and keep it from spoiling? Is he sensitive to his own body signals and responsive to the need for sleep, nourishment, and medical care? Is he aware of the benefit of physical exercise to emotional and physical health? (Comparable questions for a less able child: Will there be people near him who understand his signals and signs of hunger, weariness, and sickness? Is he learning to enjoy physical activity, and will he continue to exercise?)

Joy in Living. Does he find pleasure in some daily activities? Does he know the joy of accomplishment? Does he know how to modulate recreation to include both exercise and passive activities, neither to excess? Does he have friends?

Self-Esteem and Acceptance. Is he content with the way people treat him, on the whole? If not, how does he react to rejection? Can he be philosophical? Does he have a realistic awareness of the many different ways human beings relate to each other, varying in different situations? Is he able to recognize hints and accept them as valuable guidance rather than insults?

Freedom from Suffering and Abuse. Does he know how and where to seek help when he is in distress? Can he sense trouble, and take the necessary steps to avoid serious consequences? Is he aware that some variations in physical and mental well-being are normal rhythms, not cause for alarm?

I omitted love from the list of basic needs because it has been overburdened with the responsibility for solving all problems. True, deep mutual affection between human beings adds much to the joy of living. Benevolent love is tied to acceptance. People may suffer for lack of love. But by itself love is a word of no specific meaning which is too often promoted as if it were a mulching blanket which keeps down noxious weeds and releases nutrients.

Parents who count on the magic of love to cure autism suffer inner anguish when their child fails to bloom on schedule. "Haven't we loved enough?" they wonder. For a while they try harder. Ultimately the dissonance can only be resolved by shifting blame to the child, saying, "We loved, but he failed to respond."

This is destructive. It creates a rift between parents and child where partnership is urgently needed. The burden of the autistic disability is so great that it calls for the cooperative effort of many people working toward realistic goals. Pride in progress ought to be mutual, not competitive. Everybody deserves a share of the credit when goals are attained. The child, especially, needs clear recognition for his effort. If a child is being blamed for failing to respond to the cure-all, love, what credit does he get for going through countless hours of lessons, therapy, and behavior modification? How can he gain any confidence that he is worthy of the love being offered?

Let me now elaborate on the problems autistic people meet when they try to satisfy basic human needs. You will then understand the purpose of my guidance questions.

A PLACE TO LIVE

When Jack said he wanted to move out of the family home he was 22, with his first steady job and a car. He had no training or experience in locating a place to live, and he wanted no help from us. It was a time of turbulent relations between us, which he now asks us to forget, calling it "my adolescent rebellion." He could be right. Perhaps he reached that stage at a later age than our other three children. We know that turbulence can be a propellant. By the time an adolescent has determined to leave home and has secretly plotted the steps to independence, it is often too late for thoughtful discussions. During Christmas vacation of 1969 Jack told us he had found a room to rent. He moved his clothes and other possessions from our home. Finally, he triumphantly invited the entire family (home for the holidays) to visit his new abode.

We followed him to the center of town, to an old hotel with an unsavory reputation. Silently, the eight of us filed through the foul-smelling lobby where forlorn people were sitting on broken couches and chairs. We went up one narrow flight of stairs with carpet worn thin, then a second flight of bare wood with gaping holes. In the top corridor Jack had a key for one door. We all crowded into his tiny room. It was so hot that the temperature was surely more than 100° Fahrenheit.

When we mentioned the heat, Jack explained that his radiator was stuck in the open position. To remedy that, he kept his single window wide open. This, he pointed out proudly, provided him with a handy refrigerator on the outside ledge, and an effective stove for cooking on the surface of his sizzling metal radiator. The room had a single bed, a wooden chair, and a dresser, but no closet. He had hung his clothes on nails. Most of his other possessions were in cartons on the floor. For this accommodation he was paying a weekly rent which would add up to half the cost of a decent apartment, the sort of place he might have shared with one other person.

Not wanting to hurt his pride, we kept our dismay hidden that day. But later Jack's brothers and sister joined us in urging him to look for a better place to live. His employer strongly backed that opinion. We all inquired about rentable rooms in town. Just about anything would be better than the firetrap where he was living. When a place was found, Jack took over negotiations with the landlady. His new room, which once would have seemed very humble to me, looked magnificent. The old hotel was soon afterward bulldozed to rubble. In many cities similar hotels still operate, charging all they can get and foisting off their worst rooms on naïve people like Jack and your autistic friends.

Thinking about this episode later, I wondered how we might better have prepared Jack. He was unaware of the way most young people seek a place to live in our city. They read newspapers and bulletin boards, visit agencies, and post notices where young people gather in search of roommates. They size up the market by talking to many people. If housing is scarce, they enlist friends, co-workers, and relatives in their search.

Compare the steps of Jack's move. He decided that renting a single room would be best, logically the cheapest place to live. From family trips, he knew that the name of a place which rents rooms is a hotel. He went to the shabbiest hotel he could find because he assumed that a better one would be more costly. Once he had made that choice, he did not question the price which was quoted for a room, nor ask to see the place in advance. That seemed like rude behavior. For the same reason he did not criticize the room which was given to him. In Jack's opinion a well-bred person makes the best of hardship and focuses on any redeeming feature, like the radiator which could double as a stove.

Jack had reasoned things out on his own. What seemed to us like colossal stupidity was a thoughtful attempt to be independent, frugal, polite, and adaptable. We were as much to blame for the fiasco as he was, because we never taught him the elementary skills for independent living, adapted to his need for precise instruction.

Finding his first place to live away from home was just a start. Jack had many more lessons to learn. We began to see the pattern of his errors and to anticipate some of them. The trick was to show him how to do things without damaging his pride. I decided to write a teacher's manual on home economics for special students (Dewey, 1976) and Jack agreed to test many of the lessons. This willingness continued when I started a book on human relations (Dewey, 1978), which is an even greater obstacle for autistic people. No amount of training can completely eliminate the disability of autism, but I think our lessons helped. At least they sharpened my awareness of all Jack still needed to learn in order to get along independently.

Not every parent of an autistic person is able to continue to give crisis support indefinitely. If there is a willing parent or other relative, the partnership should be encouraged, however. Certainly it should not be made to seem like the *cause* of the autistic adult's immaturity! Therapists with this message must think that autistic immaturity is nothing more than lack of the freedom to explore naturally. Not so! In autism there is a genuine disability to process information accurately and rapidly, as needed in most social situations. After a few alarming experiences an autistic person may lose faith in himself or the world outside his narrow sphere of safety. He will be reluctant or bitter, according to how he places the blame. Sometimes blame is focused on the family, at least temporarily, and in that case it is important for the autistic person to have the minimal skills necessary for moving away.

Regardless of where an autistic adult ultimately lives, he will be a consumer of housekeeping services. Therefore I believe that every autistic adolescent should learn to perform as many of these as possible. This is not to say that they should be made into household slaves or treated much differently from their brothers or sisters. *All* young people nowadays need to know the basics of home care. Boys can no longer assume that some female will do it for them. Girls cannot expect to hire maids as readily as their grandmothers did. Though the glittering kitchens and bathrooms of TV commercials are virtually unattainable, every adolescent should learn to do what is essential promptly, and postpone other chores if necessary.

For example, if the young adult is late for work, can he leave a bathtub ring unwiped? What about a toilet which is overflowing? Would his landlord accept the excuse that he was late for work and could not tend to it just then? I am speaking of things this basic, which might put an end to independent living as soon as an eviction notice arrived. As for teaching autistic adolescents to keep brass doorknobs polished, forget it unless they are training for domestic jobs. That is a chore they might enjoy doing around home, however.

In 4 years Jack progressed from being the resident of a single rented room to being the owner of his own three-room house. He gave me a key with the understanding that I would enter only when invited, unless I had reason to expect a catastrophe. Since Jack had no training in housecleaning as he grew up, he invited me to visit his house and help clean it once a week. Don't smile. I treasured those invitations. They were a chance to teach him how to deal with problems which come up when basic home care is neglected.

My visits were a challenge to him. He noticed what I was doing and tried to surprise me the following week by having done that chore himself. This is not to say he is a fastidious housekeeper. Not by a long shot! He couldn't keep up his work and the chores of daily living if he made a fetish of cleaning. But his house doesn't look bad for a bachelor's pad, as he is fond of saying. The most persistent problem has been clutter, insidiously growing.

Negative criticism is *very* hard for Jack to accept. That's not unusual. Most people dislike being told that what they did was wrong. Yet that is the most direct way of guiding a learner, coupled with praise for correct moves. Perhaps because autistic people fail so often, and invest so much in efforts to succeed, they overreact to yet another message of failure. I have found that it works better to shape Jack by positive reinforcement.

My repeated advice to clear some of the junk from Jack's house was ignored with increasing shows of annoyance. It was his house, after all. Months passed and the situation worsened. I pointed out some good reasons for disposing of much of his useless hoard. Clutter in homes is a fire hazard and a lure for vermin. He was losing valuable living space. The house was more difficult to clean. He said sharply that he was much too busy to think about sorting just then. The matter rested. If I had pushed beyond that resistance I would have been unwelcome as a weekly visitor. One day, however, Jack took the initiative. He apologized for piles of things on his piano and table, saying he planned to sort them soon. That was an opening for positive reinforcement. It took no acting skill to approve his *plan* with enthusiasm. (You know and I know that such plans are often postponed indefinitely. With an autistic person, one must be alert to any progress in the desired direction.)

Shortly after this Jack asked me to drive by his house on trash collection day and see the amount of junk he had set out. It wasn't impressive, but I praised him, aware of the great wrench it was for him to part with anything of imaginable future use. For an autistic person, that is likely to cover everything except degradable garbage. His sorting has been going on for months now, fueled mainly by weekly praise for the size of his discard heap. I do not mind that it is taking a long time. That way, perhaps the habit of letting go of junk will be established.

I elaborated on this topic to show how an autistic person is best guided. It also shows what petty things can be their downfall if neglected too long. In teaching an adolescent how to find a place to live, and how to care for it, you have made a start. But you will almost certainly need to give continued guidance to correct insidious and unexpected problems.

The foregoing discussion may leave readers uneasy about their own messy quarters. Most of the problems autistic people face are similar to problems we all face, but autistic individuals are less able to resolve problems before they reach crisis proportions. Do you have 123 empty egg cartons, as Jack once did? I doubt it, unless you live on a chicken farm.

BODILY NURTURE

We did not know what Jack cooked on the radiator during his sojourn at the hotel. His first landlady gave us a clue about his diet by lodging three mild complaints. She wished he would wash his sticky oatmeal pan instead of leaving it soaking in the sink. She was tired of having her refrigerator smell like mackerel. And she did not like him taking so much space with gallon jugs of lemonade which he made in advance from concentrate. She told us that these three items were his steady diet.

Jack explained. The mackerel was good cheap protein which needed no cooking. At that time it cost about 10¢ a can and was sold mainly to cat owners. Lemonade satisfied his craving for a cold liquid and sugar. He thought it counted for a fruit. We had no quarrel with his choice of oatmeal to start the day. *He* did, however, when he realized he had to complete the clean-up before going to work.

As you can see, Jack has some awareness of nutrition. He also has a good instinct for economy, not present in every autistic person. But he lacked balance. He had tried to reduce eating to a simple formula and was oblivious of the impact of his habits on other people. This last trait is one of the most bothersome aspects of the autistic handicap. I will speak of it in more detail under the heading of acceptance.

To help Jack widen his diet repertoire, and to keep in touch for our own peace of mind, we issued a standing invitation to our house for weekend dinners. He might have declined out of pride, but we emphasized that we enjoyed his visits. This turned out to be increasingly true as our other children married and moved to other states.

Seeing that Jack was pressed for time, I offered to pick up for his use some of the bargains advertised as weekly specials in our supermarkets. He deposited money with me as a grocery account. (The need to feel independent was strong.) The following week I would ask which items he found easy to use and which went to waste. Gradually I learned to limit my purchases to items which needed little or no preparation and which had a low risk of spoiling.

As far as nutrition was concerned I kept the advice simple, but not because he would be unable to assimilate scientific terms. Quite the opposite. He is likely to make a fetish of seeking a better diet, going to outlandish extremes with declining health. Because he depends more on his mind than bodily signals, he is susceptible to the many fads which permeate our society. I never know when he will begin to look wan because he is trying something new from a health-food store. Fortunately his experiments do not extend to drugs.

Jack has almost as much trouble interpreting the signals of his body as he does with social signals. He can go great lengths of time without food. Yet he can consume prodigious amounts in a single meal without seeming to suffer discomfort. Recently I asked whether this had changed, because I actually have some leftovers after he dines with us. He replied, "I still do not know when to stop eating by my feelings, so I look at the amount other people eat. I judge what is enough and stop with that, though I could easily eat more."

The inability to read bodily signals extends to sleep and illness. He is able to stay up all night if he has an important project to complete. Yet he can sleep away a good portion of a weekend. We learned to watch him for symptoms of illness rather than expecting him to report when he felt sick. It seemed that he was an unusually healthy child. Now I wonder whether he did not carry around a lot of unreported misery. Once he collapsed on a Boy Scout hike and it turned out he had pneumonia. Yet until he fell he was trying to keep up. Nobody noticed his weakness because they were used to Jack's lagging and seeming out of touch with the others.

I have heard tales about other autistic children being resistant to pain. One boy I know broke a bone and did not mention it, though he was able to talk. Recently my mother returned to me a letter I had written to her when Jack was a baby. I boasted that he was the only child in the clinic who did not cry when he got his shots. How foolish I was to view this as bravery in an infant too young to know the meaning of courage! It was an early clue that something was wrong with his perception of bodily sensations.

I believe that strenuous physical exercise helps autistic people. This may be well known, but it is often overlooked. Some forms of exercise are for recreation and add to joy in living. Some exercise is work and improves self-esteem. I am talking here about the part that exercise plays in bodily nurture, especially its role in keeping emotions balanced. Since autistic children are excluded from spontaneous play groups, they miss a lot of running and romping when they are little. In team sports they are a disaster because they are unable to coordinate their moves with team-mates. As a result they may be "excused" from gym. We were lucky that Jack was directed to physical fitness programs, and swimming and other solo forms of exercise. Like many other autistic people, he uses a bicycle for transportation much of the time, even though he now owns a car.

When Jack was growing up we heard nothing about exercise causing the release of endorphins in the brain, and thus causing feelings of well-being. It was clear, however, that he felt better after a 6-mile bike ride or a session of woodsplitting. More research on the way exercise flushes toxic substances from the blood might reveal how to reduce the need for mood-altering drugs or extreme manipulations of diet.

JOY IN LIVING

Sustained bliss is not a human need. It is not even a natural state. By "joy in living" I mean the sum of small satisfactions which make life worth living for any one individual. What sources of happiness are available to an autistic person? Are any overlooked, or needlessly denied to an autistic adult because of the handicap?

The rhythmic hand or body movements of autistic people which therapists call self-stimulation should not be ranked as a source of pleasure, in my opinion. Adolescents who overcome such movements are, without exception to my knowledge, happy that they gained control over themselves. We have a picture of Jack at the age of 3 with a radiantly happy expression. His body is tense with excitement; his hands are a blur of activity close to his face. We whirled a toy fan to bring on that smile for the camera. Here self-stimulation and joy were connected.

But I remember also the two most miserable human beings I ever saw. It was 25 years ago and I was being shown through a state institution. The boys were chained to beds, wailing endlessly as they rocked and rocked and rocked. As in the case of Jack's joy, I think their bodily movement helped discharge intense emotion. By their teenage years most autistic children are ashamed of being unable to control rocking or flapping. They are embarrassed by reminders and reprimands. Lack of control makes them all the more miserable, which in turn increases the need to move.

The joy of gaining in skill is open to autistic children regardless of the extent of their handicap. A baby taking his first steps beams with pride because at last he can do it! He is not at that moment comparing himself with other babies, but trying hard to put it all together and move on his own two feet without falling. Happy as the child is to walk alone, he cannot be made to do so before he is ready.

I do not know the answer to the riddle of how to motivate an autistic person to learn a new skill. Resistance may be based on fear of failure. If so, attempt to set small goals which are sure to succeed, and to inch slowly forward, building on increased confidence. I have tremendous admiration for dedicated parents and teachers who have figured out ways to help the children in their care know the joy of gaining in skill. For each child it is an individual problem. Sometimes the lure is a chance to pursue their special interests. Sometimes it is something as simple as a drink of soda water, for a child who happens to crave that liquid. Ultimately the learning itself brings more joy than the rewards for attempting new skills.

If, as I believe, exercise is a valuable aid to reducing the anxiety of autistic children, the teaching of physical skills serves a double purpose, contributing to joy in living and to health. Few autistic children learn anything quickly. This is especially so of skills which are learned by imitation. They do not reverse movements which they see being done by somebody who faces them. Complex verbal instructions are even more confusing. Luckily there were some patient teachers in Jack's childhood who manipulated his limbs to show him how to ride a bike and to swim, and who did not discourage him by outbursts of impatience. Once he knew how to do these two things, he put both to good use. On his bicycle he studied the layout of our city, knowledge which has served him well as a serviceman. In the water he developed style and speed which astonishes people who are used to his clumsy movements on land. There is not time to teach many skills to an autistic child, but I think some which involve strenuous exercise should be included.

The joy of outstanding achievement is available to some autistic children. They are a minority, however. I will not go into detail about Jack's musical talents, therefore. The dilemma which faces parents is worth mentioning. Should they hold back on the obsessive interest to aim for "normalcy," whatever that is? Or should they actively assist an autistic child to develop a special talent? We thought it was not wise to risk making Jack more unbalanced by giving him early musical training. Only when he was 13 did we relent and provide lessons. Maybe this was a mistake. He once said he resented missing his chance to be a prodigy. Elsewhere I discuss the pros and cons of this difficult choice (Dewey & Everard, 1974).

The joy of creating does not require unusual talent. Ordinary cooking, sewing, and gardening can be creative. Working with wood or metal appeals to some autistic people I have known. Others knit or weave, taking pride in the results. As in the case of swimming and riding a bicycle, there is an initial hurdle of learning to make the right movements with the body or with tools. After that, an autistic person may pursue a creative skill to admirable lengths.

The joy of anticipation plays a large part in making life worth living for autistic people. To anticipate is to believe something is going to happen. Individuals who are distressed by the unpredictability of life need to be able to count on a few daily comforts. Many therapists have observed that autistic people thrive on structure. Living by routine eliminates painful uncertainty. Rewards are built into the daily routine of young autistic children, who have play time, song time, juice time, and even tickle time in some programs. This sort of program may continue into adolescence for some autistic teenagers, with slight modifications in the rewards. An autistic teenager who is making progress in school is likely to be overloaded with work routines, however. If no reward is built into the day's schedule, all the rest will seem hardly worth the effort. Something which is anticipated with pleasure should be included in the daily routine of every autistic adolescent.

Long-range anticipation is exceedingly important to autistic individuals. They remember traditions for years, and eagerly await special events. I would like to see research on the long-term memory of autistic people. It should not be dismissed as parent lore. The phenomenon may hold clues to the physiology of autism. I have documented evidence that at least *some* autistic individuals can store an extraordinary amount of detailed material in memory—in Jack's case, extending to years before he could talk. "How could you remember that!" I challenged him, regarding one recollection that a certain friend had brought us our fireplace grate when she had a blue car. It was the day we moved into a new unheated house, on his second birthday, but those details he did not recall. He replied that he had not known the words at the time, but it was a visual memory for which he later supplied the vocabulary. I checked with our friend and she consulted her auto-purchase records. She had indeed traded in her blue Ford just after that date. Thus he did discriminate colors and individuals and objects long before he was able to talk about them, perhaps before he realized that words represented the things he saw. Parents of mute autistic individuals have told me about the joy with which their children seem to anticipate certain familiar holidays. Even without language, they may have a clear visual memory of colorful fireworks in July, a bounteous meal in November, and tinsel and lights in December. To the extent that they can help with preparations, they should be encouraged to do so. Feeling useful and helpful adds to the joy of living, also.

You cannot deny autistic people the joy of giving, but it is a good idea to provide firm guidelines. Otherwise they may get the habit of giving away possessions or favors for approval. This leaves them open for exploitation. Certain people, certain charities, and certain occasions have to be learned, and the appropriate way to give to each. The dilemma is that in explaining the risks of indiscriminate generosity you may make the autistic person somewhat paranoid. And after all the variables have been discussed, an autistic person will still need guidance in deciding whether or not to give or lend money. A good backup rule is this: For any transaction over (a specific sum), seek advice from (a specific person). This rule once saved Jack from possible grief. Two strangers offered him a large sum of money for his car, far more than it was worth. I do not know whether or not it was intended to be a joke or a confidence game. At any rate he said he had to talk to his parents first, and did so at once; then he followed our advice to avoid the men thereafter. The same rule should apply to giving, lending, borrowing, and selling as to buying expensive items. Double-check with a trusted person before acting.

Jack brings us charity solicitations he receives in the mail. He gets many, far more than we do, so he must have responded to a few. Now he asks for our opinion of the worthiness of the organization. I am glad he does. Quite a few are highly questionable as charities. He learned his own lesson about lending money to a so-called friend. One day he ran into a young man he had known in high school. Because this person had once mingled voices with him in a choir, Jack assumed he could be trusted. He loaned him $20 in response to a hard-luck story (for that amount of money there was no promise to consult us). Weeks passed without a word from the friend. Jack decided to track him down, wasting more time than the loan was worth. That too was a good lesson. When the borrower was finally located, he apologized with more tales of woe, signing over his "latest paycheck" to Jack in exchange for the difference in cash. At the bank Jack discovered that the check had been stolen and the signature on it was a forgery. The anguish this caused him was only resolved by talking to his pastor. He let the matter drop.

You may protest that Jack's loan was not a gift and that the topic is out of place under this section, joy in living. There is a connection, however. The impulse to be generous and helpful is a beautiful thing, which can lead to happiness. I think parents and teachers should not overlook the rewards *or* the pitfalls of giving.

A feature story in the *New York Times* (Molotsky, 1978) begins, "Clarence A. Browne is on welfare, having given away most of his $120,000 inheritance to friends who, he says, do not speak to him now." The story goes on to describe a man of 51 living in the kind of wall-to-wall disarray I fear for Jack if he does not learn to discard some things. Mr. Browne was not identified in the *New York Times* as autistic. Many clues point to that conclusion, however. Because of his recent poverty he had been living for 5 years without heat, water, or electricity in his 14-room house. Autistic people seem to tolerate such discomforts because of their reduced awareness of bodily sensations. Repairs on the house were neglected. Taxes were unpaid, so that Mr. Browne faced eviction along with his treasured collection of 750,000 phonograph records. The inability to set priorities which conform to society's demands is typical of autistic people. So too is the obsessive interest in a collection of records. Although Mr. Browne is not mute, the content of his speech is naïve and guileless in a way which suggests autism. "Mama always said to help out everyone you can. I know I shouldn't have done it: I can't say no, I can't refuse anybody. At least I didn't spend it on wine, women, and song." Autistic people with speech are fond of clichés. I suspect Mr. Browne uses this one often. His gifts were, in a sense, loans of goodwill to people he thought needed help. Now he says, in his own time of need, "None of them have tried to help me. Now they turn the other way." Judgment of another person's integrity is a complex skill. It depends on recognizing many subtle cues, not just a verbal declaration of friendship. Autistic people do not have the ability to blend many social cues and come up with an accurate judgment. For this reason their giving does not always bring them joy.

A gift of service is less risky, except for sexual services. You can encourage an autistic person to volunteer for charity work, but you have to consider whether he will be more a burden than a help. At any rate, those who supervise or share the work should be helped to understand the nature of autism before a gift of service is offered.

It is too bad that I had reason to mention false friends before I added friendship to the list of sources of happiness for autistic people. Most autistic people will not control enough wealth to attract scoundrels. They count as friends all people who are kind to them, who acknowledge them as individuals. Such friends may be of any age, race, occupation, or social standing.

Jack's first experience at volunteer work was giving piano lessons to 10 retarded children. Most of the pupils appreciated his efforts and he counted them as friends. There was one girl, however, who did not endear herself when she chided him for the way his kitchen smelled on a day when he failed to take out his garbage. He quoted her remark to us, "Jack, yo kitchen smell lak a pigpen." Without thinking, I asked, "Oh, is she black?" Jack looked thoughtful for a moment before answering. "Yes, I think she is. Her twin brother is." He had imitated her accent not to mock her, but because his keen ear heard it that way, and it was his custom to quote exactly what he heard. Her race was an insignificant detail which he had not, until that moment, bothered to assess.

You may have noticed that Jack's pupil used his first name. Everybody does. This is further evidence of his lack of concern for social standing. One day I discovered, quite by accident, that he is on a first-name basis with customers all over town. I asked how this came about and he replied, "They call me by my first name so I thought I was supposed to do that." If a new customer calls him Jack and introduces herself as Mrs. Jones, he simply asks for her first name and uses it thereafter. Perhaps a few customers have been shocked by this unexpected familiarity from a serviceman. If so, they avoided calling him again. He holds on to a large following of loyal customers, however. Perhaps his assumption of social equality has actually raised him in their esteem.

Few other autistic prople have jobs which enable them to build a citywide network of casual friends. (Over the years some of Jack's customers have become more than casual friends, they tell me. He gets a great many personal messages and homemade cookies at Christmas.) Unless your autistic friends abandon society entirely, there will be people who interact with them. Autistic adolescents need help in sharpening other-awareness in order to know the joy of friendship.

There is no room for a vengeful spirit alongside the autistic handicap, and not much room for self-assertiveness. Jack follows this advice from his older brother: "Never try to get revenge, because you might be wrong." It should not be hard to remind an autistic person that he often misunderstands and misinterprets. Add to that the fact that unknown circumstances may have caused another person to say or do something offensive. Rather than risk inflicting wrongful harm on another human being, why not play safe and forget about revenge? Sooner or later most mean people do suffer for their unkindness. An autistic individual has enough to worry about without taking on the dangerous role of avenger. Early training for an autistic adolescent should aim to make this part of his life philosophy.

Failure, disappointment, and rejection are risks that go with the sources of joy I have mentioned. Achieving a balance that makes the risk worthwhile is the challenge which faces parents, teachers, and therapists.

SELF-ESTEEM AND ACCEPTANCE

In recent years self-esteem has become a talisman second only to love for its reputed curative power. There is some justification for this attitude. Handicapped people, especially, need to feel that they are valuable human beings, worth the extra effort they put into living. It does no good to tell an autistic person, "Look, why don't you face it? You are stubborn, self-centered, and incompetent. Unless you shape up, you won't make it." This kind of ego-smashing does not guide the autistic person away from self-defeating behavior. Yet mildly autistic individuals with potential for independent living get just such messages. Worse than useless, demeaning contempt destroys the will to go on.

The opposite extreme is when an autistic person is artificially bolstered by the unqualified assurance "You're O.K." Remember, we are talking about people who are pathologically literal in understanding meanings of words. The autistic person who believes he is always O.K. can only assume that when others reject him it is their fault.

Well-meaning parents sometimes tell a handicapped child that anyone who rejects him is an intolerant oaf, not worth any more consideration. For the moment that message may sooth hurt feelings. But an autistic person is likely to conclude that the world is peopled by intolerant oafs if he has no guidance in understanding how his behavior can affect others. The more an autistic person is rejected, the more he tries to get attention from the few people who have refrained from open rudeness. This increases the burden on their time. One by one they make themselves unavailable in self-defense. An autistic person without social guidance has no awareness of the way he courts rejection by pursuing acceptance in unacceptable ways. Without guidance he does not realize that hints are a face-saving clue to the need to change behavior, if he senses hints at all. Even with much guidance he is apt to come up with the wrong interpretation. There are no easy solutions. Fran Eberhardy (1970) succinctly described the social behavior of an autistic person by quoting this limerick:

> There was a young man so benighted,
> He didn't know when he was slighted.
> He went to a party
> And ate just as hearty
> As though he'd been duly invited.

I doubt that any training can completely wipe out the social handicap of autism, which stems from an innate disability to process shifting clues. No two situations are exactly alike. What was proper in one place may be offensive in another. Severely autistic people are sheltered of necessity. Those who are less handicapped learn to move in limited circles where they know how to behave acceptably. The milder the handicap, the greater the range of activities for which they must learn specific rules of behavior. At any level of handicap, achieving self-esteem and acceptance is an elusive goal for autistic people, achieved one day and dashed the next.

Over many years an autistic person may pick up enough concepts to almost take the place of social intuition. How many specific lessons will accomplish this? Thousands, at least! Talking about mistakes after they occur is more painful than preventing them. You cannot point out to an autistic person every single social error he commits. The sheer number of them is overwhelming. The effect of teaching by correction is a barrage of negative remarks. However, to the extent that an autistic person wants social guidance and asks for it, you may be able to point out what he is doing wrong. Sometimes Jack describes a puzzling social experience and asks us to explain the course of events. Here is one example:

Jack was asked to tune a piano at the summer cottage of a customer. This was far from town, and by the time he finished the work it was too late to drive home. Therefore the customer invited him to spend the night. The next morning Jack wanted to leave, but nothing was said about his fee. Apparently we had taught Jack that asking for money is rude, and he had carried this early training over to his adult work. Up to this point there had been no conflict, because his employer sent bills or private customers said "What do I owe you?" At the cottage he did not dare be so rude as to *ask* for his pay. So he lingered. The customer served him breakfast and he took a swim. After lunch he wandered around the lake a while. Nothing had yet been said about his pay at supper, so he ate that meal also, and slept in the same bed another night. On the third day he decided he must be rude and asked to be paid so he could leave. The customer replied, "Don't you think we are about even, with all the meals?" Humiliated, Jack settled on a low fee and left. He was unhappy about the lost time and income, and wanted to know what he did wrong.

We said, "Surely you had some hints that they wanted you to leave earlier. Didn't they start to act cool?" He said they did seem unhappy about his presence sometimes, but he thought that was due to family tensions. At such moments he did what seemed prudent, going outside to swim or walk. From this example you can see that family training and role-playing episodes cannot totally prepare an autistic person to deal with different people in various settings. Jack unhappily accepted our opinion that he had overstayed his welcome, and wrote a note of apology to his hostess. We did commend him for lowering his fee in response to her hint that he was indebted for the meals.

According to Jack, having a skill which people value adds much to his self-esteem. Finding a job for an autistic person is not easy, even after intensive training. It makes good sense for parents to be broadminded about many options: sheltered workshops, part-time work, and apprenticeship at low pay, for example. Sometimes a niche in a family business offers a start. Other parents of handicapped children can be understanding employers. They are more likely to give the autistic employee a second chance. But, sadly, it takes just one big blow-up to spoil it all. In the work situation the importance of early training in impulse control is magnified. Therefore a high degree of self-control is directly related to self-esteem and acceptance for autistic adolescents. By that age the time for indulging explosive emotional reactions is past, if it ever has therapeutic value for an autistic child. I doubt that it does. "You're O.K. We love you. We care about your feelings." These are important messages for any human being. Parents want their autistic adolescents to hear these words, but they want even more for their children to be able to inspire genuine love and acceptance.

FREEDOM FROM SUFFERING AND ABUSE

In giving autistic people the protection they need, it may be necessary to restrict the total freedom they crave. Every parent of an autistic person I know is haunted by fear of the future. It matters not whether the degree of the child's autism is mild or severe. The parents can imagine realistic situations in which he would suffer and be helpless to change the situation by himself. This is as true of the mildly autistic who live in the community as it is of the severely handicapped in institutions. There are hoodlums on the street who know a likely target for attack, and there are human vultures like those who swooped down on the estate of Clarence Browne.

Parents daydream of an ideal situation, one in which the autistic adult will have personal freedom yet be supervised in a benign way. The degree of freedom which can be handled differs from one individual to another. The way in which supervision is accomplished also varies. When parents continue to provide this service, they risk seeming unnaturally protective in view of the age of their "child." It may seem to some observers that the autistic adult is socially immature *because* the parents keep in close touch beyond the usual age of leaving home. When I said that parents want understanding, it included understanding of their own adaptations to the handicap of their child. Casual observers with simplistic solutions such as "Treat him like an adult and he'll act like one!" simply do not understand the nature of autism. To the extent that a person with a severe handicap like blindness or autism can cope with the disability, it *does* help to treat the person as if he were normal. But when assistance is needed, somebody with sight (or insight) had better be available! Otherwise the helpless person may suffer or be abused.

Our arrangement with Jack works well, for the present. It suits his degree of independence and his need for occasional advice. He eats dinner with us on weekends and holidays, and I visit his house once a week for 2 hours of housework. In addition, Jack sometimes phones us to ask for advice. My heart does not sink when he begins "I have a problem." I know from experience that Jack does not discriminate well between trivial and serious problems, and that the majority of his perceived problems would be no problem at all to other people. On the other hand, if a strange voice asks whether we are Jack's parents, I fervently hope that it is just somebody who wants to locate him for a piano tuning.

Not long ago Jack came to us with a sober expression. Two bad things had happened to him that day, he told us. He needed advice at once. While he was napping, somebody had knocked on his door. It took a while for Jack to dress, so he kept the person waiting. It was the postman, who was more than a little annoyed by the delay. This was Bad Thing #1, the anger of the postman. No doubt, the fact that he wears a uniform similar to a policeman's increased Jack's worry. Bad Thing #2 was in the insured package which was delivered to Jack. It was a brand-new watch, from a company which had repaired and returned his old watch months earlier. Due to some snafu they sent him a new one, with no explanation. Jack thought it was a matter of honor for him to send money for the watch which he did not need. The crisis was easily resolved. We helped him write a letter telling the shippers to send postage within one month if they wanted the watch returned. (Nothing happened, and he had a nice gift for his brother.)

Some things which have happened to Jack since his childhood have been more serious. He prefers that I not mention them. I am grateful for his permission to use the examples in this chapter. We both hope that the invasion of his privacy will be more than offset by the value of his experience to other people.

Looking back, I can see things we might have done differently to avoid our worst experiences. Yet I know that Jack's present adjustment rests on what he has learned from painful lessons as well as some good guesses in plotting his way of living. Who knows whether this house of cards would have risen to its present height if any card at a lower level had rested on a different premise? Therefore we would do nothing different for Jack. But starting with a different autistic child today, we would have less hope for a cure, and would focus more on helping the child live with the degree of handicap which was evident.

A few years ago we heard the phrase "reaching the highest potential" applied to all kinds of learning disability. If this is taken to mean that an autistic person is expected to *sustain* the highest level of performance and social adjustment achieved under guidance, it is a cruel ideal. Who *can* continue an achievement which calls for the utmost concentration and effort? Not I! Freedom from suffering includes finding a way of life which can be continued comfortably, without constant stress. Setting high standards for a handicapped person is not in itself abuse. But holding him to his highest achievement with threats of humiliation or worse punishment for slipping back borders on abuse. Autistic adolescents should be taught that they, like all people, have moods and abilities which fluctuate. It seems to me that some of the panic that grips an autistic person in distress is the belief that he has permanently lost all he worked so hard to achieve. Parents share the fear that one lapse of effort will topple it all. This was evident in my phrase "house of cards" for Jack's present adjustment.

So I will end my chapter as I began it, with a plea for better understanding of the nature of autism. A blind person does not live under the fear of punishment for failing to see. A deaf person is not threatened with humiliation for not hearing. Both are taught to compensate for the sensory skills they lack. Temporary dulling of their ability to deal with their handicap is not seen as total failure. More likely it is viewed as a result of sickness or fatigue. Similar fluctuations occur with autistic people of all ages. This understanding should be common knowledge to autistic individuals and their helpers, to reduce their well-founded fear of failure.

SUMMARY

Parents of autistic adolescents want wider understanding of the problems they face. They need help in preparing their fast-growing children for an adulthood which provides the basic human needs:

1. A suitable place to live, knowledge to care for it, provisions for the future
2. Good bodily nurture, including health care, exercise, and food
3. Sufficient joy in living, self-esteem, and acceptance to make life tolerable
4. Freedom from suffering and abuse

Providing examples and opportunities is not sufficient for an autistic person. He or she needs help and assistance to achieve any of these basic needs. Most autistic people need continued supervision in adulthood. They should therefore be taught that willingness to consult other people is a sign of strength.

Because they head for goals with single-minded determination they are easily tripped. Because they misinterpret social cues they often intrude on other people and are hurt by the response that meets them. Because they do not recognize subtle social hierarchies they fail to make adjustments in familiarity from one situation to another. This is just a sampling of the reasons autistic adolescents need a great deal of training and guidance to prepare them to get along well in any living situation which lies in their future. Provisions for the future will vary according to the severity of their handicap, yet all humans have similar needs. Awareness of these needs should guide efforts to help.

REFERENCES

Dewey, M. *Teaching home economics to special students.* Portland, Maine: J. Weston, Walch, 1976.

Dewey, M. *Teaching human relations to special students.* Portland, Maine: J. Weston Walch, 1978.

Dewey, M., & Everard, M. The near-normal adolescent. *Journal of Autism and Childhood Schizophrenia,* 1974, *4,* 348–356.

Eberhardy, F. The view from the couch. *Journal of Child Psychology and Psychiatry,* 1967, *8,* 257–263.

Eberhardy, F. *Proceedings of 2nd Annual Conference,* National Society for Autistic Children, San Francisco: Panel III, Parents of Young Adults. Public Health Service Publication no. 2164, 1970.

Molotsky, I. A. penniless heir fears for his record collection. *New York Times,* Feb. 1, 1978.

15

Legal Needs

LAWRENCE A. FROLIK

As an autistic child approaches adulthood his parents are almost certain to experience anxiety and apprehension over the inevitable upcoming events in an adolescent's life: the child's reaching legal adulthood, the real or feared physical decline of the parents, and the eventual death of the parents. When the child becomes legally emancipated, either at 18 or 21, the parents will no longer be the child's natural guardian and the child will become an independent adult.

The maturation of the child also signals the aging and eventual death of the parents. The demanding task of caring for an autistic child may become an increasing burden to the aging parents, who themselves may require support and assistance. The eventual death of the parents raises the troubling question of who is to replace them in the care of and concern for their child.

The law provides three major avenues of recourse to the parents of an autistic adolescent. The first is the use of advocacy, which impinges very little upon the independence and autonomy of the child. Advocacy should be considered before resorting to any more drastic measures that might inhibit the growth and development of the child. Second, guardianship with its attendant loss of autonomy may, however, be necessary if the severity of the disability requires a formalized caretaker for the child or his property. Finally, the law allows parents to dispose of their property at their deaths in the manner that will best benefit their disabled child.

LAWRENCE A. FROLIK • School of Law, University of Pittsburgh, Pittsburgh, Pennsylvania 15260.

LITIGATION AND ADVOCACY

An autistic adolescent on the threshold of adulthood has needs that extend beyond physical support and emotional care. With adulthood will come an increasing interaction with various state and federal authorities as well as with private businesses and enterprises. That involvement will likely give rise to the need for professional assistance. Few if any of us are capable of proceeding through life without having occasion for such assistance in an increasingly complex world. Almost everyone at one time or another has need for an advocate or a lawyer to assist him in obtaining rights or privileges that should be his but which he is unable to obtain on his own.

For most individuals the need for such assistance may be sporadic or infrequent, but for the disabled individual the need may be regular and frequent. Although judicial decisions and legislative enactments have established many rights and legal benefits for the disabled, it remains for the individual disabled person to secure his receipt of those rights and benefits. To do so will often require the assistance of an advocate or a lawyer.

For every court case which appears on the front page of the newspapers or for every law that is passed, there are literally hundreds of small victories for the disabled as advocates and lawyers pursue the rights of their clients. What is needed are not earthshaking new developments but the translation of past judicial and legislative victories into day-to-day realities. Lawyers are aware of the long step between the passage of legislation or a victory in the courts and the enforcement of the rights so won. It should come as no surprise that repeated advocacy and litigation are often necessary to convince bureaucrats, private employers, and elected officials that the rights of the disabled as expressed in a case or statute are not empty words, but are to be translated into literal behavior.

Traditionally lawyers have translated vague general rights into specific benefits for their clients by lawsuits or merely by threat of suit which causes the opponent "voluntarily" to behave in an acceptable manner. Since many of the rights of the disabled are either granted or enforced by local administrative agencies, it is natural that lawyers are hired to represent the individuals before such administrative agencies. Whenever the disabled individual has a problem, either in having his statutory rights enforced or in having the definition of his rights clarified, it is appropriate to turn to a lawyer for assistance. However, most lawyers are not cognizant of the rights, needs, and expectations of the disabled. Therefore it is not enough to say to a disabled individual that he needs a lawyer.

What he needs is a lawyer expert in the law of the particular disability. The number of lawyers who are qualified in the law of disability is, however, relatively limited, and it may require a rather diligent search to find a knowledgeable one.

Use of a lawyer is not the only possible solution. In many cases the disabled individual's legal rights are clear; what is needed is pressure to enforce those rights. Where there is little doubt as to the legal rights involved, but there is a failure of effective delivery or enforcement of those rights, then an advocate might be appropriate. An advocate, as the term implies, speaks for the rights of the disabled individual. An advocate might be a lawyer, but he could just as well be a social worker, a psychologist, or any interested party who is sympathetic and knowledgeable about the needs of the disabled individual. Parents are perhaps the best examples of advocates. They are motivated by love, but other advocates could be motivated by financial rewards if necessary. Whatever the motivation, it is always appropriate to consider who, if anyone, speaks for the disabled person.

If the parents feel that they are no longer capable of acting as an advocate, they ought to make arrangements for a volunteer or paid professional to be the child's advocate. Ideally the advocate would provide assistance and emotional support to the disabled individual in his dealings with the outside world. The advocate does not have supervisory authority over the individual, but is akin to a friend or relative (Kopolow & Bloom, 1977).

Whenever possible the disabled individual ought to participate in the selection of the advocate and in the definition of the role that the advocate should play. The advocate and the disabled person should work together and reinforce each other in obtaining the rights and benefits legally belonging to the disabled party. An effective advocate should thereby minimize the need for assistance in a more intrusive form, e.g., a guardian.

An advocate, however, will only have the authority to act as a legal agent if the disabled individual is legally competent. As the agent of the disabled individual the advocate has the legal authority to speak on behalf of the disabled individual and cannot be dismissed as merely being a meddlesome interloper. Even if the advocate is not an acutal legal agent, for example if the disabled individual lacks the legal capacity to appoint an agent, the advocate may still perform valuable functions. In many instances advocates will be allowed to speak for the interests of the disabled individual even though they might lack any actual legal authority. However, in some situations, such as a serious medical treatment decision, the advocate's lack of legal authority may prevent him from participating in the decision-making process. A court-appointed legal guardian therefore may be unavoidable if the disability is so severe that the disabled individual cannot legally empower an advocate to act on his behalf.

GUARDIANSHIP

At one level guardianship is rather straightforward: it is the grant of legal authority for one adult to make decisions concerning the person and property of another adult. Commonly, the disabled adult in need of such assistance is referred to as the ward, while the adult acting as the caretaker is the guardian or, in some states, conservator. The scope of the power or authority of the guardian is governed by state law; there is no federal law of guardianship. State guardianship laws and practices are fairly similar, but any generalization about guardianship may be incorrect as to any particular state.

Guardianship laws trace their origins to the feudal law of England when the king was the guardian of "orphans, idiots, and lunatics." Idiots were those born without reason (mentally retarded) and lunatics were those who lost their reason (mentally ill). As the United States was settled the colonies adopted the English practice of the state as the protector or guardian for those unable to care for themselves. The responsibility of the state was of course not limited to orphans, idiots, and lunatics, as the destitute and poor were also thought to be the responsibility of the society, which acted through the local village or town government. But the responsibility of the state to the disabled differed in a most significant manner from its self-imposed duty to the poor. The latter were given sustinance and shelter in return for having their lives subjected to supervision and regimen designed to encourage their return to self-sufficiency (Rothman, 1971). Yet in spite of extensive state interference in their lives the poor remained in legal (if not physical or actual) control of their lives, and they were free to reject the proffered state assistance. The disabled, in contrast, had no such choice, for the very nature of their need for state assistance (being mentally incompetent) barred them from voluntarily renouncing it.

The identification of a mentally disabled individual was, at common law, highly significant, for if one were mentally disabled one lacked reason. Lacking reason meant that the individual was incapable of caring for himself or making decisions concerning his life, because it was only through the power of reason that man could govern himself. An individual who lacked the power of reason could not be left to his own devices. Yet if an individual lacked reason and could not make decisions for himself, who was to care for his property and person? English common law found the answer in the creation of a relationship to the disabled that was analogous to that between parent and child.

Definition of Incompetence

Under traditional common law the parent was the natural guardian of his child, meaning that the parent was responsible for caring for the person and property of his child. As a corollary the minor child (at common law a child was a minor until age 21) was not legally responsible for his person or property, nor did he have any legal rights to choose how he might live. The control of the parental guardian over his child was complete, with all the power resting in the guardian and none in the child. The absolute and unambiguous nature of the parent–child relationship reflected the value that the common law placed on having an individual's legal status clearly and unequivocally defined. A minor was, by definition, one who lacked any legal control of his life. Not believing in ambiguous solutions, the common law could only conceive of a parent–child relationship as one in which the child had no independent legal rights over his own life. Yet the anomoly was that at the child's 21st birthday the legal status was turned on its head. At age 21 the child was legally emancipated, became an adult, and came into complete control of his life. The parents, who had up to that day had complete dominance and control, suddenly lacked any legal authority over the child. From a legal standpoint there was (and still is) no gradual entrance into adulthood. One moves from the total protection of childhood into the complete freedom and autonomy of being an adult.

The parent–child relationship became the model used by common law in providing care for the mentally disabled. Acting under the belief that reason was an either/or situation—one either had it or one did not—the common law classified all adults as either competent, having the power of reason, or incompetent, lacking the power of reason. If an individual was competent he was allowed to control his own life, even if he were to act in a foolish or irresponsible manner. But if he were mentally disabled he would not be allowed to control his own life because he lacked the reason that was the crucial element of self-goverance. Therefore, just as the child was under the total control of the parent, so was the disabled, incompetent adult under the total control of his protector, the guardian. The disabled, incompetent adult was a ward of the guardian, and as such his status was that of a person wholly lacking in civil or personal rights. Any and all decisions concerning his life were the providence of the guardian. The logic of the common law demanded this total and complete transfer of decision-making from the ward to the guardian, because by the logic of the law the ward, being incompetent, could not make rational decisions, and therefore could not be allowed. if only for his own good, to make any decisions. At the common law there was no gray area: an individual either did or did not control his own life.

The legacy of this rigid common law view of the world is with us still and explains why the parents of an autistic child must fear the day he reaches adulthood. For when the child becomes legally of age (depending on state law, either at age 18 or at age 21) the parents lose their status as natural guardians and therefore their legal right to control the child's life without regard to the capabilities of the child. Legally the child is considered to be a competent adult and fully in charge of his own affairs.

Weighing the Need for Guardianship

What can parents do when faced with a legal status that conflicts with the actual abilities and needs of the child? First, the parents must decide what legal status will best enable the child to control and shape his own life to the extent that he is able. This is determined by considering how much assistance or control the child requires from the parents. Once the parents have a fairly clear picture of the role that they wish to play in the life of the child, they can choose the legal relationship they require vis-à-vis the child. If the child is reasonably independent and capable of caring for himself, the parents may wish for little more than an advisory role: the opportunity to be close to the child so that they might serve as an advisor or advocate. Should that be the case the parents need ask very little of the legal system. Essentially the child will act as an independent adult whose relationship to his parents is based not on a legal status but on love and respect (unless the parents act as formal, legal agents for the child; see the preceding section on advocacy). If the autistic child should suffer from a more severe mental disability, then the parents may reasonably believe that the child will continue to need a guardian or protector even though he is legally an adult. Should that be the case the parents may well want to seek legal authority to continue to act as the child's guardian.

As noted, the parents' legal status as the natural guardians of their child ceases the day that the child reaches legal adulthood. The only way for the parents to reestablish their authority as guardians is to file a petition with the appropriate court asking that they be appointed guardian. The standards that govern whether a guardianship is legally appropriate vary from state to state, but in general a court will only appoint a guardian if adequate proof exists that the child is incompetent. Some states avoid the use of the term "incompetent," and instead use the phrase "incapacitated person," or "disabled person." The standards used to define these terms vary fairly widely, but in the end almost all states attempt by statute to define a class of disabled persons for whom a guardian can be appointed. Typically the statute will speak of a person who "lacks sufficient understanding or capacity to make or communicate responsible decisions concerning his person," (Uniform Probate Code, 4th ed., 1975, vol. 8, sect. 5-101[17]). The purpose of the judicial hearing is to determine if the alleged incompetent is legally incapacitated.

Because the appointment of a guardian requires a judicial hearing, it is necessary that someone initiate proceedings by filing in court a petition requesting the appointment of a guardian. The court, which will determine whether a guardian is needed, cannot initiate the proceedings. It is a passive body that awaits action on the part of someone concerned enough about the disabled individual to take the trouble to file a petition of incompetency. Hence even an obviously incompetent person will be considered legally competent until someone initiates proceedings to cause a court to declare him incompetent.

The guardianship hearing is usually a relatively straightforward affair. In most states the hearing is held without a jury, with a single judge deciding whether the disabled individual is mentally incompetent. In many states the alleged incompetent need not be present at the hearing if his presence would be harmful to his health or his well-being. Often the hearing is fairly brief, with the testimony of a physician or psychiatrist being the most telling, if not the only, testimony offered (Regan, 1972). Generally the party who filed the petition seeking a finding of incompetency will also have asked to be named the guardian. In the absence of anyone requesting to be named guardian, the court will select an appropriate individual. Some states require the appointment of relatives as guardians unless they refuse.

The guardian remains accountable and answerable to the appointing court, and the guardian has no powers greater than those granted to him by the court. The disabled individual is a ward of the court whose care is the responsibility of the guardian.

Just because the disabled individual is legally under the care of the court does not mean that the court necessarily keeps a close eye on the ward. In fact the reality is often just the opposite: the court has almost no idea what the guardian is doing or whether he is doing anything at all. Personal guardians often report only infrequently to the court, and it should not be assumed that the court's review of the guardian's report is either imaginative or thorough.

Hence in considering the wisdom of seeking a declaration of incompetency and the appointment of a guardian, only modest court supervision should be assumed. Certainly the guardian will be almost totally on his own as to day-to-day events. The desirability of this relative lack of effective supervision depends on one's confidence in the guardian. The more certain one is that the guardian will be a sympathetic, caring, and responsible individual, the more likely one is to be content to use a guardian. However, if no qualified guardian is at hand, then the use of guardianship should be seriously questioned.

Conservators

If the parents have decided that the condition of their child warrants their seeking appointment as guardian, they must decide what kind of guardianship to seek. Guardians are of two types: guardians of the estate and guardians of the person. In addition one may serve as both the guardian of the estate and of the person, which is known as a plenary guardian. In some states the guardian of the estate is referred to as a conservator. Whether called a guardian of the estate or a conservator, the duties are the same: to assume possession and control of the property of the disabled person. The conservator takes charge of all the wages, savings, governmental benefits (e.g., Supplemental Security Income) or anything else of value owned by the ward. The duty of the conservator is to act as a fiduciary or trustee; that is, he is under the legal obligation to protect and conserve the financial resources of the ward. The conservator is accountable (generally annually) to the court that appointed him as to how the money was invested and spent, with the primary duty being one of fiscal conservatism. The conservator is expected to ensure that the assets of the ward are secured in risk-free investments, and to spend amounts as needed for the support and comfort of the ward.

The conservator may be an individual, but in the majority of cases it is a corporate entity such as a bank. If an individual is appointed he may be required to post a bond or pay for sureties who will insure any losses that might result from his negligence or theft. In recognition of the burden of being a conservator, states allow the appointing court to pay reasonable compensation to the conservator, and to repay the conservator for any expenses he might incur. For example, if the conservator is an individual or an institution which provides room and board for the ward, then the court will authorize payment for those expenses. All such payments come from the assets of the ward, so that he bears the cost of the management of his property. Normally the cost of a conservator is rather modest, but it is a drain on the limited resources of the ward and to that extent the wisdom or necessity of a conservator should be carefully considered. Moreover, if circumstances require a conservator, relatives of the disabled individual might consider having one of themselves named with a view to not accepting any fees and thereby conserving the limited assets of the ward.

The conservator, who has total control over the assets, wages, and property of the ward, has no power over the person of the ward. That is, the conservator cannot dictate where or how the ward is to live, or what he is to do with his life, or decide how the ward should care for himself. The conservator cannot substitute his judgment for that of the ward as to any personal matter, e.g., medical treatment decisions. To be sure, the power of the purse allows the conservator significant control over the life of the ward, for if the ward lacks control of any assets his range of choices is severely limited. In practice the life of a ward will be maintained by the conservator very much as it was carried on before the appointment of the conservator, or at least to the extent permitted by the finances of the ward. So long as the status quo is maintained the ward will be granted relative freedom to live as he chooses in regard to day-to-day affairs, while the conservator attends to the financial concerns. But should circumstances demand a change in living arrangements, for example, or should the health of the ward fail and consent be needed for proposed medical treatment, then the conservator's scope of authority may prove to be too limited and a personal guardian might be required.

Personal Guardians

Guardians are often granted authority over both the person and the property of the ward, and in such cases they are called plenary guardians. Both a personal guardian and a conservator will be used if the court is unable to locate an individual willing or capable of serving as a plenary guardian. In those instances the court may appoint a corporate conservator (a bank) to provide professional management of the ward's property and an individual as personal guardian to care for the person of the ward. (Corporations, i.e., banks, are rarely appointed to act as personal guardians.) The use of both a conservator and a personal guardian may also occur if a conservator was initially appointed and only later did the need for a guardian arise. At that point the court might not wish to disturb the continuity or experience of the conservator, and therefore may appoint a guardian with powers limited to the person of the ward.

In many instances, however, the guardian will have the combined authority over theperson and property of the ward, i.e., plenary power. In such cases the guardian has complete control over all aspects of the life of the ward, who by reason of the finding of incapacity has no legal right to make any decisions concerning his own life. In some cases such total control may be a necessary solution, but in many other cases, and particularly when dealing with an autistic adult, such total control and resulting dependence may be unnecessary and destructive of the adult's reaching his full potential. Fortunately in many cases use of a plenary guardian can be avoided.

The court may be empowered by state law to appoint a limited guardian who does not have complete control of the ward's life. The limited guardian has only those powers granted to him by the court. The ward is considered only selectively incompetent, being legally incompetent only in regard to certain areas of his life, but in those areas where he is competent he is left in control and is free to act as he chooses. Hence to the extent feasible the ward is allowed to care for himself and control his own affairs. Ideally the goal of limited guardianship is to create a guardian who assists the ward, rather than one who completely supersedes the ward's own decision-making powers. At present only a handful of states permit the appointment of a guardian with limited powers, but there exists growing pressure for the amendment of state laws to allow its use in all states.

The recently enacted Washington state guardianship statute is a good example of a limited guardianship. The statute states that the intent of the legislature was to recognize "That disabled persons have special and unique abilities and competencies with varying degrees of disability" (Revised Code of Washington, 1980, vol. 16, Title 11, sect. 11.88.005). To that end the statute permits limited guardianship for disabled persons without the need for a determination of total incompetency and "the attendant deprivation of civil and legal rights." Hence the ward retains all his civil and legal rights except those specifically set forth in the court order which established the limited guardianship. The primary duty of the limited guardian is to care for and maintain the disabled individual, assert his rights, and to provide consent to necessary medical procedures.

As a corollary to limited guardianship some states prohibit the guardian from undertaking certain activities without the express prior approval of the court. Typically the guardian may not "voluntarily" commit the ward to a mental institution; nor consent to "voluntary" sterilization of the ward; nor consent to psychosurgery or electroshock treatment; nor consent to amputation. Even in states which have not yet established limited guardianship it is not uncommon to find either statutory or case-law prohibitions on the right of the guardian to approve such procedures without specific prior court approval. In deciding whether to apply for a declaration of incompetency and the appointment of a guardian a parent should be aware of the potential limits, if any, on the power of the guardian. The fewer limits on the guardian, the more hesitant the parent ought to be in opting for a guardian.

Another factor that should be weighed in the decision as to whether to seek a guardian is the availability of less restrictive arrangements that might meet the needs of the disabled individual. If, for example, the disabled adult receives Supplemental Security Income or social security payments (or will receive them upon the retirement or death of one of his parents), a representative payee might be used to receive the monthly checks and handle the disbursements. A representative payee can be appointed merely upon the presentation of a doctor's statement that the recipient of the SSI or social security is disabled, and does not mean that he is incompetent of lacks capacity. Naturally the representative payee has no control or power over any other aspects of the disabled individual's life.

Another possible solution is the use of a general power of attorney whereby the autistic adult voluntarily turns over control of his financial affairs to a third party, either to a professional such as a bank or to another individual. The power of attorney can be revoked at any time, and it can be a limited power whereby only certain degrees of financial control are turned over.

A third possibility is the use of a trust established by the disabled adult whereby the management of some or all of his assets is turned over to a trustee, either corporate or individual, who controls only the assets transferred to the trust by the disabled party. The power of the trustee is governed by state law, and the creator of the trust may further limit the power of the trustees. The trust instrument, as written by the creator (called the settlor), will provide how, when, and to whom payments out of the trust are to be made. A trust may be revocable at any time, or for a term of years (e.g., 10), or may be irrevocable and for life. Naturally the use of a power of attorney or trust presumes that the individual's disability is not so great as to call into question his capacity to grant the power of attorney or create the trust. The trust or power of attorney would not be valid if it were later determined that the individual was incompetent at the time of the creation of the trust or the grant of the power of attorney.

The need for a guardian can also be greatly reduced if the living arrangements for the autistic child have been carefully planned. Studies indicate that individuals living in group homes often lack a guardian, limited or otherwise (Mesibov, Conover, & Saur, 1980). Apparently the group home supervisor assumes the role of caretaker or advisor for the day-to-day needs of the inhabitants of the home. Even if the individual does have a guardian, the group home supervisor is often unaware of the fact and thus acts in a capacity as titular guardian.

Of course groups homes are not the only answer. Continued residence with the parents generally reduces the need for a guardian. Still the parents are likely to predecease their autistic child, or it may be undesirable for any number of reasons for the autistic adult to continue to live with his parents. Relocation of the child may also be necessitated by the death of the parents. If it is not practical for the autistic adult to move in with another relative, then the need for a competent decision-maker to determine where he is to live may well trigger an incompetency hearing and the appointment of a guardian. Hence the importance of the parents' having provided for an orderly and predetermined living arrangement for their child after their deaths.

Another factor to be considered is the availability of someone to serve as a guardian after the death of the parents. As stated, banks frequently serve as conservators and thus, unless the assets of the ward are too small to bear the cost, a conservator can normally be found. Even in the absence of a bank, someone is usually willing to serve as a conservator since the amount of assets in question will be fairly small and the expenditures tend to be relatively routine, e.g., the regular payment to a boarding home for room and board. Finding a personal guardian, on the other hand, may prove more difficult. With the exception of relatives, most individuals are reluctant to accept the responsibility to act as a personal guardian. Relatives may do so out of a sense of personal responsibility, and sometimes a friend or neighbor will come forward, but all too often the individual's need for a guardian arises in part from his misfortune in having no one willing to look after him.

Where no suitable individual exists to act as guardian the choices open to the court depend on state law. Some states, e.g., Ohio (Page's Ohio Revised Code, 1980, vol. 20, sect. 2110.10), permit the court to appoint a nonprofit organization to act as a guardian, while other states, e.g., Minnesota, have what are known as public guardians (Minnesota Statutes Annotated, 1980, vol. 17, sect. 252, A.11, 20). The latter is a public agency whose function is to serve as guardian of last resort. At present nonprofit corporate guardians and personal guardians are permitted in only a minority of the states, but there is a growing recognition of their desirability and in the future more states can be expected to adopt these alternatives.

PARENTAL ESTATE PLANNING

The death of the parents may not only necessitate appointment of a guardian or conservator, but may also mean that arrangements will have to be made for the financial support of their autistic child. To be sure, parents are free to decide who should become the owner of their property after their deaths. They have no legal obligation after their deaths to support their children even if they are disabled or minors. But most parents of disabled children want to provide financial support for their child for fear that the child will not be able adequately to support himself. Even if the child is capable of supporting his normal needs, his disability may create extraordinary expenses, or the disability may at some future date prevent him from being self-supporting. Hence there is a special need for effective estate planning by the parents of an autistic child.

A parent, of course, need do nothing with his assets and they will still be distributed at his death. Dying without a will causes one's property to pass by intestacy. Each state has its own law of intestacy which determines who will take the deceased's property. Generally state laws provide for some level of support for the surviving spouse and then the rest of the property is divided equally among the children. If there is no surviving spouse, almost all states provide for an equal division of the property among the surviving children without regard to their financial capability or need. Therefore the only way to ensure that one's property will be distributed with a view toward the particular needs of the children is to write a will.

Wills

The first aspect to consider when drawing up a will is whether the autistic child will be able to support himself financially throughout his life. If he is capable of supporting himself and is capable of handling his own financial affairs, then presumably there is no need for special financial planning for him. However, if the child is likely to need financial assistance, then the parents must determine whether they will have sufficient assets to be able to support the child throughout his life. If they cannot, then government assistance will be required. Should that be the case the wisest choice may be for the parents to disinherit the child.

As stated earlier, the law allows a parent to disinherit a child, even a disabled one. Disinheriting the child may be desirable if that would qualify the child for greater government benefits. Many federal government benefits, i.e. Supplemental Security Income and Medicaid, depend on a financial needs test. If the child inherits money from his parents, he may be disqualified from SSI and Medicaid until the inheritance has been exhausted. Similarly, most states base their assistance to the mentally disabled either on a financial needs test or on ability to pay. The latter means that the individual is expected to pay for benefits provided by the state in accordance with that individual's financial resources. Therefore if the individual has assets he will have to pay for services which would otherwise have been provided free. Leaving an inheritance to a disabled child under these conditions does not really assist a child, but only serves to supplant otherwise available state or federal assistance. Therefore a parent with a relatively modest estate and other demands upon it might consider disinheritance of the disabled child and leave a small, yet personally meaningful gift to indicate the parent's love and concern. Naturally no one should disinherit a disabled child without careful consultation with an attorney who is knowledgeable about estate planning for parents of disabled children.

In lieu of complete disinheritance, the parent might leave property to another individual with instructions that the property be used for the benefit of the disabled child. This is known as a "morally obligated gift" (Frolik, 1979). The use of such a gift will not affect government benefits since technically the disabled individual does not own the gift. But it has risks. The individual receiving the gift owns the property outright and, except for his sense of obligation to the disabled child, need not use any of it for the benefit of the child. The instructions that accompany the property are not legally enforceable since the gift legally belongs to the one who received it, not the disabled child. Hence there is no way to ensure that the gift will be used to benefit the disabled child. Moreover, even if the morally obligated recipient does use the gift for the benefit of the disabled child, there is no guarantee of continuity of care or support, because the individual who has undertaken the obligation might die or otherwise become incapable of carrying out the obligation.

Trusts

If the parents have sufficient assets, then serious consideration should be given to the use of a trust. A trust is a written legal agreement which allows property to be owned and managed by one person, called the trustee, for the benefit of another, the beneficiary. The assets in the trust are called the principal or the corpus, which is invested and earns trust income. Trusts may have one or more beneficiaries and they may have one or more trustees. The trustee may be an individual or a corporate entity, e.g., a bank.

The trust agreement is a written document that creates the trust. It represents an agreement between the creator of the trust (the settlor) and the trustee which spells out the purpose of the trust and the duties of the trustee. At the termination of the trust, which is determined by the settlor (for example, at the death of the beneficiary), the property that remains in the trust is distributed in the manner designated by the settlor as stated in the trust agreement. The trustee can never use the trust principal or income for his own benefit and may only use the assets in the manner provided for in the trust agreement.

Trusts have several advantages, including the fact that a properly drawn trust will not disqualify a disabled child from government benefits even though the child is the trust beneficiary. The child does not legally "own" the assets in the trust; the trustee is the legal "owner" of the trust assets. Moreover, unlike arrangements supported only by a moral obligation, a trust creates a legal obligation. A court can compel the trustee to perform in the manner required by the trust agreement.

A trust may be either *inter vivos* or testamentary. An *inter vivos* trust is one created during the settlor's life. It may be funded and put into operation immediately or it may remain unfunded and inoperative until the settlor's death, at which time it will be funded under provisions of the settlor's will. An *inter vivos* trust agreement is a private agreement between the settlor and the trustee, and the contents of the trust and trust agreement are not matters of public record. A testamentary trust is one created in the settlor's will to take effect after his death. Because a deceased person's will is a matter of public record, the trust will appear in the court records and be open to public inspection. Whether *inter vivos* or testamentary all trusts are subject to the jurisdiction of the court and the trustee is subject to the supervisory control of the court. Any questions concerning the proper operation of the trust will be answered by the court.

Trusts may be mandatory or discretionary. A mandatory trust is one which requires the trustee to make distributions of income or principal to the beneficiary. For example, the trustee might be required to pay $1000 a year to the beneficiary or to pay all of the educational expenses of the beneficiary. A discretionary trust leaves the amount and the timing of income or principal distributions to the judgment of the trustee.

A mandatory trust may not be advisable for a child receiving state and federal benefits or services. The trustee has no choice as to when or why distributions occur, and therefore the distributions may disqualify the child for government benefits or cause increased liability for state-provided services. A discretionary trust avoids this problem by allowing the trustee to determine when each distribution should take place.

The purpose of the trust should be stated clearly so that the trustee can carry out the intention of the parents, and should also state that the trust is to supplement and not to replace otherwise available government aid. The trustee could be directed to finance advocacy for the child or pay a lawyer to enforce the child's legal rights. The trust should grant the trustee the power to accumulate income rather than distributing it, should that be in the beneficiary's best interest. The settlor must name a remainderman who is the person or persons who will receive the remaining trust assets at the termination of the trust. Finally, the trust should contain a spendthrift clause which will prevent the beneficiary's creditors, including the state, from reaching the trust assets (Frolik, 1979).

CONCLUSION

Parents of an autistic adolescent face serious decisions concerning the use of guardianship and in planning their estates. Correct answers are difficult to come by, and are problematical at best. Yet the growing maturity of the child signals that time waits for no man, and that action must be taken no matter how uncertain the choices. Parents should seek out professional assistance from a lawyer who is familiar with the problems of autism (or at least mental disabilities) to aid them in evaluating the options open to them. The one choice not available is to do nothing.

REFERENCES

Frolik, L. A., Estate planning for mentally disabled children. *University of Pittsburgh Law Review*, 1979, *23*, 323–325; *26*, 327–351.
Kopolow, L., & Bloom, H. (eds.), *Mental health advocacy: An emerging force in consumers' rights*. Washington, D.C.: DHEW Publication No. (ADM) 77–455, 1977.
Mesibov, G., Conover, B., & Saur, W. Limited guardianship laws and developmentally disabled adults: Needs and obstacles. *Mental Retardation*, 1980, *18*, 221–224.
Regan, J. J. Protective services for the elderly: Commitment, guardianship, and alternatives. *William and Mary Law Review*, 1972, *9*, 603–605.
Rothman, D. J. The discovery of the asylum: Social order and disorder. *New Republic*, 1971, *4*.

IV

Social and Community Programs

16

Social and Interpersonal Needs

LORNA WING

The question of the specificity of the classic autistic syndrome as first defined by Kanner (1943) is still under discussion. Some workers believe it to be a separate entity while others consider it as part of a wider range of handicaps involving abnormalities of language and social communication. Wing and Gould (1979) used an operational definition to cover autism and autistic-like conditions—that is, absence or impairment of comprehension and use of nonverbal and verbal communication (especially the former), of two-way social interaction, and of imaginative development, with the substitution of repetitive, stereotyped activities in place of flexible pretend play. The present chapter will be concerned with adolescents with these problems, regardless of intelligence level or presence of other handicaps, or of underlying cause, since whether or not autism is eventually proved to be unique and specific, all the syndromes that fit the more general description given above present many similar problems of management. There are differences in behavior and in prognosis between individuals with these handicaps, but these are more clearly related to factors, to be discussed later, other than the presence or absence of all the features of the classic autistic picture. The word "autistic" will be used for convenience, but in this chapter will cover the whole range of related conditions.

SOCIAL BEHAVIOR IN ADOLESCENCE

Adolescence produces physical and psychological changes with which all young people, whether handicapped or normal, have to cope. Many

LORNA WING ● Medical Research Council Social Psychiatry Unit, Institute of Psychiatry, London   SE5 8AF England of these changes affect social and interpersonal behavior. Increasing size and strength, especially if the adolescent becomes larger than his parents, make management of behavior problems considerably more difficult. Whereas a small screaming child can be picked up and removed from an embarrassing situation, this is not possible with a large teenager. Even the most handicapped autistic adolescent seems sooner or later to realize the implications of this change, and becomes more determined to have his own way.

The increase in self-awareness that occurs during adolescence usually brings with it a desire to be independent of parents and others who have exerted control in the past. Children, however stubborn they may appear at times, have a basic amenability to adult authority, presumably related to their physical and intellectual immaturity and dependence on others for care. By early adult life this amenability tends to be replaced by a desire to be free of such controls. The equivalent feelings can be seen in autistic people, especially in those of higher ability, though the manifestations are likely to be odd and unexpected (Wing, 1980).

Involvement with the peer culture increases in normal adolescents. The impairments of social interaction interfere with this aspect of development in most autistic people, but those who are more able and who have become more sociable with increasing age may try to imitate their peers. This also tends to be shown in a variety of inappropriate ways.

Adolescence leads to a fading of interest in childish toys and games. In the normal teenager these are replaced by age-appropriate social, intellectual, sporting, and practical activities. One of the saddest problems of the more handicapped autistic person is that the childish pursuits which, though simple and repetitive, previously filled his time no longer hold his attention when he is an adolescent, but his handicaps prevent him developing more adult occupations. The latter need social awareness, imagination, and the ability to understand a range of concepts, all of which are available in a limited way only to the small proportion of the most intelligent autistic people.

The implications of developing sexual maturity are a major worry for many parents of autistic children. This topic was dealt with in Chapter 9; here, only the aspects which particularly affect social relationships will be touched on.

The special problems of the autistic adolescent arise from the continuing presence of the handicaps underlying autism, even though their manifestations may change with increasing age. The problem which most affects social relationships is the impairment of the normal human ability to approach and respond to others appropriately, in the context of the situation—to be aware that other people have thoughts and feelings which are expressed nonverbally as well as verbally, and to adjust one's comprehension and use of language in the light of the social context (Weber, 1980).

CLINICAL CLASSIFICATION

Although autistic and autistic-like people share the same underlying impairments, there are wide individual variations which make it difficult to generalize about problems of management and provision of services. The task becomes a little easier if some system of subclassifying is used, related to the reasons for the individual differences. There are many factors that affect the clinical picture in each case, but in the present author's experience three appear to be of particular importance: the quality of social interaction, the potential for developing useful skills, and the characteristics special to each person which are collectively referred to as his temperament or personality. It is not suggested that this is the only or even the best way of subgrouping, but it is chosen here because it provides a framework for a discussion of autistic adolescents' social and interpersonal needs that, in the author's experience, has proved useful in practice and has been found helpful by parents, teachers, and professional care givers.

Social Interaction

The quality of social interaction is by definition abnormal in an autistic person, but the abnormality is shown in different ways in different people. Wing and Gould (1979) described three types of impaired interaction which can be recognized and have practical significance. First, the aloof child or adult has no pleasure or interest in social interaction. He may approach others in order to obtain his needs or for simple physical sensation or comfort, even a rough-and-tumble game, but he does not seek social contact for its own sake. Other people may be pushed away or avoided if they come too near. Such a person often has a close dependence on his parents and siblings and perhaps one or two other adults who have cared for him, but this is shown by turning to them for basic needs rather than in more usual sociable ways. This is the classic autistic aloofness as originally described by Kanner (1943). Second, there is the passive group. Those who fit this category do not make any active approaches, but are content to be approached and led by others. They can be drawn into simple activities such as singing and miming games, and will even take a passive role in pretend play, such as the patient in a game of doctors and nurses. Finally, the third group can be best described as "active but odd" for want of a better term. They do make spontaneous approaches to others, but these are one-sided, repetitive, and confined to their narrow range of interests. Their speech and behavior is not affected by any suggestions, made verbally or nonverbally, by the person who is approached. Repetitive questioning, for example, about other people's ages and dates of birth is particularly common in this group.

These categories are not distinct entities but shade into each other. A child may change his group as he grows older, though few if any changes occur after the later years of childhood. Some are difficult to classify on this dimension because, depending on the situation, they show behavior which may be characteristic of more than one of the groups. However, the system of subgrouping can in most cases be applied in a rough-and-ready way in practice in autistic children and adults.

Level of Ability

The potential for developing useful skills can be measured to some extent by standardized intelligence tests. The term "level of intelligence" is best avoided when describing the abilities of an autistic person since, even if he scores in the normal or superior range on the available tests, he lacks the imagination and the understanding of social rules that are important components of intelligence in the normal person. The most useful tests for autistic people are those that measure their visuospatial and rote memory skills, which are usually the areas in which they function best. The results are highly correlated with prognosis (Rutter, 1970). The level of ability can range from no skills at all up to a sufficiently wide range to allow independent living as an adult, though this outcome is seen in only a small minority.

Temperamental Characteristics

Autistic people have their own individual personalities even if they are handicapped. These can be discerned in the most as well as the least severely affected. As originally pointed out by Bartak (personal communication) autistic children often resemble one or other parent in psychological characteristics as well as in physical appearance, just as do normal children. These characteristics affect the way each person reacts to his handicaps. Someone of a placid and amenable disposition will be much easier to manage if autistic than someone who would have been determined and headstrong whether or not he was handicapped. It is a mistake to assume that everything one observes in an autistic person can be explained by the autism. This attitude makes the differences between autistic people harder to understand.

SOCIAL PROBLEMS OF DIFFERENT SUBGROUPS

Each of the three factors mentioned above can vary independently of the others. Though there is a strong tendency for social aloofness to be associated with low levels of ability (Wing, 1978) this is not invariably the case. Since the variables are dimensions or axes and not composed of discrete categories, they can be arbitrarily divided into any number of subgroups and a classification based on a combination of the factors could contain any number of classes. For the purpose of the present discussion, the different types of social interaction will be considered in turn and the influence of the two other axes mentioned within this context.

The Aloof Group

The aloof group are by definition those who appear most cut off from social contact with others. With appropriate education and management throughout childhood they may gradually learn to tolerate being with other people, but most of them continue to want and need a place of their own to which they can retreat at fairly frequent intervals, especially if exposed to larger numbers of other people than usual, or to strangers. The tendency to reject unsolicited physical or social contact may remain into adult life, even though the person concerned may enjoy such experiences for a brief time if he himself initiates them.

Despite the outward appearance of withdrawal, the aloof autistic person tends to be very dependent on a few familiar figures and he may become disturbed in behavior if the care givers change or if too many different people are involved.

Social aloofness tends to be associated with severe impairment or absence of verbal and nonverbal communication, so those who work with people in this group receive little or no direct evidence that their care is appreciated. At times their attempts to help are rejected, perhaps with physical aggression. The care givers have to learn to understand the idiosyncratic signs by which an autistic person expresses his attachment—perhaps by a particular facial expression or a special sound, or by the choice of one individual rather than another to approach when wanting food or physical comfort. Parents or caring staff also have to learn to interpret the indications of different needs if these cannot be expressed in words or manual signs. Autistic people of this kind require love and understanding given without thought of reward. Piecing together the story of Victor, the "wild" boy with autistic behavior found wandering in the woods of southern central France at the end of the 18th century who was educated by the physician Itard (Lane, 1977), it seems that Itard's housekeeper, Mme Guérin, gave Victor this kind of unqualified affection. Perhaps the surprising thing is that autistic children and adults do have the capacity to call forth instincts of compassion and the desire to help in so many people, despite their strange and difficult behavior. On the other hand their inability to communicate and defend themselves makes them especially vulnerable in settings with too many residents and too few overworked and undertrained staff.

There are a small number of socially aloof autistic adolescents with a range of useful skills. Except in very special circumstances, such as an employer willing to make special arrangements, such people are not able to obtain work on the open market. It is, however, important for their quality of life for them to be able to exercise their skills in a sheltered setting. The work supervisors need to understand the nature of the autistic handicaps, and to be calm, confident, and patient. The most satisfactory environment is one in which the autistic person has his own special place, where he can arrange his working tools in the way he prefers, and where he can be part of the group at times but can move away when he chooses.

Behavior disturbance such as aggression, destructiveness, screaming, wandering, self-injury, and so on are particularly common in the aloof group, especially those with very low levels of ability (Gould, 1976). Also, simple repetitive activities, including rocking, arm flapping, self-spinning, object flicking, are a marked feature (Wing and Gould, 1979). These abnormalities are off-putting, even frightening, to others, including the non-autistic mentally retarded, and add to the problems of social relationships.

The handicaps of the aloof group are so severe that they tend to obscure the effects of individual differences in temperament. However, even among this group it is still possible to detect those who, had they not suffered from the brain dysfunction causing autism, would have been friendly and amenable people, others who would have been loners, and yet others who would have been active, determined, perhaps irritable, in their social interactions. A sensitivity to these underlying traits is helpful in creating the environment most suitable to the individual concerned.

The Passive Group

The passive autistic people are the easiest to manage and to integrate into a social group. Unlike the aloof children and adults, most of them are able to imitate other people's actions to some extent, although the quality of the imitation shows that there is little or no understanding. The author has observed that some go through a stage in childhood in which they "echo" other people's gestures, in a way which is equivalent to the immediate echoing of speech. Despite the lack of comprehension of the movements that are copied, the ability provides a useful basis for teaching a range of activities, including the imitation of other children's pretend play. Perhaps because they can copy others and therefore have something positive they can do, passive autistic people are willing to be drawn into group activities and obtain pleasure from being involved.

In general the passive group have higher levels of skills than those who are aloof. The relatively less able settle down well with the sociable mentally retarded in school or, later, in a sheltered workshop. They enjoy the activities available in such settings. The only problem is that they might be left out because they do not take the initiative or push themselves forward. The staff can ensure that this does not happen if they are aware of the tendency. They also need to know that sudden, unexpected changes in the familiar environment or routine may cause temporarily disturbed behavior in a person who has hitherto given no trouble.

Adolescents and adults in the passive group who have high levels of ability are the most likely to become independent as adults, though even among them it is the minority who do so. They are usually well liked by their workmates, and if they have some outstanding skill may come to be regarded with special affection as the "eccentric professor." Nevertheless there are a number of problems that may arise. The amiable passivity in social situations may be mistaken for lack of enjoyment so that no more invitations to join in group activities are given. This can cause great distress, which the autistic person is unable to express, so the situation is not remedied. Autistic adolescents with some social awareness often want to have friends, but not understanding the nature of friendship will assume that everyone who speaks to them is a friend. If they go on to make incorrect assumptions about the degree of intimacy a relationship allows, this can lead to rebuffs and hurt feelings. Attempts to find partners of the opposite sex are especially fraught with misunderstandings, as discussed elsewhere in this book.

Occasionally a young autistic adult with some high-level skills and the wish to copy and join in with his peers may decide to leave home because this is what others in his age group are doing. Actions of this kind undertaken on impulse usually end in failure. In most cases independent living, if it is possible at all, can be achieved only gradually, with much support from parents or others in the background.

Although this type of autistic adolescent likes to take part in (or rather, be present at) opportunities for social interaction, he can become overtired and confused if intruded upon too enthusiastically by others, and expected to enter into conversations or other activities that are beyond his capabilities.

In the case of the passive autistic group the type of social interaction is closely linked to the temperamental characteristics. However, successful integration into a group, whether in sheltered or in open conditions, is easier for the adolescent who is calm and equable rather than timid, shy, and anxious.

The "Active But Odd" Group

The autistic adolescents who make "active but odd" social approaches are the most difficult group of all. Unlike the others, they demand social attention because of their lengthy monologues or repetitive questioning or, if lacking in conversational speech, their physical touching or clinging, which may turn into physical aggression. This is unpleasant and wearing for those approached because the normally sociable person feels impelled to reply, but is disconcerted to find that the more he responds the more the same demands are repeated. Sometimes the content of the repetitive speech is bizarre or horrific and this can increase the difficulties of organizing any form of social life for the autistic person concerned.

On the whole, people in this group have more skills than the aloof group, but their behavior interferes with achievement so they do not do as well as the passive adolescents. At all levels of ability a major problem is the tendency for parents and professional workers to underestimate the severity of the handicaps, mainly because of the apparent sociability and talkativeness. For this reason there is often a history of a series of school placements that have failed. Each time the teachers begin by being convinced they can teach the child and end by rejecting him. Sadly, the same pattern may continue into adult life, making it difficult to find a suitable placement.

Social interaction with such people has to be organized with particular care. The natural desire to encourage social approaches and to answer questions has to be controlled so that responses are made once only to each remark and repetitions are ignored. New topics of conversation and social interactions are encouraged, but the stereotyped talking and actions are not rewarded.

Autistic adolescents of this kind usually want to take part in group activities, but can become disturbed and disruptive unless their behavior is carefully managed by someone who knows them well. From the outside it appears that they are driven to approach other people, but when they do the level of excitement rises until it spills over into aggression, destructiveness, or some other undesirable activity. They need social experiences, but these have to be organized with care until behavior is more reliable.

Personality characteristics have an effect in this group also. Someone who is basically friendly and cheerful is easier to tolerate, even if he pesters, than someone who is by temperament demanding and irritable.

PSYCHIATRIC PROBLEMS

Disturbed Behavior

Clinical experience is beginning to show that increases in behavior problems are relatively common in autistic adolescents, though the proportion likely to be affected is not yet known. These difficulties may be due to the physical and psychological changes in adolescence mentioned earlier. It sometimes appears that they are a response to too much pressure to learn new skills, or exposure to too much social stimulation. On the other hand failure in attempts to make social contact and consequent social isolation may precipitate a breakdown, especially in a more able autistic person with some awareness of his handicaps. Medication such as major tranquilizers may diminish the severity of the problem, but does not solve it. Although no systematic work has been done in this field, it is possible that anticipation of the onset of adolescence, and a gradual change to less schoolwork and more practical, domestic, and physical activities, might prove helpful.

Psychiatric Illnesses

In some cases it appears that the behavior disturbance is due to an identifiable psychiatric illness (Wing, 1981). Clinical symptoms of depression or anxiety, or a mixture of both in mild, moderate, or severe form are relatively common in autistic adolescents, though no studies of prevalence have been published. They can occur in association with any of the types of social interaction, but affective problems are easier to recognize in people who have enough speech to describe their symptoms. The depression often appears to be associated with dawning awareness of the implications of the autistic handicap and failures in personal relationships, especially with the opposite sex.

Treatment includes medication if the clinical picture makes this appropriate, but for the more able autistic person with some insight, help from a counselor who understands the autistic impairments is equally important. This must be geared to the level of understanding of the autistic adolescent, and consist mainly of discussion of problems, simple advice, and reassurance as to personal worth in spite of handicaps.

Other psychiatric conditions can be superimposed on autism in adolescence and early adult life, but these are less common than depression. Psychoses of the adult type with delusions and hallucinations, including typical schizophrenia, have been reported (Wing, 1981; Wolff & Chick, 1980) which exacerbate the difficulties of social interaction. These need treatment with the appropriate medication and a careful analysis of the precipitating factors, which may sometimes include too great a degree of pressure to perform well in a social group.

Severely or profoundly retarded autistic people with little or no speech may, when they reach adolescence, develop swings of behavior with periods of excitement and overactivity alternating with periods of apathy. The lack of communication makes it difficult to know what feelings accompany these changes, but those who know the person concerned will often feel that cheerful elation goes with the excitement and depression and misery with the apathetic state. These behavioral changes may be the outward manifestations of mood swings. They have a profound effect on social life, because at either extreme the behavior interferes with social interaction even on a simple level. In these cases antidepressive medication may help, but care is necessary in case unwanted side effects or even worsening of the behavior problems occur. The severe communication impairments make counseling an impossibility. Behavior management techniques are difficult to apply because it is usually not possible to discover the reasons for the marked fluctuations—they appear to be related to internal rather than external states. It is the author's impression that they tend to become less intense with increasing age.

IMPROVING SOCIAL SKILLS

The Severely Handicapped Group

For those with autistic impairments in marked form, especially if accompanied by severe general retardation, the possibility of joining in social pursuits is as limited in adolescence and adult life as it was in childhood. Careful control of behavior problems remains important, as does repeated emphasis on simple rules, such as the need to take turns, to accept the proximity of others, and not to take other people's food or possessions. Opportunities for social mixing have to be chosen with care to ensure that the autistic adolescents enjoy at least some aspects of the occasion and are not exposed to strange situations for longer than they can tolerate. Planning and organization are even more important than with children because adolescents are less willing to accept direction from others. If they have no interest in becoming more sociable, of if they find social contact distressing, there is little point in pushing them. For people of this kind it is better to allow them to be on their own when they feel the need, even if it means disappearance as soon as visitors arrive, than to press them into staying in a highly stressful situation.

The More Able Group

Helping more able autistic people who themselves wish to improve their social skills presents a different kind of challenge. There is no lack of motivation, at least to begin with. The problem lies in the autistic person's difficulty in grasping the subtle rules that underlie social inter-action. To an even greater extent than with language these rules shift and change with the context, and unlike the laws of mathematics they cannot be stated in absolute form. For example, the conventions concerning the use of surnames versus given names vary with age, sex, class, degree of familiarity, and from time to time, and between groups even within the same cultures.

Although it is a daunting task, the only way to help an autistic person is to try to teach him as many of the rules as possible, and in as simple and concrete and safe a form as possible; for example, it is better that a handicapped adolescent should use surnames too often than that he should be too familiar with others. Everyone concerned, parents as well as profes-sional workers, should help in this process, taking every opportunity of explaining the most appropriate way to behave. This must be done with tact and understanding, giving praise whenever possible. Most autistic young people who have some insight are sensitive to failure and easily give in to black despair over seemingly minor setbacks. As emphasized before, they also have the adolescent's resentment of authority if it is shown in too heavy-handed a way.

Psychologists and others who are beginning to work in this field use techniques such as acting out everyday social encounters with the autistic person taking different roles; videotaping interactions, real or acted, so that problems can be discussed in detail; and regular discussions of the day's events, with constructive suggestions for future behavior (Argyle, 1973).

Progress is usually very slow. Rules that are learned by rote can easily be misapplied. For example, a young man came into the office of the director of the unit he attended without tapping on the door. After being reminded, he apologized politely, turned around, and tapped on the inside of the door. This story demonstrates the way in which an autistic person, however well motivated, understands the letter but not the spirit of the laws he learns. However, patient effort on the part of the autistic person and his helpers does show some results eventually. Even though a lifetime is not long enough to learn by rote all the rules of social conduct, a large number can be accumulated over many years. During the learning process continual encouragement will be needed. It is also helpful to explain that many nonhandicapped people are not particularly sociable, but can still be valuable and respected members of the community.

For some autistic people, as already mentioned, the problem is too much rather than too little social contact. Parents of young autistic people who make inappropriate approaches to others often worry about discouraging them in case they revert to the aloofness of former years. This does not seem to be a real problem. Tactful explanation and teaching of more appropriate behavior can be as helpful with this group as with the more withdrawn autistic person.

In addition to the rules of social interaction it is also useful for the more able autistic adolescent to develop skill in any sports or games that he is willing and able to learn. These include outdoor pursuits such as horse riding, swimming, walking, climbing, team games, athletics, and indoor activities such as table tennis, card games, chess and other board games. For many, poor coordination limits the range of possibilities, but it is worthwhile trying to find some area in which the individual concerned can achieve at least adequate performance. All these pursuits facilitate social contact without the need for conversation. They can help fill the leisure hours, which are especially difficult times for an autistic person. Becoming a member of a club organized around a particular activity can be a source of support and satisfaction. Musical or artistic skills may also be a key to joining a group of people with similar interests. As mentioned earlier, the school program needs to be modified as adolescence approaches. Systemic efforts can be made to explore each child's capabilities and structured teaching given in the areas in which he shows some aptitude.

For all kinds of autistic people care must be taken not to apply too much pressure, but to give enough encouragement for some progress to occur. This process is like walking a tightrope, so narrow is the divide between over- and understimulation. Experience and a sensitive understanding of each individual are the only guides.

Personal Friendships

Most autistic people, because of the severity of their handicaps, are not able to initiate or take an active part in a friendship. They depend on the care and concern of parents and other care givers for emotional support. In some families a nonhandicapped brother or sister becomes closely attached to the autistic sibling, who may respond with pleasure, shown in his own peculiar way, to this special relationship. In schools or units for adolescents and adults two autistic people may show some preference for each other by choosing physical proximity or appearing to be unhappy when parted for any reason. Rather more often, in a unit for mixed handicaps a sociable retarded person will become fond of someone who is autistic and will help in caring for him and try to involve him in social activities, sometimes in the face of strong resistance.

More able autistic adolescents often wish to have a friend, but most fail to form a satisfactory peer relationship. Some, however, are more fortunate. Partnerships between people who are both autistic do occasionally develop, and, more rarely, friendships between an autistic and a nonhandicapped person. There may be a considerable age gap in either direction. Autistic people are characteristically unaware of the social implications of differences in age and social class.

None of these relationships can be planned or organized, but they can be most valuable when they grow spontaneously, giving pleasure and satisfaction to both members of the pair. Care is needed to ensure that on the one hand the autistic person is not dominated or pushed too far and on the other that the nonautistic partner is not wrapped up in the one-sided friendship to the exclusion of other activities. Parents, teachers, and other professional workers need to be sensitive to the existence of these relationships, fostering them when they are of benefit, giving advice when asked, and intervening with tact if problems occur.

PROVISION OF SERVICES

Models of Care

Many different models for residential and day services for autistic people have been tried and all have their successes and failures (Baker, Seltzer, & Seltzer, 1977). There is no one solution to all the problems, since there is such variation in need even among those who have in common the basic impairments of autism. The greater the range of provision, the more likely one is to find a suitable place for each individual.

The question of the value of mixed units versus those specializing in autism is often raised, the defendants of the former arguing that socially withdrawn people must exacerbate each other's problems of social interaction. In practice it is found that both types of provision have their place. Specialized units with experienced staff who make opportunities for social experiences for the residents provide a better environment for withdrawn autistic people than a mixed unit where none of the activities provided is of the kind in which an autistic person can join. On the other hand a mixed unit in which the needs of autistic people are studied as carefully as those of sociable residents may be able to provide a satisfying life for both. The staff in specialized units should ensure that there are opportunities for appropriate activities together with nonautistic people, and staff in mixed units should recognize the need for autistic people to be protected from too much social intrusion.

There is also controversy concerning the place of sheltered, usually rural, communities, as opposed to group homes within the normal community. Those who prefer the latter feel that the sheltered communities deprive the residents of the benefits of normal social life, but others are of the opinion that they have special advantages for autistic people. In the United Kingdom, the National Society for Autistic Children has been involved in the establishment of both kinds of service in the belief that both are needed. The former offer residential care and suitable occupation. Sites are chosen with adequate grounds so that the residents have as much freedom as possible without interfering with or suffering interference from other people. Leisure activities outside as well as inside the sheltered community are organized so that the residents are not cut off from the normal world. Accommodation in small group homes within the normal community is most suitable for the least handicapped autistic people who can take advantage of the opportunities for a more normal social life. For those who cannot go out on their own, and especially those with behavior problems, small group homes can, paradoxically, mean isolation and confinement as opposed to the relative freedom of the sheltered community. The difficulties for this group are exacerbated if there is no day center or other facilities for sheltered work in the vicinity.

A third unsolved question is whether it is best to mix or segregate people with different degrees of severity of handicap. Those who favor mixing point out that the levels of attainment and quality of life of the most severely or profoundly disabled individuals are raised by association with those of higher ability, whereas segregation produces further deterioration. On the other hand the proponents of separation according to level of function are concerned that the more able people will be adversely affected by the more severely handicapped and that the quality of their social life will suffer. The argument is most relevant when considering the best model of care for the behaviorally disturbed. The problem is that there is truth on both sides. The result is that services tend to go through cycles of segregation, followed by mixing, and back to segregation again, because of the disadvantages of each model.

From the author's observations, even day and residential centers set up by parents' associations with the initial intention of accepting autistic people of all levels of handicap gradually change until segregation is practiced by the exclusion of the more severely handicapped or disturbed people. In order to ensure that the latter are cared for, admission policies have to specified in advance, and the staffing, the physical amenities, and the daily program organized to suit the special needs of this group. If a unit with a wide range of severity of handicap is envisaged, then the needs of those of all levels of ability have to be considered in detail. It is particularly important that applicants for posts on the caring staff should be made aware of the unit policy and only those accepted who are in sympathy with the aims.

On balance it is hard to say whether mixing or segregation produces more problems. One answer which is possible in a residential community is to have segregated living units for different types of people on one campus, with social mixing carefully organized for some of the daily activities. But constant vigilance is needed to ensure that the standards of care in this type of service do not slide down to become institutionally rather than individually oriented (King, Raynes, & Tizard, 1971). It should also be remembered that decline in standards can also occur in small group homes in the community unless care is taken to avoid this.

Organization of Units

Whatever the general form of the service, there are certain factors which are particularly important for autistic people. First, at least some of the staff providing care should be experienced with and understand the nature of the handicaps. Second, there should be enough staff to allow for some individual attention. Third, each living or day unit should care for a small group, even if there are a number of such units grouped together on one campus. Fourth, the physical size and shape of the unit should allow for appropriate management of behavior problems, and also provide a place for each autistic person at times to withdraw from social contact and indulge in solitary activities, such as listening to his own records. Finally, each small living unit should have a substantial degree of autonomy so that staff and residents can choose furnishings and decorations, cook their own food on the premises, buy and launder the residents' clothing, and arrange their own daily routines. External supervision is needed to ensure that standards are maintained and that the unit is run in accordance with the philosophy of the service and to the benefit of the residents, but such supervision can be given while still allowing a high degree of independence for each group.

The provision of opportunities for social experiences has been emphasized in this chapter. Autistic people are more likely to enjoy these and to behave well if they have a clear role to play which is within their capacity. For example, the tasks of opening the door to guests, taking their coats, helping and serving at tables, taking around drinks, clearing and washing dishes can be divided among the autistic adolescents, tactfully supervised by the staff. This type of functional role can give much pleasure, whereas taking part in party chatter is a severe strain or an impossibility. Experienced parents and other care givers know how important it is to cut short social outings once the formal organized proceedings have ended.

The above comments apply to sheltered accommodation and occupation. Autistic people who become independent and live on their own can become lonely and isolated because there is no one to organize their leisure time for them. Some, who have a special hobby such as playing chess or collecting train numbers, find a group of people with a similar interest and organize their own leisure time. There are others, however, who do not find such pursuits for themselves. They may accept, even prefer, their lonely lives, but a number eventually break down with depression or bizarre behavior and have to be found a more sheltered way of life. The possibility of this sort of outcome consequent upon living alone poses a dilemma for parents and professional workers when deciding whether or not to encourage an autistic person to try for independence. Factors such as a special interest which can be pursued in the company of like-minded people, good self-care skills, including knowing that clothes need changing and laundering regularly, and a calm, equable temperament are factors suggesting that the attempt may be successful. Without these positive attributes it is wise to be cautious when advising an autistic person about his future lifestyle.

The social and interpersonal needs of autistic children are in most cases best met if they live with their own families and attend a school that can cater to their problems, although for many different reasons this may not be best for the rest of the family so that other forms of care have to be found. However, by late adolescence and adult life the situation has changed. At this time it is to the advantage of both the autistic person and his family for him to move away from the family home, usually to some sheltered residence, but in a few cases to independent accommodation. Close contact with the family should if at all possible be maintained, but it is best for all concerned for the young autistic adult to adjust to his new life while his parents are still around to help him through the difficult early stages. At the moment this ideal is hard to attain for large numbers of autistic people because of lack of services. Encouragement of the development of suitable provisions for adults, for both accommodation and occupation, is one of the priorities of all those concerned with the well-being of autistic adolescents.

REFERENCES

Argyle, M. (Ed.). *Social encounters*. Harmondsworth, England: Penguin, 1973.

Baker, B. L., Seltzer, G. B., & Seltzer, M. M. *As close as possible: Community residences for retarded adults*. Boston: Little, Brown, 1977.

Gould, J. Language impairments in severely retarded children: An epidemiological study. *Journal of Mental Deficiency Research*, 1976, *20*, 129–146.

Kanner, L. Autistic disturbances of affective contact. *Nervous Child*, 1943, *2*, 217–250.

King, R. D., Raynes, N. V., & Tizard, J. *Patterns of residential care*. London: Routledge and Kegan Paul, 1971.

Lane, H. *The wild boy of Aveyron*. London: Allen & Unwin, 1977.

Rutter, M. Autistic children: Infancy to adulthood. *Seminars in Psychiatry*, 1970, *2*, 435–450.

Weber, S. *Aspects of the language of autistic children: A study in linguistic progmatics*. Zurich: W. Schneider, 1980.

Wing, L. Social, behavioural and cognitive characteristics. In *Autism: A reappraisal of concepts and treatment* (M. Rutter & E. Schopler, eds.), New York: Plenum Press, 1978.

Wing, L. *Autistic children: A guide for parents*. London: Constable, 1980.

Wing, L. Asperger's syndrome: A clinical account. *Psychological Medicine*, 1981, *11*, 115–129.

Wing, L., & Gould, J. Severe impairments of social interaction and associated abnormalities in children: Epidemiology and classification. *Journal of Autism and Development Disorders*, 1979, *9*, 11–29.

Wolff, S., & Chick, J. Schizoid personality in childhood: A controlled follow-up study. *Psychological Medicine*, 1980, *10*, 85–100.

17

Benhaven

AMY L. LETTICK

OVERVIEW

Nature of the Program

Benhaven is a day and residential school community which was founded in Connecticut in 1967. It has an intensive program, demanding of teachers and students, individualized and time-intensive, with the goal of achieving optimum development in each student through maximizing the potential for independence and competence in vocational, residential, and recreational skills, and thereby avoiding custodial institutionalization in adulthood.

Benhaven offers a combination of a flexible individualized program, a time span of services running from childhood into adulthood, and the availability, within its own physical boundaries, of a variety of environments—urban, suburban, school, workshop, residence, and farm—that can accommodate a wide range of intellectual, physical, and vocational aptitudes and of behavioral deviance.

The Benhaven Philosophy

When the school opened, a working philosophy was developed that has shaped the program over the years. Its main points are:

AMY L. LETTICK • Benhaven, New Haven, Connecticut 06511.

1. Special education, not psychotherapy, is our tool; we are educational and behavioral in our orientation.
2. We cannot wait for relationships to develop before we begin work; through work, relationships will be formed.
3. We must individualize programs, with continual measurement and adjustment.
4. There is no one way; we must use all the methods that will work.
5. Learning, for the handicapped, is not always pleasant for the teacher or the student, but temporary stress is worth the ultimate gain. Extreme disability often requires extreme measures for remediation.
6. Education and socialization must be accompanied by vocational training and must continue into adulthood.
7. Families must play a positive role in the program.
8. All children should leave home by young adulthood, and this should be viewed positively, as is the departure of their normal brothers and sisters.

Population

Approximately 90 students have been enrolled, for periods ranging from 1 to 15 years. Presently there are 50 enrollees, 19 of them 21–28 years old, the remaining ranging in age from 8 to 21. Although we have had a starting age of 6, we now accept younger students.

Virtually all have autism as their primary handicap, with accompanying emotional disturbance and retardation. A few are also deaf or legally blind. Approximately half are mute and have learned to communicate in sign language. The other half have varying levels of speech. No student has totally normal language. Two students are neurologically impaired without being autistic. Three-quarters of the population are in adolescence. Approximately one-quarter have occasional episodes of aggression or self-abuse. One-third receive medication to control seizures or to improve behavior. One-quarter are female. Three-quarters come from Connecticut, one student comes from Mexico, and the rest from other parts of the United States. There is only one with normal intelligence. One or two have areas of exceptional skill, counterbalanced by glaring lacks in other areas. All but a few of the younger children are involved in prevocational or vocational programs.

There is no cut-off age in our day program. Enrollees can remain at Benhaven as long as it is the least restrictive and best program available to them, and as long as funding is available.

Physical Plant

The headquarters is a 22-room house located atop a small hill in a residential neighborhood of New Haven. A gymnasium and small playground are in the rear. Seven miles away on our farm campus, a 35-acre plot straddling the borderline between North Haven and East Haven, are two barns, a farmhouse, a greenhouse, a ranch house, a swimming pool, and our new residential unit. The farmhouse and ranch house serve as residences for seven of our students.

The new residence, opened in February 1981, is a V-shaped, one-story duplex with two self-contained wings joined by staff quarters, which occupy the angle of the V. Each wing has its main entrance at one end of the V and contains sleeping accommodations for six students. Screening shrubbery in the angle gives each wing the feeling of a small house.

Kitchens, bathrooms, and laundry rooms are extra large, to accommodate teaching activities. All rooms can be shut off from each other, to eliminate distraction during lessons; for the same reason, picture windows are eliminated except in staff quarters. Corridors are extra wide so that staff members can walk alongside the students to provide both control and companionship.

In each wing there are two bedrooms for students and two for staff members, plus a small single bedroom. There is a fifth staff bedroom for a floating staff member. One staff bedroom is large enough to accommodate a spouse who may live with us but work elsewhere.

The staff quarters, with quick and easy access to each wing for emergency and social relief, provide privacy and comfort for the staff while remaining close to student quarters, directly in communication with residents. An office provides storage space for records and research equipment. The staff living room contains cooking and dining facilities for use on nights off. Staff members and their guests can enter and leave without going through student quarters.

This 7,000-square-foot house is financed entirely by private funds. Residential fees, along with tuition fees for school-age children, are paid by the towns or school districts where parents reside. This house is licensed as a group home by the Connecticut Department of Mental Retardation; adult residents are thus eligible for funding of residential costs by the state Department of Mental Health.

PROGRAMS AT BENHAVEN

Benhaven offers residential and day programs for children and has an adult division that is licensed by the U.S. Department of Labor as a

Work Activities Center. Day and residential clients are provided with academic training, sex education, and vocational training. The day program is supplemented with home programs, and families of day students are also offered respite services. The adult division, using guidelines from the Department of Labor, offers vocational training and employment to those over 21 years of age.

Day Program

The school day runs from 9:30 A.M. to 4:30 P.M. Monday through Saturday, all year, with Sundays and six holidays off. During the summer, all academic, fine motor, and vocational work is conducted in the morning at the school. Afternoons are spent at the farm, where the entire student body engages in the vocational and gross motor components of each program. This summer clustering of activities frees certain staff for half of the day to develop individualized programs for each student for the following academic year.

Each student has an individualized program. Five half-hour periods in the morning and in the afternoon are interspersed by snacks and lunch. As the attention span allows, periods are combined into larger blocks.

Behavior, communication, and socialization are not regarded as isolated areas of instruction; they are carried on through the activities of the other areas. We do not teach "good behavior" as a separate activity. Behavior modification, combined with manipulation of the program and environment, occasional medication (supervised closely by our Medical Review Committee), and consistency among all involved, including the parents, are the tools for encouraging normal social interaction.

Academics. Readiness, reading, numbers, writing, and language are taught. The language and testing areas are supervised by a clinical psychologist and speech pathologist. Although a few students approach normalcy in math, the academic achievements of most are limited, so we spend more time on self-care and functional academics connected with vocational training.

Sex Education. Benhaven's program on sexuality and social awareness is discussed in Chapter 9. The program was developed for students who display no capacity for forming social attachments, those who cannot benefit from already-developed successful methods of teaching about, and encouraging, normal social interaction. This program is inappropriate for a more highly socialized person; it is simply another alternative in a range of services. The curriculum units deal with identification of body parts, menstruation, masturbation, physical examinations, personal hygiene, and social behavior. These units are carried out with close involvement of parents.

Vocational Training. Only three of our students are under the age of 12 and too young for formal prevocational training. Most of the others are engaged in either prevocational or vocational activities. In prevocational training we present simple tasks associated with the vocational activities to follow later (Freschi, 1974). What is paramount is that a student learn to perform the task the right way from the beginning, and work without a behavioral blow-up. If he can attend to a task and maintain a steady effort, it is likely that he will be able to work in a group later. When he can work for an hour independently he is eligible for promotion to the vocational program.

In the vocational program the teacher assumes the role of workshop supervisor, teaching, assigning tasks, recording work accomplished, striving always to keep the student growing in ability to work, relate, and behave. Student work teams are put together for jobs requiring combined effort, such as lifting and carrying. The repetition involved with the work we choose is an important factor in our success with our students. Their satisfaction in repetitive tasks and their compulsion toward sameness make it pleasurable to complete tasks repeatedly. These traits, otherwise considered handicaps, become marketable skills and assets in the workplace.

For our farm work we frequently consult the nearby agricultural experiment station. We find it best to have a teacher who knows our children develop our program, however, and then to get technical advice, rather than to start with a technical expert. The outside expert is usually dismayed at the limitations of our labor force, and does not have the inclination or imagination to adjust the process to the needs of the population. Our goal is not successful enterprise as such, but the development of human beings. As a board member says, "We use plants to grow people."

Successful vocational enterprises include:

Button making. This is, by far, our most enduring successful activity. All our students are able to do some or all.

Horticulture. We have completed a second greenhouse to accommodate the vocational opportunities available. This area, like button making, offers a variety of tasks involving levels of skill, with repetition.

Agriculture. We farm approximately 1 acre of land. A problem we faced was the lack of organization and perception in our students. Some could not distinguish plants from weeds, cultivated areas from walking spaces. Our farm coordinator solved this by planning for a yard-wide strip of grass between each row of plants. This substituted easy mowing for weeding. Instead of furrows, he developed mounds of enriched irrigated soil. The combination of raised furrows and green walking space provides clues for both feet and eyes. We don't expect to expand beyond this 1 acre; operating a large farm would require the total time of our students, and would limit variety in their programs.

Poultry raising. We maintain three to four dozen chickens. The chicken coops are designed and organized so that students take care of the operation almost independently. Wire-mesh floors on a slight angle roll the eggs to a trough from which the students can pick them up without risking a pecking. The combination of mesh floors with elevated coops make cleaning of the droppings possible without entering the coops. The feeding troughs are filled from outside. The poultry raising operation undergoes continual refinement and improvement.

Furniture refinishing and woodworking. Students in the workshop wear protective clothing, and only the most capable are allowed to work with chemicals or electrical equipment, under close supervision. If a student cannot produce work that meets the normal competition, we must find other work for him.

Mailing. We process the school's bulk mail; we also do subcontract work for a local letter-mailing shop. Two of our students work half days at that shop, and one has done so for over three years.

We have been unsuccessful in some of our vocational enterprises. For example:

Bread baking. We can't eliminate the need for judgment.

Printing. Our students can set type and hand-print, but the process is too slow to guarantee delivery within a reasonable time.

Bookbinding. A few students can and do handle this, with thin books. But a thick book offers too many opportunities for error, thus requiring too much supervision.

The Adult Division

Vocational activities take up more and more of the day as the student gets older. The last 6 months of his 21st year is a transition period to the adult program.

We started our adult division in 1978, becoming licensed as a Work Activities Center by the U.S. Department of Labor. As of 1982, we are licensed and supervised by the Connecticut Department of Mental Retardation, with the day program for adults paid for by the state-funded Community Sheltered Workshop Program.

In the adult program, the focus is on vocation-related activities, with less time devoted to formal academics and gross motor training.

There is one positive aspect to reducing the scope of the program. The lack of pressure in academic and motor areas has resulted in less explosive, more contented adults. They are comfortable in their programs, know what is expected, and can do it. This makes us wonder whether we are perhaps pressing too hard, too much, when they are younger. From that pressure, however, has come the competence without which they would still be sitting in a corner somewhere, tranquil perhaps, but incompetent. So we feel that early pressure is justified if it results in calm, competent adults. We continue therefore to press for maximum growth while they are young.

Though adults have a half hour of recreation in the gym at lunchtime, they are no longer in the school building classrooms—they are in the workshops or at the farm.

We limit our adults to graduates of our day school. This restriction is necessary if we are to assure placement for the steady stream of our own students as they turn 21.

The staff ratio during teaching is 1:1. Supervision afterward is 1:3. Nearly all need individual instruction when learning a new task, or need 1:1 during a brief episode of poor behavior. Some 1:8 periods allow us the 1:1 necessary for individualized help when it is needed.

We never keep a student at the same task for more than 2 hours. If he worked at the button workshop in the morning, he may be assigned to the greenhouse or furniture refinishing workshop in the afternoon. We don't lock him into one vocational slot just because he is good at it. This policy often prevents us from accepting orders for quick delivery, because of lack of labor. We sometimes get around this by subcontracting.

Residential Living

Benhaven began its residential program in 1972. In each house—and in the case of our newest residence, in each wing—live three, sometimes four or five students. A minimum of two staff members lives in each house.

Residents are occupied all day. They have half an hour of free time when they come home from school or work at 5 P.M. At that time they are free to rock, sit, pace, to do anything they prefer that is harmless, under the gaze, but not constraint, of the staff. This applies only to students who show no possibility of eventual integration into the community.

We are more restrictive of bizarre behavior in those who will lose from it.

At 5:30 they resume their schedules, some preparing dinner, others cleaning, doing their laundry, until the evening meal is served between 6:30 and 7:30. Student capability early eliminated the need for a hired cook-housekeeper.

When after-dinner chores are finished recreation begins, extending until bedtime preparation and bed between 10 and 11 P.M. Recreation is geared to the skills of individual students. For some, evening lessons in reading or cooking are recreation. Residents sometimes spend the night in one of the other residences as a form of vacation.

Residence staff members regard themselves as teachers, not parents. Tasks must be analyzed, goals and objectives quantified, evaluation methods prearranged, and data collected daily. The staff members are usually promoted from within, with a year's service as a teaching assistant on a per-hour basis providing an apprenticeship and observation period before selection. Each evening and Sundays, live-in staff is augmented by an equal number of hourly-paid staff, who are often teachers from the school itself. As a result of such after-school work the school staff becomes familiar with the homelife of the students, and can be more aware of their needs. Residential staff is encouraged to work parttime at the school, or at least to visit, for the same reason. The coordinator for residence/school helps both staffs to coordinate their programs.

Our desire for normal living rules out having three staff shifts with one shift awake during the night. We recognize that there are risks, but feel that the benefits of a noninstitutional setting are worth the risk. (This is discussed more fully in Chapter 9 on sex education at Benhaven.) In our new residence we have installed a sensitive, selectively activated intercom and alarm system which alerts the staff member on duty to all students' whereabouts. Without serving as jailors or constant observers, we can protect student privacy yet safely allow independence.

We encourage regular phone calls and frequent visits by family. Home visits occur only when parents feel there is something the child could enjoy at home, and are planned with great care. We do not make parents feel guilty if they are not willing to have the child visit at home. Staff members frequently accompany students on initial home visits, to see that the child maintains newly learned good behavior and also to demonstrate to parents means of fostering tranquil, happy visits. This results in highly successful subsequent home visits.

Religious holidays, which are observed in school only as vehicles of language and fine motor learning with comprehending students, are all observed in our residences.

With little opportunity for extended evaluation of students before admission, we have had to trust in sometimes unreliable, incomplete reports, which have left the staff unarmed for behavior they could have handled more effectively had they been alerted to its likely emergence. To avoid this, we make staff preenrollment home visits when indicated, and meet with the child's parents, observe the child at his present situation, and if possible talk with his teachers.

Home Programs

To sustain continuity with the school programs we require all parents of day students to be involved in a home program concerning behavior, self-care, or acts of daily living. The program is developed and supervised by the child's team, the school social worker, and the parents. We do not overwhelm the parents with too many objectives and we are careful not to rate the parents' results, lest they become discouraged or resentful.

Parents, as the years stretch out, get tired and are less enthusiastic about beginning or maintaining such home programs. Those with the oldest, most difficult children are most apt to peter out without constant support. One can only wonder how long we can expect parents of autistic children to be enthusiastic teachers or child-care workers. They have had unremitting stress, little or no relief, and no reward of instant cure dangling before them. What becomes the reward for our parents is the possibility of residential placement at Benhaven, where younger, capable, and enthusiastic people take over the job. Parents look forward to quitting, if they can do so with a clear conscience. One can't blame them. Meanwhile we can offer respite to make life easier.

Respite Services

All Benhaven day students are eligible for respite service at our residences. We urge that families plan for visits when there is no crisis, so that they can be anticipated as well as enjoyed. We usually take a student for 2 or 3 days at a time, more in some crisis cases. Acceptance for respite is always left to the discretion of the residential staff; if there are behavior problems with the permanent residents or if there is a new resident settling in, no vacation respite student will be admitted. With four houses, we usually have one in which a crisis visitor can be accommodated. Payment is on a sliding scale, wholly determined by the parents.

The only successful way we have found to handle respite for severely autistic children is to take them one at a time, integrating them with a relatively stable living arrangement in which the respite visitor is the only variable. Even this way the person is a threat to the living pattern of a group that is tenuously developing an orderly, predictable living sense. But the existing pattern, schedule, and procedure support the residents against the unfamiliar behavior of the respite visitor. The combination of a well-known daily routine, a familiar setting, familiar staff members, and careful preliminary conferences and planning make our respite visits highly successful.

Before respite, house staff talk with the parents at length about home patterns of eating and sleeping. We frequently arrange to have on hand the very staff members who are the child's teachers in the day school so that the only elements of strangeness are the sleeping and the hours spent with the resident students in the evenings or on Sundays. Our residential staff also observes the respite prospect in his day program at school.

The visits of even our most difficult children are surprisingly good. Children seldom seem to display the sustained difficult behavior often reported at home. A tranquil visit prevents returning home in an excited state, which would make subsequent home life more difficult.

Outpatient Clinic

Our Outpatient Clinic serves those who live too far away, who are too young, or for whom we have no room. At the initial visit we evaluate motor skills, perception, cognitive skills, language, and behavior. The student, his parents, and teacher return a month later, at which time they go over the written evaluation and the program developed by the Benhaven team. Benhaven serves as consultant thereafter. Students usually return every 6 months.

Additional Components of the Program

Professional Training. We offer professional training at Benhaven. As described later in this chapter, Benhaven trains its own staff by initial orientation, apprenticeship, and ongoing seminars. For professionals who work elsewhere, however, we operate our Professional Training Institute, an informally structured endeavor tailored to the needs of the enrollees. Training is provided by the day, often paid for by Developmental Disabilities Technical Assistance funding. In 1979 we also began an exceptionally valuable form of professional training in collaboration with Southern Connecticut State College: we train house parents, in connection with their formal 4-year course.

Research. We are frequently approached for permission to conduct research on students. If the project interests the staff, the proposal is screened by the Professional Advisory Board members who constitute our Human Investigations Committee. Considerations of students' time, health, and eventual benefits are weighed against possible risk or inconvenience. Teams from Yale University, under the direction of Donald J. Cohen, M.D., have recently carried out research projects on attentional response and on adjustment to group residential living.

STAFF

The executive director supervises the overall operation, future planning, and the Outpatient Clinic. The assistant director in charge of programs is responsible for the day-to-day operations and for hiring of staff. The assistant director for financial matters also oversees the vocational and residential programs.

Benhaven presently has 13 full-time teachers and 20 full-time teaching assistants. All staff have a minimum of one college degree, and upon hiring are required to acquire special education certification. Promotions usually come from within, providing an incentive for good performance and continuity. Length of staff employment varies from 1 to 15 years, with an average of 3 years. Staff move around within the job framework, shifting jobs as inclination and needs arise.

A new teaching assistant is evaluated after 2 months and again after 6 months (Lettick, 1978). If his work is merely satisfactory he will be fired. In our staff evaluation system, staff members set up their own goals and objectives within time frames. They meet periodically with their supervisors and choice of peers to discuss progress. Regrettably, limited staff time makes it difficult to conduct evaluations on a frequent, regular basis.

We prefer not to hire couples. One member of the couple is usually stronger professionally, so in order to maintain the necessary level of performance the stronger one usually takes on some of the duties of the weaker spouse, thereby increasing his own burden and perhaps lowering his own proficiency. If we want to fire one, we lose both. Their understandable desire to have the same time off limits the flexibility of scheduling for both. Their loyalty to and support of the spouse requires more than usual delicacy on the part of other staff in discussions or evaluations of professional work, and hampers the free and uninhibited exchanges which ordinarily accompany staff interaction.

The senior staff members teach, train their own assistants, prepare lesson plans, programs, and reports, and collect data. They help choose their colleagues, since they must work closely as teams. They are encouraged to develop innovative programs. Our educational supervisor oversees the programs and provides in-service training in behavior management and educational techniques to staff and parents.

Each senior staff member has three to six students for whom he is an advocate. These are generally students who are in his daily area of instruction. The advocate is responsible for seeing that his student has a suitable program and that reports are done on time; he attends meetings with the school system, develops and supervises the behavioral and social programs, attends parent conferences, often accompanies the child on dental or hospital visits. He conducts the team meetings on his child.

We serve as an unofficial laboratory school for the Yale Child Study Center, providing a field for research, observation, and training. Yale professors serve on our general and professional advisory boards. Benhaven's two top administrators hold faculty appointments to the staff of the Yale Child Study Center. In 1975 Yale University conferred an honorary doctorate upon Amy Lettick, for founding Benhaven and for her work with autistic children.

Southern Connecticut State College, Yale University, and half a dozen other colleges and universities send us work-study students or psychology, speech therapy, and special education students, who carry out their field work as teaching aides on a nonpaid basis. This relationship with area institutions of higher learning allows for an exchange of ideas similar to that available at a teaching hospital, and is mutually beneficial.

We pay our staff to attend bimonthly early-morning in-service training seminars at which Yale faculty members speak or staff members explain their areas of work to other staff members who do not otherwise have time to see what their colleagues are doing. We also fund training courses and staff attendance at conferences.

TEACHING TECHNIQUES

Self-Contained vs. Departmentalized Classrooms

After trying both systems we have chosen to be departmentalized, for the following reasons: Although self-contained classrooms allow for more easily maintained continuity and relevance in the program, and for greater teacher awareness of students' progress through the day, they also require a teacher's equal interest and competence in all areas of the curriculum. They eliminate the fruitfulness of a team approach and the number of teacher–student relationships that can build slowly. Most important, they confine a teacher to the same students all day. Facing an entire day with a student with a serious behavior problem is more wearing than facing a day with a variety of students with a variety of problems. Departmentalization means that we can develop teachers who are specialists in areas. Fresh teachers can cope better with a misbehaving student. The classmates of a misbehaving student are not confined to his presence all day. Teams of teachers bring more expertise, and eliminate the disruption that occurs when a staff member leaves.

Behavior Modification

Behavior modification is used effectively throughout our program. There are times, however, when the typical response–reward paradigm is either too slow, too impractical, or less immediately effective and simple than alternatives which are therefore employed instead. For example, for some students the demonstrated command "Do it this way" would be as effective as, and faster than, shaping a student's behavior by rewarding his approximations or suggesting that he try another way. Some children may not have enough imagination to think of another way. Physically "putting a student through" an activity when he doesn't know he can do it (but you do know it) may be the alternative to eliciting and rewarding approximate behavior. These alternatives will still employ behavior-modification theory but skip steps, or are more teacher-directed.

If positive means exist for changing behavior, we prefer to use them. With some children we can find no positive means, and with others time to discover possible positive means is limited by the immediate danger of behavior we are trying to eliminate. We use aversive methods when positive measures are not possible, when the alternatives available are worse than the aversives proposed. Our Human Rights Committee, composed of professional advisory board members, scrutinized and approved, line by line, our 50-page handbook, *Benhaven's Manual for Handling Severe Aggression and Self-Abuse* (Lettick, 1980) to assure that our policy in no way violates the human rights of our students. A 3-page version of the policy on use of restraint is studied and signed by parents before their child's enrollment. The main points are: physical restraint is an individualized, temporary measure, used only when positive alternatives have failed and other aversives are worse; it is not intended to inflict pain, and is used not as a punishment but for defense, or to make teaching possible. No procedure is used without prior written parental consent, except for a one-time emergency in a life-threatening situation. Parents witness the procedure whenever possible and there is daily recordkeeping and frequent evaluation. A restrained person is never left alone.

Developing Lesson Plans

In developing lesson plans we have learned two important things: (1) Our students cannot always learn to do a task most easily in its natural setting. They learn best in a structured, undistracting environment. The elements that make it difficult in its natural setting can be added after the routine aspects of the job have been mastered (Freschi & Wood, 1974). (2) Steps are not necessarily learned best in their natural sequence in the task, whether forward or backward. The practice of backward chaining, while aiming for successful conclusions, does not take into consideration the relative difficulty of steps.

In the task of hand-washing, for example, the last step could be, according to the teacher's analysis of the task, either wiping the hands or hanging up the towel. If the backward chaining method were employed, then that last step would be the first one the student would be taught and expected to perform. Certainly, however, the step of rinsing off the soap by holding one's hands under the water faucet is a simpler task than either wiping hands or hanging up a towel, and one more likely to be achieved successfully and quickly. If we want to begin with an easy step to ensure initial success, then rinsing the hands would be taught before the harder step. Our steps are generally learned in the order of difficulty, no matter where in the sequence they occur. The sequence is maintained by the teacher or the student with teacher assistance, with the student's solo performance inserted at the appropiate places. In some versions of the teaching sequence the student's performance establishes the relative difficulty of steps. In other versions of our lesson plans the teaching sequence is predetermined by the teacher, and is indicated in alphabetical order alongside the numerical order of the performance sequence. Thus Step 2 in the hand-washing analysis in Table 1 may have alongside it the letter A, to indicate that while it is the second in the performance sequence, it should be the first step taught.

Table 1
Analysis of Teaching Order and
Sequential Order in Hand-Washing

Teaching order	Sequential order[a]	Student will:
F	1	Turn on water
A	2	Wet hands under running water
C	3	Pick up soap
J	4	Lather palms with soap bar
	etc.	

[a]Each step can be broken down further if necessary.

Precision Teaching Techniques Combined with Task Analysis

Task analysis produces the objectives in logical steps; precision teaching provides data for measurement of progress in each step, and consequently direction for further teaching. Unless such specific analysis and data lie behind it, a teacher's estimate that a student "is doing better" or "can perform 50% of the bed-making task" gives no indication as to where in the sequence the difficulty lies or what steps need to be worked on. Also, as a round figure "50%" is misleading, since the average may be derived from such a scatter as to mask a truly unusable pattern of performance.

A drawback: Task analysis makes no provision for consistency in presentation or individual teaching style, and at a school like Benhaven in which lesson plans are often carried out by more than one staff member over a period of time, this is a weakness. The "how" of teaching must be presented in one chunk at staff orientation lessons, to be adapted and generalized throughout the lessons, and this does not ensure consistency. What led to the present lesson planning is the economy and precision of drawing new objectives from task analysis and the present staff accent on the "what" rather than the "how" of teaching.

Reports

Reports are prepared collaboratively by the senior staff, with the supervision of the assistant director and the supervisor. Past and future objectives in each area are measured and prescribed quantitatively. Reports range from 5 to 25 pages, and go out three times a year to parents and school systems. (For a typical set of reports, see Lettick, 1979b.)

Total Communication

Since January 1971 total communication has been taught to all Ben-haven students who do not speak reasonably well (Lettick, 1979). All our nonverbal students have learned to communicate in sign on a level commensurate with the rest of their development. We use signed English. Finger spelling has virtually been eliminated as the signing vocabulary, supplemented by signs we invent, is adequate for all the communication needs of our students. Parents and siblings are encouraged to learn and use signing at home. We begin total communication as soon as a student comes to us. If a student shows signs of developing speech, then sign is discontinued. Three students developed their first speech between the ages of 10 and 12. Of these three, two of them, now 12 years old, are developing rudimentary, primitive language. The third, now in his 20s, learned to speak in sentences within 4 months of his enrollment at the age of 10.

A large proportion of our students do not show aptitude for developing normal speech patterns. For them we have developed a functional language program centering on acts of daily life (Rumanoff-Simonson, 1979). All our students have learned to communicate either in sign or speech at one level or another.

Group Socialization and Recreation

Handing play equipment to low-functioning autistic children usually results in its misuse or inappropriate use, and in no increase in socialization of the children. Socialization and play must be taught, and can be taught, to varying degrees. Through our methodical program we have changed "loners" into persons who play baseball, volleyball, badminton, relay races, and circle games.

In totally individualized programs students are taught first about their bodies and what they can and cannot do (laterality, ocular management, body part discrimination, etc.). They are concurrently taught splinter skills for future games, along with the language involved. Groups are then formed for using the splinter skills together with the appropriate language.

One way used to instill the idea of groupness is through tying three to five students with a length of rope from waist to waist during gym activities. Subsequently the rope tied to them is replaced by a rope held voluntarily by the students. Eventually this is replaced by the voluntary touching of the next person, which is succeeded by a visual contact with the person ahead or alongside. At this point a sense of groupness has been established.

It is at this stage that the awareness of and pleasure in play can develop. The ideas of winning, losing, your team, my team, are taught, along with the language of team play. Gradually, after learning the splinter skills and getting help in combining them with other children, some children acquire the sense of a game and enjoy it. Others can never understand or care about winning or losing, but we find that in their own limited way they show they want to be part of the group and the activity. They get their own pleasure out of group socialization. Skills are meanwhile improved in dual play such as table tennis and badminton, and solitary play such as bike riding or roller skating.

WHAT HAS NOT WORKED

The Cure of Autism by Acquisition of Language. Being able to communicate does not eliminate the essential lack of relatedness; rather, it serves to corroborate and emphasize it. (See Caparulo and Cohen, in press.) One has only to listen to the autistic children who do speak to realize that their language mirrors the greater problem still lying within them. Verbal autistic people tend to talk *at* each other rather than *to* each other. Undoubtedly, being able to speak eliminates the frustration that comes from not making needs known, and life is easier all around, but it does not provide the cure for autism.

Lasting Jobs in the Community. Our students have held jobs as custodians, stock clerks, kitchen assistants, and greenhouse workers. One, after 2 years, was offered a full-time position as a custodian in a plant where we had found him a trial job before he "graduated" at age 21. Regrettably, at that time he passed out of our jurisdiction and the job was not pursued or secured by succeeding advocates. Eight or nine have held part-time jobs for periods ranging from 2 months to 3 years. Only two are still holding those jobs; despite goodwill on the part of co-workers and employers, bursts of inappropriate behavior in most eventually cost them their positions. These young adults are now filling similar jobs at Benhaven, where their occasional regression does not keep them from their tasks the rest of the time. We try to provide an environment that will be the least stress-provoking.

Day School as a Substitute for 24-Hour Care. For some students even the time-intensive day program we offer is not enough; they need the consistency and safety of the round-the-clock program of the residence. The benefits of staying home are outweighed by the deterioration of family life. One-third of the students who are no longer with us had to leave because they could no longer be kept at home and we had no room for them in our residences.

Parents as Teachers in Our School. We do not use parents as teachers in our school. Parent-taught programs have evolved from lack of other available education, lack of funds for professional staff in small schools, and the need for training in the preschool years and for home maintenance of school programs later. Parents should take an active part in securing and ensuring a good program for their child; they should be trained to maintain continuity with the day program when the child is home; but they should not be obliged to teach, any more than the parent of a normal child is obliged to teach.

A parent is not innately endowed with ability to provide a program in such a difficult area of expertise. Knowing one's own child is no guarantee of competence in dealing with other autistic children with other problems. Along with the understandable parental motivation for teaching comes emotional involvement and strain—no help to a teacher. Parents themselves invariably prefer to have a professional teacher rather than another parent teach their child.

Benhaven does not use as teachers parents who are also professional educators. After having employed some very capable ones, we found that the staff could never be sure whether they were discussing that teacher's child or his pupil. The staff felt constrained in discussing that child in the presence of that person. There is the possible violation of the rights of privacy when the teacher/parent is free to know details of another parent's problems.

Being the parent of an autistic person should not determine and monopolize the life of a parent, although it often does. Parents of severely handicapped children need the relief of being separated from their problems for part of the day. We advise that they get jobs unrelated to their problems.

Volunteer Help. We use nonpaid help which can be called "volunteer" help in connection with college field training. In these cases there is an obligation to work for grades. The volunteer help we do not use is the person who has no commitment, no sustained effort. For such a person, volunteer work is something to do only if everything is going well and there is nothing better to do. But for us, when a teacher's aide doesn't show up there is a child left teacherless and we have to scramble to reschedule. It just isn't worth the work of training the volunteer.

Provision of Residence for All Our Adults. Our original plan called for unterminated residence at Benhaven. If we followed this policy, the first generation would fill the houses and there would never be room for new students. Without a flourishing day school the adult program cannot exist, since it relies on the physical plant and staffing of the day school. So the adults in residence must give way to new school-aged children. To make this possible we have encouraged our parents to form a corporation whose purpose is to establish Department of Mental Retardation-licensed group homes near enough to Benhaven so that residents can continue in the adult day program. At the age of 21 residential students must shift to a Benhaven alumni group home. We hope that the first of such homes will be in operation within the year.

Teaching Machines. The machines in themselves present too much of a distraction, and many are also usually programmed for higher functioning students. Common machines, such as typewriters, tape recorders, and calculators, are used in individual cases.

GENERAL ISSUES

Possible Achievement of Severely Handicapped Autistic Adolescents

Positive achievements to be expected for an adolescent in a good program are the acquisition of functional communication skills, increased independence in acts of daily living, ability to play and engage in team games, happy school years, ability to move from one-to-one to group work, progress from prevocational to vocational activity, and the ability to hold part-time work for a limited period of time.

There have been some steady areas of social integration with the retarded, but they must be qualified. It is not integration with the retarded that has been achieved; it is a version of "parallel play" at functions designed for the retarded. Our advanced students attend holiday parties run by the Regional Center for the Retarded or by civic groups. They attend weekly recreation sessions run by the special education students at a nearby college. And what we have is space in the community awareness and consciousness. Again, for any autistic children who can benefit or enjoy it, this is good and we encourage it. For most it is not really integration because of their own inability to integrate.

We can expect a decrease in behavior problems. The longer students are with us, the less frequent their behavioral upsets and the milder the episodes. This is occasionally countered by cyclical regression over which we have no control and no understanding. A student's increasingly good behavior often lulls staff members with false assumptions of his relative normalcy, until he has an unexplainable behavioral outburst. Then the shaken staff, who now catch a glimpse of the immutable disorder under-lying, realize that it is only Benhaven's structure and environment that are creating, supporting, and maintaining the superficially normal behav-ior. And they realize then how essential structure and environment are for the student's lifetime expectations and happiness.

We can expect a decrease in bizarre behavior. Bizarre behavior can be reduced or changed, but its total or permanent elimination would re-quire unending effort on someone else's part. We try to change it to more acceptable forms, or confine it to specific times and places. If it interferes with work, we can provide alternative behaviors in the work itself. It can be a soothing pastime or a reward. Bizarre behavior makes our students conspicuous in the community, and for that reason we try to minimize it in all, particularly those who move about more frequently in public places, but since most of our students will never live in an unsheltered world, we do not have to fear loss of jobs because of the behavior. Bizarre behavior is not the aspect of autism that will make the biggest differences in the life of the student. We have students who exhibit no bizarre be-havior; although they are less conspicuous, their other problems are more limiting. It is not the finger-flapping that keeps them from integrating with the community.

Personal and Family Problems

With adolescence, personal changes take place. The cuteness that elicits public tolerance for misbehaving children vanishes in adolescence. Aggression often appears or increases. Tantrum or antisocial behavior in full-grown people is uncomfortable and frightening. We understand that. When our adults can behave, they are regularly brought to libraries, stores, theaters, and restaurants. But we do not inflict misbehaving adults on the community, any more than we favor inflicting normal misbehaving chil-dren on the community.

Although vocational and social competencies keep improving, and we see growth in the ability to work together, there is a plateauing of intellectual development in later adolescence, with one-to-one teaching still necessary in learning of new skills or knowledge.

No matter how much improvement we can achieve, it is possible that, under stress, the student regresses. Since it is impossible to eliminate stress entirely, it can be expected that at some times a student will display unacceptable behavior publicly, which can lead to his expulsion from a group or situation. We accept this, work to reduce it, and do reduce it to a minimum, but never eliminate it completely.

With the aging of the autistic child and his parents, home life, seen as so beneficial in early childhood, now takes on a different view, one lacking stimulation, companionship, consistency, energetic supervision, physical safeguards, and round-the-clock care and education. The initial parent dread—placing one's child away from home—diminishes before the greater dread—not having a place in which to place one's child away from home.

Autism erodes family happiness and health. Parents as well as their other children need training, respite, and counseling. Parents need to be helped to see that residential placement is the logical aftermath of the early home years, to be sought without guilt. It is not the white flag of poor parenting; it can be the supreme act of good parenting, and can result in the rescue and rehabilitation of an entire family. Parents must be encouraged to compartmentalize their joys and sorrows, and not sacrifice all for the handicapped child.

Parents who work can keep autistic adults home only if there is a day program available. Unless there is a martyred sibling to continue to operate the parental home after the parents die, the autistic adult eventually has to leave his childhood home. Therefore we must view adult-living-at-family-home-with-day-care as a time-limited arrangement before the adult leaves, either for an institution or a group home. Since group home residence, like living at home, is also impossible without an available day care program, assuring involvement in a good day program is the key, and takes priority in family planning for the autistic member even over group home residence itself.

Transportation

A major problem at Benhaven today is the lack of transportation to our adult day program. It's not money; transportation costs for adults can be included in the daily reimbursable rates. But that does not set up the *system* that must be available to provide the service. Because our clients live far apart, even one or two pickup arrangements for adults could not possibly collect all of them within a reasonable time. When they were children their towns transported them. There are perhaps 20 carriers bringing children to us daily from all parts of the state. This is undoubtedly where the solution must lie. But meanwhile this is not available to adults, except for a fortunate isolated few whose earlier carriers still bring them. As for the rest, they cannot travel alone. Presently parents bring a few; one is picked up by an obliging staff member. For those who face age 21 in the future, lack of transportation may mean the end of their years at Benhaven. For so many, a place to go is the problem; for ours, getting to that place is the problem.

Integration with the Community

Shelter vs. Mainstreaming. For the severely impaired autistic person, mainstreaming is highly questionable as to its usefulness, practicality, or desirability. It assumes a satisfaction from and awareness of participation in community life which is absent in the most severely impaired autistic people.

Mainstreaming calls for the least restrictive environment. At our city facility we must always be concerned with keeping our students from trespassing, with protecting them at street crossings. Placing them in the midst of neighbors, even those as understanding as ours, imposes on the staff the stress of acting as buffer, protector, and interpreter.

At our farm, on the other hand, space dissipates noise, keeps danger at a distance, and instills serenity. We can send a student alone from one building to another across the meadow without worrying. Students are allowed more independence because of the sheltered, safe nature of the farm. So the shelter, not the mainstream, is the least restrictive environment for the severely impaired.

Deinstitutionalization. Some believe that deinstitutionalization and total integration with the nonhandicapped provides the optimal environment for the autistic, and should be the only setting acceptable. If a person cannot presently function in that setting, they state, it is the fault of the community in not accommodating and providing adequately for his needs, and so the imperative is to improve the community and desegregate all. Presently such a welcoming, suitable community does not exist, to serve either as a model or proof of the validity of this belief.

Integration into a group of normal students is unavailable as well as inappropriate; as for integration into groups of people with other handicaps such as the mentally handicapped, placement with disturbed people with normal intelligence is unsuitable because of the lower level of functioning and unsociability of the autistic persons. They are never admitted to such houses, nor would we recommend such placement.

Placement of the severely autistic in group homes for the retarded, if allowed, causes scheduling and staffing problems. The inability to function as part of a group for sustained periods requires extra-high, usually prohibitive, staffing costs. Without adequate staffing, either the severely autistic person withdraws, in which case he will be allowed to remain, at little advantage to himself, or else he will regress under stress, be disruptive to the group, and be expelled, with justification.

Autistic people are not usually invited to live in such homes unless the level of their disability is so mild as to be almost unrecognizable. To the present time we have had only two students who have ever been accepted into group homes for the retarded. The first, one of our highest functioning alumni, more sociable and less autistic than most of our students, is, after a 4-year wait, in such a home for about a year now, and doing very well. The other student, also a mild-mannered, relatively high-functioning one, was expelled from his group home within a year because of his lapses into bizarre behavior.

Even more impossible is the attempt to lump the autistic with the physically handicapped with normal intelligence. The latter need independence of mobility (achievable through modified public transportation), jobs, and community acceptance. Given these, they need no constant supervision. For the autistic, independence without judgment is a danger, work opportunities in an unsuitable setting are impossible to maintain, and acceptance into the community is a meaningless goal or state. For the mildly impaired such goals may be meaningful or attainable, but one cannot set those as desirable goals for all mentally impaired people, particularly not for all the autistic.

While a small portion of the autistic population may be able to function in a nonspecialized setting, the majority require a range of alternative settings, from small group homes to local, benign, small institutions. Just because the legal right to community integration exists does not mean that it must be exercised at the expense of the individual (not to mention the class of normal children whose own learning conditions can be radically disrupted by the presence of the severely handicapped). Benhaven has demonstrated the effectiveness of a small, benign institution. In a follow-up study on autistic children the Yale Child Study Center learned that the only parents who felt that their children's needs had been met and were being met were the parents of students at Benhaven (personal disclosure from one of the researchers; see Provence, Abelson, Naylor, & Gerber, 1979).

There are many mildly autistic students who never need the services of Benhaven but who find it difficult to get or hold a job in the outside world. Benhaven has provided a good solution for a few. We have hired two of them to be staff assistants at our farm. They need to have their tasks structured, and need supervision and understanding of their real incapacities. These young men do not identify themselves with the student body. They drive our trucks and do our errands. As far as they are concerned they are a part of the staff. Their parents say they have never been happier.

Behavior and Independence

Steady behavior and independence, not relatedness or language, are the keys to the future. We have students who are mute, who have bizarre mannerisms, who go no further than signing their basic needs, but who fill key positions on work crews, who take care of themselves with minimum supervision, who enjoy life and give pleasure to others. They are partially self-supporting, can work for 1 or 2 hours at a time with little or no supervision, and, severely autistic though they may be, are welcome members of a group home at Benhaven, where occasional regression is tolerated and overlooked, where provision for structure and stability are routinely made.

Right vs. Need

It takes much money to provide the staff ratio and individualized treatment needed by severely autistic persons. Just because they need that expensive treatment, do they have a right to it? If they don't have the right to the treatment, and therefore nobody has to provide it, what happens to people like this? They don't simply disappear; they eventually have to be institutionalized. And this is where the bleak fact emerges— it costs more to institutionalize them than to provide the expensive treatment to which they apparently don't have a right.

Presently at Connecticut's mental hospital it costs $68,000 per year to maintain and provide education to a severely autistic child. If, instead, a child can be enrolled at Benhaven's day program and live at home, it costs his town and state combined $19,500 per year. If he is enrolled in the residential program, which includes the 6-day school program, it costs $44,500. Appallingly large as this sum is, it is still less than it would cost the state to institutionalize him, and at Benhaven he is learning, becoming partially self-supporting and partially independent. Even if at some time in the future he must leave Benhaven, his training there may have made him able to fit into a group home rather than the costlier state institution. Early residence in the state institution, on the other hand, is a dead end.

We find that by the time our students reach adulthood and graduate from Benhaven, many of them are far more independent, and therefore less burdensome to care for. So it is to the ultimate benefit of the state and the individual to provide the best treatment available, *early,* to avoid the expensive care later on. Perhaps what we should say is that rather than the right to expensive training our students are entitled to a chance to reduce the state's cost of supporting them for life. Their inability to learn to function well without training makes their need, combined with the state's obligation to reduce costs, a powerful argument for providing good services at the most fruitful time.

The problems of the world outside may not be solvable. But within Benhaven's benevolent and varied environment we have developed a world that meets the needs of our population. We see this as the best answer at this time. We shall continue to change that world to meet the needs of the future.

REFERENCES

Caparulo, B., & Cohen, D. J. Developmental language studies in the neuropsychiatric disorders of childhood. In *Children's language* (K. E. Nelson, ed.). New York: Gardner Press, in press.

Freschi, D. *Experimental prevocational training project for autistic, neurologically-impaired children.* New Haven, Conn.: Benhaven Press, 1972.

Freschi, D. *The Benhaven staff evaluation system.* New Haven, Conn.: Benhaven Press, 1974.

Freschi, D., & Wood, L. *Vocational education lesson cores.* New Haven, Conn.: Benhaven Press, 1974.

Lettick, A. L. (Ed.). *The Benhaven policy handbook, 1978.* New Haven, Conn.: Benhaven Press, 1978.

Lettick, A. L. *Benhaven then and now.* New Haven, Conn.: Benhaven Press, 1979a.

Lettick, A. L. (Ed.). *Benhaven at work.* New Haven, Conn.: Benhaven Press, 1979b.

Lettick, A. L. (Ed.), *Benhaven's manual for handling severe aggression and self-abuse.* New Haven, Conn.: Benhaven Press, 1980.

Lieberman, D. A., & Melone, M. B. *Sexuality and social awareness.* New Haven, Conn.: Benhaven Press, 1980.

Provence, S., Abelson, W., Naylor, A., & Gerber, B. W. *A follow-up of autistic children in Connecticut: Interviews with parents.* New Haven, Conn.: Yale University Child Study Center, 1979.

Rumanoff-Simonson, L. *A curriculum model for individuals with severe learning and behavioral disorders.* Baltimore: University Park Press, 1979.

18

The Jay Nolan Center
A Community-Based Program

GARY W. LAVIGNA

FORMATIVE FORCES

The best introduction to the Jay Nolan Center is a brief discussion of the factors that led to its conception and development. These include the relevant research, the principles of normalization and developmental programming, parent advocacy, and previous attempts by others to provide appropriate and meaningful programs.

Relevant Research and Treatment Issues

Research and the development of treatment programs has primarily focused on younger autistic children. Few studies have addressed the characteristics and treatment of these children when they have grown into adolescence and adulthood. Long-term follow-up studies of autistic individuals are not encouraging. Our understanding of this literature led us to conclude that institutionalization is not as much a function of behavioral excesses and deficits as it is of society's present inability to provide appropriate community-based residential programs designed around the principles of normalization and developmental programming.

Eisenberg (1956, 1957), in an outcome study of Kanner's original cases, concluded that 50%–75% had future prospects that were very poor.

GARY W. LAVIGNA ● At the time of writing this chapter, Dr. LaVigna was with the Jay Nolan Center, Newhall, California. He is now at the Behavior Therapy and Family Counseling Center, Van Nuys, California 91401.

They had not "emerged" from autism to any great extent and their functioning was markedly maladaptive, characterized by apparent feeblemindedness and/or grossly disturbed behavior. Three decades ago, at the time these studies were carried out, Eisenberg found virtually no positive effects of treatment on outcome.

In England, one decade later, Rutter, Greenfeld, and Lockyer (1967) followed 38 of their original patients who at the time of follow-up were 16 years of age or older. While their findings concerning outcome were similar to Eisenberg's, they also found grounds for limited optimism: (1) there were a few who made substantial progress even with inadequate provisions for education and treatment; (2) there was evidence that the amount of schooling received by the child influenced later social development; and (3) there were several examples of children who gained initial speech after 5 years of age and made fair progress. In all cases the later acquisition of speech occurred at a time when the child was receiving good schooling and/or speech therapy. This and future studies established structured education as an integral part of treatment.

At the time of the Rutter follow-up the behavioral treatment of autism was in its infancy. While earlier studies had reported success with specific treatment targets, it was not until 1973 that a major follow-up study of the long-term results of behavioral treatment was published. In their landmark report, Lovaas and his colleagues (Lovaas, Koegel, Simmons, & Long, 1973) found that treatment gains were either maintained or improved for those who remained in settings with parents or staff trained to use behavioral procedures and who provided structured programming. For those who ended up in institutions where such programming was lacking, earlier treatment gains were lost. They concluded that at the present time structured programming appears necessary for both the establishment and maintenance of treatment gains.

These results suggested that this population requires continual intensive programming and behavior modification to meet their training and behavior management needs, and that in adulthood and adolescence these needs may be largely independent of previous treatment programs. Without proper structure the gains obtained in previous programs would not generalize and accordingly would not be reflected to any great extent in present functioning. The generalization of treatment gains across time as well as across responses and across stimulus situations is a problem which has implications for the living arrangements provided for autistic adolescents and adults. As long as treatment gains can only be maintained in settings which provide structured programming, residential settings ought to have this capability. This problem is an important one since most families eventually reach the point where, for one reason or another, placement outside the home must be considered. While institutions typically, and perhaps inherently, seem unable to meet this challenge, it could be met by "teaching homes" with professional "teaching parents" (Lovaas, Reference Note 1).

A major factor which has led to the eventual institutionalization of most autistic adolescents and adults may be the general lack of constructive, alternative living arrangements, i.e., the lack of noninstitutional settings in which these individuals could continue their development toward independent, productive living. Based on the hypothesis that institutional placement is primarily a function of the unavailability of community-based programs and not of training needs and behavior problems which can only be met in an institutional setting, the Jay Nolan Center for Autism was established.

Normalization

Another important influence on the Jay Nolan Center was the growing impact of the principle of normalization (Wolfensberger, 1972) on treatment and programs for those who have disabilities. The essential idea is that a person's developmental problems do not justify isolation and segregation from the community and the elimination of opportunities to interact with nonhandicapped peers and engage in age-appropriate activities in age-appropriate settings. While the ideal of a normal lifestyle can only be approximated, our goal is to maximize it to the greatest extent possible.

Accordingly, our largest living arrangement has only six clients living in a small group home located in a suburban community no closer than 1 mile to any of our other group homes. There are no indications on the house that show it is different in any way from other homes in the neighborhood. Clients dress and groom in an age-appropriate manner and care is taken to minimize the negative attention they may attract, as the goal is social integration and participation in the community. To contribute to a normal lifestyle, our school-age clients attend public school and our adults attend our occupational training program which is located in an industrial park.

This trend toward normalization and deinstitutionalization has made increasing moneys available from local and private agencies to establish less restrictive, community-based programs. Our major problem has been to keep up with all the opportunities we have had to start new programs and services, rather than to attract start-up money. This may be partially attributable to the emphasis we place on the principles of normalization and the concordance of this approach with the current objectives of various funding agencies.

Developmental Programming

The long-range goal for our clients is nothing less than independent living and productive functioning as fully participating and valued members of the community. This sounds ambitious for some of our people, and it is. Our focus, however, is not so much on independence and productivity as on the process of becoming independent and productive, for we believe that dignity and happiness come not necessarily from the state of being independent or productive—or from *being* anything else for that matter—but rather from the active participation in the process of *becoming*. Accordingly, our focus is on the design and provision of a learning environment that actively engages our clients in the process of becoming. We believe that this process never has to end for our clients. Each day, week, month, and year can find them more independent and productive than the one before. To this end we apply our technology and our efforts; with this intent the Jay Nolan Center was established.

Parent Advocacy

The establishment of our center was the direct result of action taken by a parent advocacy group. In 1975 the Los Angeles Chapter of the National Society for Autistic Children (LANSAC) wanted to do something directly about establishing programs and services for those who had the problem of autism. Their decision was to launch a free-standing, not-for-profit corporation called Programs for the Developmentally Handicapped (P.D.H.), Inc., with a separate board of directors appointed by them. That corporation is now doing business as the Jay Nolan Center.

Given this historical beginning, and the relationship that continues between LANSAC and the Jay Nolan Center, we consider ourselves a consumer-based organization. The majority of people on our board of directors are parents of autistic children, and this ensures our continuing consumer orientation. Accordingly, while professionals design and administer the Jay Nolan Center, our organizational goals and objectives and our governing policies are established by a board of directors who are primarily secondary consumers.

An Analysis of Past Failures

The intent in establishing the Jay Nolan Center was to establish something permanent. It was therefore important to understand why other programs which had been established with a similar intent had failed. We discovered that success was determined by something more than excellence of program. That is, to be successful beyond a demonstration period treatment effectiveness was a necessary but not a sufficient factor. We learned that competent management and administration were of crucial importance. For example, we learned of one well-funded program which had to close because it ran out of money. In spite of its adequate funding level it had neglected to develop a budget and had managed its finances out of a checkbook. The Jay Nolan Center has a board-level Finance Committee, chaired by a C.P.A., which oversees its financial operations. Each year we develop a monthly budget projection by line item for each program component. Monthly financial statements are prepared by an outside accountant and compare our actual expenditures against our projected (budgeted) expenditures. We are also discovering that the bigger we get, the more formal we have to become in establishing policies and procedures in areas other than financial management such as program services, personnel administration, and property management.

We have learned, however, that there is an area even more important to long-term success than technology and the management and administration of an organization. This involves the political/social arena and addresses such issues as board–staff relations and extra-agency relations with funding sources, regulatory agencies, the community, and other outside groups. Relations in these areas must be considered as of fundamental importance if an organization wishes to survive. Graziano (1975), in his book *Child Without Tomorrow,* describes how a good program was fatally affected by problems in these areas. Liberman (1979) argues that behavior analysts must address these broader systems issues to assure that contributions survive beyond the demonstration phase. They both argue that an organization remains viable only to the extent that it is successful along a hierarchy of three levels of importance, with technology being only the "tip of the iceberg"; increasing importance must be attached first to internal systems of management and administration, and then to external systems involving board–staff relations and extra-agency relations.

PROGRAM DESCRIPTION

The Jay Nolan Center

The Jay Nolan Center has the long-range goal of developing a full continuum of residential, vocational, recreational, and educational services and programs for autistic children, adolescents, and adults regardless of their level of need. In addition we plan the development of comprehensive research and training programs. We are functionally organized around our present programs and services.

We currently serve approximately 500 client families with a variety of services and programs. These include small group homes, apartment units, occupational training, Saturday recreation, intensive intervention, in-home respite, and an extended-year program that bridges the gaps in the public school schedule. While the focus of this chapter is our adult group homes and associated occupational training programs, the concept of a *continuum* of both residential and nonresidential services should not be lost. No single service or program can meet the range of needs this population presents.

Our present programs and services were established to meet the objectives set during our annual planning process. This process is jointly carried out, with staff input, by the boards of directors of both P.D.H., Inc. (the Jay Nolan Center), and LANSAC. As a result of this planning process, for the next two years our focus is shifting from an emphasis on expansion to an emphasis on consolidation as the top priority for the organization as a whole.

Each program and service of the Jay Nolan Center has its own goals and objectives as well. The major goals of the small group home and occupational training program are:

1. To provide a learning environment that will give our clients the competencies needed to be contributing members of society, where their services and/or products will be in demand
2. To provide a learning environment that will maximize their ability to (a) take care of their own personal needs; (b) structure and enjoy their own leisure time; and (c) get around the community independently
3. To provide the support services which will encourage and enhance their ongoing relationships and involvement with their families
4. To have a research program which will (a) develop more effective methods and procedures to be used in teaching the skills they need; and (b) develop more efficient service delivery systems

Site Selection Criteria

Having established the opening of a small group home for adults and associated occupational training program as one of our earliest objectives, an important question for us was the home's location. We had all of Los

Angeles County to consider. We believe that the criteria we developed to select a location have contributed significantly to whatever success we have had. While these criteria may not apply directly to other areas, analogous considerations may be helpful to others. The primary point, however, is that the location plays an important role in the group home's success or failure. Accordingly, the decision on location should not be left to chance, but should be based on as many explicit criteria as possible.

Cost and Availability. Since we were planning to open subsequent homes, the cost availability of housing in general was an important point for consideration. These factors varied considerably since Los Angeles County has widely divergent areas ranging from exorbitantly expensive housing to low-cost housing in deteriorating neighborhoods. Also, some appropriate areas simply did not have any properties on the market. Because we anticipated opening subsequent homes, we felt that cost and availability of more than just the first home had to be considered.

Local Agency Support. Depending on location, we would have had to deal with one of seven possible regional centers in Los Angeles and one of several possible school districts. Regional centers are the funding agencies in California and play a key role in negotiating program approval and rates with the state Department of Developmental Services. We interviewed the directors and support staff of the seven regional centers in the county in an effort to assess both their ability (i.e., their level of organizational stability and sophistication) and their willingness to assist and support our effort. We also interviewed key administrators in the various public school districts to make a similar assessment concerning public schools, because we anticipated opening future homes for school-age students. The community we selected fell into the catchment area of a regional center that was capable of helping us get started and had expressed a strong desire for the opportunity to do so. This was also true of the school district which served that area. We strongly recommend that other organizations assess the agencies in their areas before deciding where to place their group homes.

Community Acceptance. The nemesis for many group homes has been their failure to obtain community acceptance. While there is no way to guarantee this before the fact, we believe the criteria we used in community selection maximized the likelihood of a good outcome. This likelihood was further maximized by the steps we took after the purchase of the home.

We did not want to locate our first group home in a community that had a negative history concerning group home operations. Such communities were eliminated from consideration. We also interviewed community leaders concerning their feelings and opinions about the Jay Nolan

Center's establishing a group home in their area. We felt that if members of the city council, chamber of commerce, rotary clubs, and similar groups were in favor of our presence, they would be more likely to support us if a future controversy arose. Finally, we sought a community that had not been significantly or visibly impacted by other group home operations. We anticipated that the flocking together of increasing numbers of group homes in a single community would eventually cause an accepting community to become a rejecting one.

After we selected the community and purchased the home we held an open-house event for the immediate neighbors before the arrival of any clients. This was an opportunity to explain who we were, what autism was, and what they could expect to occur. Two messages seemed particularly important in getting people to relax about our presence. One was that there was nothing inherent in autism that presented any danger to them or to their children, and that this was further assured by the *continuous* professional supervision that was going to be available around the clock at an exceptionally high staff-to-client ratio. The second was an unrelenting responsiveness and sensitivity to their concerns and complaints. We responded to every request made and problem raised concerning noise, traffic, property maintenance, and the like, with nondefensive openness and as much compliance as was reasonably possible. We made every effort to avoid a defensive or adversarial position with any of our neighbors.

In retrospect these policies have served us well. We have opened four homes and have had no community difficulties except for a very few isolated problems with individual neighbors. Most of our neighbors have been either actively or passively accepting of our presence. We have experienced no organized or community-wide opposition.

Licensing and Zoning Considerations. Licensing of small group home facilities in California is greatly facilitated if all the bedrooms are on the ground floor and are at least 130 square feet (for two clients). This suggested an area with a supply of custom-built ranch-style homes. Areas that offered only tract or multistory housing were therefore avoided.

When we first opened, group homes were often required to get zoning variances by many local planning commissions. Since then California law forbids local agencies from requiring variances or anything special from group homes serving six or fewer people with a developmental disability. Expecting to have to deal with the old laws, we sought to locate in an unincorporated part of the county to avoid dealing with a local body. We anticipated that it would be easier to deal with a centralized county body which typically would not have any local people serving on it, and therefore would be in a better position to give unbiased consideration to any request for a zoning variance should a variance have been required.

Proximity to Generic Services. Since we planned for a large part of our program to include the development of client competencies in the community, it was necessary to locate in an area which had proximity to stores, shops, movie theaters, bowling alleys, restaurants, etc. Accordingly, we did not consider rural areas that required a "trip to town" in order to have access to these training environments.

Staffing Patterns and Preparation

Our 24-hour, residential, adult group homes provide 14 hours a day, 7 days a week of what we have termed specialized training and behavior modification, with a continuous, minimum staff-to-client ratio of 1:2. Monday through Friday, from 9:00 A.M. to 4:00 P.M. this program takes place in our Occupational Training Center. Three occupational trainers are assigned for every six clients. They provide task-analysis training to teach vocational skills as targeted in the client's individualized program plan. The qualifications we attempt to meet in filling these positions include at least 1 year of training and/or experience in providing a formal behavior-modification program and at least 1 year of experience in providing professional services to persons with autism and similar problems. We seek comparable qualifications for all our direct-service staff.

The balance of the program takes place in the homes and surrounding community. Each home has a full-time residential manager who arranges staff schedules and supervises personnel assigned to the home. Managers provide or arrange for backup coverage when necessary to maintain minimum staff/client ratios. They schedule individual client training sessions and assure that they occur. They assist and train home program specialists and behavior technicians in providing a functional, developmental program for the residents encompassing basic self-care skills, independent living skills, recreation and leisure skills, community skills, and communication skills. We attempt to fill these positions with people at the masters degree level or those who have comparable skills, training, and/or experience.

Reporting to the residential manager are home program specialists, behavior technicians, and behavior specialists. Home program specialists possess the necessary skills to deal effectively with the day-to-day problems of living with our clients and have a demonstrated ability to increase their skills in independent and productive living. Their responsibilities include the day-to-day delivery of specialized services and behavior modification for the residents. They are responsible for daily recordkeeping and for writing regular progress reports for each client. Four are assigned full-time responsibilities for each of our homes. Each team of two works a 3½-days on and 3½-days off schedule. During their 3½ days on they have on-call responsibilities while the clients are in the occupational training program.

Behavior technicians are typically hired on an hourly basis to supplement the home program specialist staff to provide the minimum 1:2 ratio. Their program responsibilities are similar except that they do not have sleep-over responsibilities, nor are they responsible for handling money or medication.

Each home is assigned a half-time behavior specialist. This person is not calculated in the 1:2 ratio. The behavior specialist maintains a complete written record of behavioral interventions and baseline procedures for each resident over time, accurately cross-referenced to summary data graphs, to illustrate changes in behavior as functions of treatment conditions. She or he assures consistent and reliable data collection procedures across settings by performing periodic reliability checks, and trains staff on data recording procedures for each intervention until adequate reliability in observation and implementation has been achieved.

Our preservice and continuous in-service training programs include the following topics: orientation ot autism; introduction to the Jay Nolan Center; maintaining healthy environments and providing emergency care; fire and safety considerations; administrative responsibilities; normalization; managing behavior; leisure and recreational time; educational considerations; individualized program planning; community placement; relationships with natural families; thoughts on sexuality; and managing assaultive behavior. We have been increasingly dissatisfied with what we consider to be decreasing quality of training with increasing size. We have been particularly unhappy with the way we have met the training needs generated by staff turnover. Accordingly, we have designed and are about to launch a training system that utilizes self-instructional materials, including written material and videotapes, with stated instructional objectives and pre/posttests for each instructional unit.

Budgeting

Our operating budget for an ongoing adult group home and associated occupational training program is displayed in Table 1. The budget for staff includes a salary allocation for the director of group homes, who is the immediate supervisor of the residential managers, and the assistant director, whose responsibilities include staff recruitment and the assurance of compliance with licensing and other regulations. The workshop allocation includes the staff costs for the occupational trainers, rental of the occupational training site, and other associated costs.

Table 1
Annual Operating Budget for Adult Small-Group Home

Budget items	1st month	12th month	Total
Income			
Fees for service	$16,680	$16,980	$202,860
Total Income	$16,680	$16,980	$202,860
Expenses*			
Adv. and Pub. Rels.	$ 100	$ 100	$ 1,200
Auto expense	500	500	6,000
Clothing	30	30	360
Consultants	100	100	1,200
Dues and subscriptions	25	25	300
Duplicating	30	30	360
Payroll overhead	1,072	1,299	13,784
Food	821	821	9,852
Insurance—property	240	240	2,880
Insurance—other	50	50	600
Interest	745	745	8,940
License and taxes	20	20	240
Medical	25	25	300
Repairs and maint.	200	200	2,800
Replacement purchases	100	100	1,200
Staff	7,655	8,766	98,450
Staff development	125	125	1,500
Supplies—home prog.	300	300	3,600
Telephone	50	50	600
Utilities	250	250	3,000
Workshop allocation	4,082	4,272	48,464
Total Direct Expenses	$16,520	$17,988	$205,360
Administrative Overhead	1,796	2,292	20,245
Total Expenses	$18,316	$20,280	$225,875
Net Income (Loss)	($1,636)	($3,300)	($23,015)

*All expense categories remain constant for the year, except payroll overhead, repairs and maintenance, staff, and workshop allocation.

Start-up costs amount to between $135,000 and $225,000, depending on whether the house is purchased or leased, and if purchased, on the amount of the purchase price and down payment. Other significant factors that go to make up this amount include the purchase of a vehicle, the cost of furniture, and the costs attached to training a staff for a full month before clients arrive. This amount also covers operating costs until all the clients are enrolled and fees for service are being received. We start clients one at a time, 7–10 days apart. Once all clients are enrolled and fees for service are being received we are still left with a monthly operating deficit of approximately $2,000. We are seeking to renegotiate our state-approved rates to cover this amount. Meanwhile we must seek compensating contributions from the private sector.

Client Selection

Selection of clients for the homes is based on the recommendations of an advisory committee to the Jay Nolan Center. This committee consists of two representatives from the Regional Center, one community-based professional, and three consumer representatives nominated by LANSAC. All appointments to the Advisory Committee are confirmed by the Board of Directors of P.D.H., Inc.

The committee makes its recommendations based on case presentations of all the applicants by the executive director. Cases are designated by a code number and presented anonymously to contribute to the objectivity and impartiality of the selection process. As part of the referral packet we require a current medical evaluation, social evaluation, and psychological or developmental evaluation/assessment. We also ask for assessment information concerning the applicant's self-care, language, and behavioral functioning.

The selection committee considers the referral information in the light of the selection criteria and the ability of the applicant to benefit from 14 hours a day, 7 days a week of programming and behavior modification. Our selection criteria are listed in Table 2. They are not very exclusionary. For this reason the Advisory Committee is instructed to seek a balance for the home. It may be possible to serve one or two people without language and basic care skills or with a really severe behavior problem involving self-injury, aggression, or property destruction, but it would not be viable to serve six such people in a single home. The decisions of the committee are reached by consensus. Representatives from direct-service staff participate in the selection process in an advisory capacity. This advisory role is particularly crucial for the issue of balance. As required by law, the executive director retains the right of veto over a client if in his opinion the client would not be appropriately served if accepted into the program. Largely because of the process we follow the veto right has never been exercised.

Because of the large numbers of applications we receive for residential placement in our group homes (we currently have approximately 150 applications on file), it has not been practical to schedule a preplacement visit for each person before selection. Accordingly, selection by the Advisory Committee is made conditionally, pending the outcome of a pre-

Table 2
Selection Criteria

1. Candidates must be 12 to 21 years of age to be considered for the adolescent houses, and over 18 years of age to be considered for the adult homes.

2. Candidates must need and be able to benefit from intensive 14-hours-a-day, 7-days-a-week programming and behavior modification.

3. Candidates must have an early development history consistent with a diagnosis of autism. For this purpose, the official definition of autism published by the National Society for Autistic Children will be used.

4. Funding, either through a Regional Center or through another source, must be identified prior to acceptance.

5. Candidates must be available for a preplacement visit to the Jay Nolan Center prior to acceptance.

6. A complete referral packet must be submitted for each candidate including a current medical evaluation, social evaluation, and psychological or developmental evaluation assessment.

7. Candidates requiring care for severe medical conditions cannot be considered at this time since the Jay Nolan Center is not licensed to provide such care.

8. The adequacy and appropriateness of a candidate's current placement and current placement options will be considered in the selection process.

9. Since an important part of the program at the Jay Nolan Center will be the enhancement of continuing family contact and involvement for those candidates for whom the family is still present, previous participation in the candidate's programs and programming will be considered.

10. Acceptance into the program is based on the information provided in the referral packet and on the basis of the preplacement visit. The first 6 months in the program are to be considered probationary and are to confirm the satisfaction of the above criteria.

11. If, despite programming, the client remains a danger to himself or others, it may be necessary to seek placement in another program.

12. When the client demonstrates or reaches a level of functioning which requires less intensive programming and behavior modification, placement in a less restrictive setting and program will be sought.

placement visit. This visit has the primary purpose of assessing the validity of the case information in the application packet which provided the basis for the selection. The Advisory Committee designates alternates as part of the selection process in case information made available during the preplacement visit invalidates a selection.

Occasionally it is necessary to reject those who obviously, and sometimes desperately, need the program simply because there are more qualified applicants than spaces. Sometimes it boils down to incredibly difficult choices. Nevertheless by maximizing objectivity we are in a better position to deal with the disappointment and bitterness that often follows from rejection. We are also better able to handle individual board member expectations and pressure from states and local agencies to accept a particular applicant.

Client Description

The clients selected for our first group home, which opened in October 1978, are typical of the clients selected for our subsequent settings. Following their descriptions we report the results of our first 2½ years with this initial group.

All six were men in their early 20s. (Through chance, no females were selected for this first home, as they have been for our other homes.) Four of the six came from the autism program at Camarillo State Hospital. Their language skills ranged from muteness to functional speech. Behavior problems ranged from high rates of stereotypic behavior to serious aggression, self-injury, and property destruction. All met our entrance criteria and had received an independent diagnosis of autism by at least two other agencies. Additional specific client information is as follows:

The first resident was 21 years old when he came to the Jay Nolan Center, after having been placed at Camarillo State Hospital at age 4, University of California at Los Angeles, Neuropsychiatric Institute (UCLA/NPI) at age 7, back at Camarillo at age 8, until he was transferred to their teaching home program in January of 1978 when he was 20. He entered the Jay Nolan Center with most self-help skills, some written language abilities, and quite an extensive verbal vocabulary. He manifested a variety of behavior problems before coming to the Jay Nolan Center including temper tantrums, operant vomiting, and screaming. The latest available psychological testing provided an IQ score of 59 on the Stanford Binet Intelligence Test.

Our second resident was medically diagnosed as autistic at age 10, at which time he was exhibiting tantrum behaviors, bizarre mannerisms, and self-stimulatory behaviors, especially when he became angry or upset. He was enrolled in private schools, was hospitalized for a short time for violent behavior, then returned home where he had been for the previous 3 years until coming to the Jay Nolan Center at age 20. He communicates quite well but may talk of subjects irrelevent to the present conversation. He keeps to himself and rarely interacts with others. During tantrums he threatens, pushes, and hits others. Noncompliance usually precedes tantrums. He received a Full Scale score of 70 on the Wechsler Adult Intelligence Scale (WAIS).

Diagnosed as autistic at age 3 while at NPI at UCLA, our third and fourth residents, twin brothers, were admitted to Camarillo State Hospital when they were 6 years old. They came to the Jay Nolan Center from the hospital when they were 20. Our third resident communicates at a nonverbal level using some signs for needs. He overreacts to loud noises. He likes to rock and will bite his hand when upset. Socially he behaves well below developmental norms. His latest standardized testing showed a social age of 2.1 on the Vineland Social Maturity Scale (VSMS) and a developmental age of 3.9 on the Denver Developmental Screening Test (DDST).

Our fourth resident was described as needing assistance with all the self-help skills. He communicated only at a nonverbal level even though he could repeat a limited number of single words. He occasionally grabbed staff members with bone-bruising force during seizures which may be psychomotor in origin. His latest standardized testing showed a social age of 3.0 on the VSMS and a developmental age of 4.2 on the DDST.

Our fifth resident came to us after spending 4 years at Camarillo State Hospital. He had a long history of abnormal development and behavior problems extending back to infancy. At age 7 he was diagnosed as a childhood schizophrenic with autistic tendencies. For the next 10 years he remained at home participating in community educational programs. His teachers were always impressed with his academic skills, but because of his inability to tolerate frustration he manifested severe aggressive/ destructive behaviors in the classroom and at home. Because of these behavior problems his ability to take care of himself was greatly impaired. He sometimes engages in obsessive conversations about morbidity. He speaks quite well about concrete things, but often lacks comprehension of abstractions. He seldom aggresses, but when he does he can go to extremes (e.g., attacking people with broken glass). He appears to be "in his own world" at times. He received a Full Scale score of 75 on the WAIS.

The last resident in our first adult group home came to the Jay Nolan Center directly from his natural home, possessing some self-help and general home-care skills. He had been involved in several community programs and special education programs. He echoes things said to him and to others, often at a much later time. He also watches and appears to like television to an extreme. He has tantrums occasionally, which include biting himself, destroying property, and flailing his arms. He prefers to stay isolated from others. His latest standardized test results showed a social age of 2.5 on the VSMS and a mental age of 2.5 on the Stanford Binet.

Residential Programming

We recognize the extreme behavior management and training challenges presented by a person with autism. The program has been organized to meet these extreme needs in an effective but humane way that clearly recognizes the right of the individual to lead as normal a life as possible. For this purpose we use small group homes staffed by home program specialists and a support staff who have the primary teaching responsibility. These staff coordinate the residents' activities inside and outside the home.

Our residents entered the home sequentially rather than simultaneously. This method allowed us to facilitate the home's operation during the first few weeks and get each resident's programs off to a solid start.

The home program specialists, behavior technicians, and the residential manager plan the daily schedule of each resident. On weekdays they work at the Occupational Training Center from 9 A.M. until 4 P.M. A more flexible schedule exists on Saturdays and Sundays for community recreational activities, family involvement, special events, and other activities, with training in these areas and in home care.

Staff carries out training programs in independent living skills which are developed in consultation with the director of group homes. Training in independent living includes, but is not necessarily limited to, toileting, personal hygiene, dressing, grooming, housekeeping, groundskeeping, leisure time, and community activities.

For each individual in the program the home staff develops an Individualized Program Plan (IPP) based on the results of all assessments, behavioral observations, and individual (or parental) requests. In each area of independent living the staff lists the individual's strengths and needs. From this short list the staff generates long-term goals, short-term objectives, and training strategies. The staff, the individual (and his/her parents), and the Regional Center representative form the Interdisciplinary Team which meets to discuss the plan. The team modifies and establishes priorities for the IPP. Finally, they agree on responsibilities for implementing the plan.

Assessment

When a person first enters the home we assess his or her ability and independence on each of 32 self-help, home-care and cooking skills by observing and scoring performance on each step of a particular task. For example, a skill such as bathing would be broken down into a series of sequential steps on a data sheet and each step marked as independent or not, with a plus or minus sign respectively, depending on the person's performance. We observe and score performance for 3–5 trials depending on variability. On the basis of the results of these trials we calculate a percent correct score for the skill involved. This score is marked on an assessment profile which illustrates the person's score for the 10 self-help, 12 home-care, and 10 cooking skills we so assess. We reassess ability across all 32 skills after 6 months in the program and then annually thereafter. A sample assessment profile is provided in Figure 1.

Training Procedures

We schedule data-based training sessions for those areas that are targeted on the person's IPP. This represents a subset of all the skills that are initially assessed and then reassessed periodically. Our training is based on Mark Gold's (*Try Another Way*) task-analysis procedures (Gold, 1976). Accordingly, tasks are broken down into sequential steps. During what is typically a whole-task presentation the trainer then provides the minimal assistance needed for the trainee to complete each step successfully. That is, if a trainee does not successfully complete a step, he is first

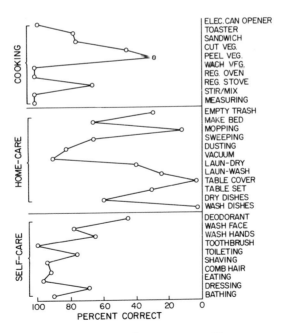

Figure 1. Sample assessment profile.

encouraged to *"try another way."* If that doesn't work he is given a *specific verbal or gestural cue.* If that doesn't work he is given a *physical prompt* to initiate the step, and finally, if needed, a *hand-over hand* prompt to complete the step.

On the data sheet we record a number which represents the degree of power which may have been required for each step. Accordingly, we score each step with 0, 1, 2, 3, or 4 (0 represents independence and 4 represents the need for a hand-over-hand prompt to start *and* complete the step). We calculate the total possible power for the task by multiplying the total number of steps in the task by four, the highest power possible for a single step. The *degree of power* for the trial is then calculated by dividing the total possible power for the task into the actual power used for that trial, that is, the sum of the power actually used for each step in the task. The degree of power is graphed by trial. Accordingly, learning is portrayed by a downward slope on the graph which reflects the need for decreasing power as the learner becomes more independent.

We consider this to be a more sensitive measure of learning than a percent correct score. For example, if before training someone needed hand-over-hand prompting to successfully complete every step in a task, this would be represented as either 100 degrees of power or 0% correct depending on the scoring system used. If after 3 months of training the person needed a specific verbal cue to do each step, this would be scored as 50 degrees of power, indicating that considerable learning had taken place, or 0% correct, indicating that no learning had taken place. We prefer to use the more sensitive measure. However, we should point out that 50 degrees of power should not be interpreted to mean half the power of 100 or twice the power of 25. It simply represents the need for less or more power, respectively.

Data Collection

In addition to the assessment/reassessment data sessions, the home schedules between 600 and 800 data-based training sessions a month. Summary graphs are maintained and kept current to within 3 days. This amount of data keeping has been criticized by some. We believe it is valuable for a number of reasons. First, by examining the daily training graphs the client advocate (a full-time staff person is assigned this responsibility for each client in the program) is soon aware of ineffective training and program revisions can be made accordingly.

Second, we can hold ourselves accountable to funding agencies with the documentation of training we are providing. This degree of documentation has been well received by the agencies to which we are accountable, and although we are among those receiving the highest rates in the state, the funding agencies feel the state is getting its money's worth. Finally, the data system acts as a management tool for communicating to staff the need for a continuous, consistent structure for the clients and a means of ascertaining the extent to which that structure is provided.

Reliability of the Data

Reliability is calculated for the scores obtained during all assessment and reassessment trials. To accomplish this the data sheets for two independent observers are compared and this total number of observations is divided into the total number of agreements to calculate an index of reliability. For example, during an assessment, four observation trials of a 25-step task would produce a total of 100 observations. This number would be divided into the number of agreements actually obtained by the two independent observers over the 100 observations. In this manner reliability was obtained for approximately 400 assessment/reassessment trials for each client representing many thousands of step-by-step observations.

Indices of reliability have ranged from 0.92 to 1.00, 0.91 to 1.00, 0.82 to 1.00, 0.81 to 1.00, 0.81 to 1.00, and 0.93 to 1.00 for the six clients over the course of the assessments and reassessments carried out during the past 2½ years. This high degree of reliability can probably be attributed to the specificity and explicitness of our task analyses.

Results and Discussion

Figure 2 shows the cumulative number of skills mastered by our first six residents over their first 2½ years in the program. These skills represent the independent living areas of self-help, home care, and cooking. The total possible is 192 (or 32 skills for each of six clients). Overall the clients mastered 105 skills in the 30 months from December 1978 to June 1981 (or an average of 18 skills per client). Mastery was measured by a score of 95% or better on the assessment/reassessment carried out most recently prior to the dates indicated.

Figure 3 shows the improvement in independent living skills by these clients as measured by the average assessment/reassessment scores obtained at initial assessment, after 6 months, after 1 year, and after 2 years in the program. We see a picture of continuous developmental growth. In fact these data provide some evidence of response generalization, since only a small subset of these skills was focused on as part of the data-

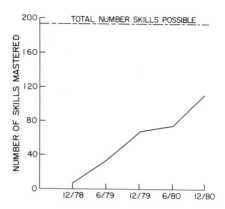

Figure 2. Cumulative number of skills mastered for six residents in the home-based program.

based training schedule. A small group home setting and associated data-based program may provide an environment that promotes response generalization. This will be an important possibility for us to investigate, since response generalization has been elusive for this population and has represented one of the major problems in the behavioral treatment of autism.

   We also have plans to collect social validation data to substantiate further the gains these people have made. Documentation of treatment gains may not be sufficient to maintain funding without such outside validation of its value and relevance to society. Such social validity will be ascertained by means of questionnaires and videotapes administered to staff, parents, and community representatives to measure the accept-

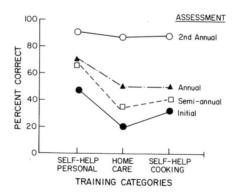

Figure 3. Average assessment scores for six residents in self-care, home care, and cooking skills over a 2½-year period.

ability of behavioral objectives, intervention strategies, and outcomes. Segments of client behaviors, taken periodically, will also be scored for overall appropriateness and client independence. Two of these clients have already improved enough to be placed in a Jay Nolan Center group home that is targeted within the year to provide a 1:3 staff/client ratio versus a 1:2 ratio.

Occupational Programming

This program occurs at an industrial plaza. Its goal is to further develop through mutual trainer–learner agreement a viable service and/ or skill marketable in the competitive working world.

Specific objectives are:

1. To develop a dignified working environment (a) by the selection of an industrial plaza within the community; (b) by presenting meaningful tasks and jobs that give each learner the opportunity to begin earning a living from the first day in the program; (c) by utilizing a schedule that represents a typical occupational work day; and (d) by having the staff present themselves as co-workers
2. To further develop existing expertise of each individual by (a) concentration on performance at industrial standard; (b) increasing the repertoire of skills related to various fields of possible employment; and (c) pursuing the skills needed to interact socially and competitively, to follow instructions, to be dependable, etc.
3. To present alternative career choices based on supply/demand features of the working world, by selecting realistic areas to choose from
4. To develop a written plan for each learner within 3 months of entry into the program by (a) composing a strength/need list; (b) deciding on objectives; (c) defining a methodology for training; (d) establishing specific criteria, for the tasks.

All training is specifically for the purpose of adding to the individual's repertoire of skills necessary for employment. Additional emphasis is placed on the use of sophisticated machinery, making it realistic for the individual to earn at least the minimum wage. For example, training in the machine shop area includes the use of a drill press, vibratory tumbler, media blaster, and a variety of other pieces of industrial equipment. Through careful study of the now-existing machine shops throughout Los Angeles County, it was discovered that these skills would indeed make an individual highly employable and able to earn a decent income.

As an individual demonstrates the ability to maintain a competent level of performance, job placement is pursued. Job placement occurs either through self-employment in something such as a grounds maintenance service, the acquisition of a position in private industry, or continued employment at a Jay Nolan Center site working 40 hours a week for at least the minimum wage.

Assessment

We do not at the present time carry out a general assessment in our occupational training program. The program includes a number of courses of study such as woodworking, grounds maintenance, building maintenance, and industrial machine work. Each course teaches a variety of tasks. For example, the course on grounds maintenance includes instruction in the tasks of raking, watering, and cultivating. Each task is further analyzed into a series of sequential steps in the Marc Gold (1976) manner. The hierarchy of power is used as described earlier, and the person's performance is scored accordingly.

We have learned that acquisition is more rapid for occupational tasks than it is for the tasks taught in the home and community. Obviously we have more latitude in selecting occupational tasks than we do in selecting self-care, home-care, or community skills. We can decide to teach somebody to rake or mow rather than to sell vacuum cleaners or to do bookkeeping. On the other hand reality imposes on us the necessity to teach them to bathe, brush their teeth, cook a meal, etc. Accordingly, having identified a course of study for a client and having targeted a number of tasks as instructional objectives for the IPP, our assessment is based on the performance of the client's doing those tasks during the initial trial only. An initial assessment based on multiple trials would undoubtedly reflect the learning that would take place during that process. Reassessment data, however, do consist of three to five trials at three subsequent points: at mastery, during a check on generalization across people and across settings, and for a follow-up 30 days or more after mastery to assess generalization across time.

Training Procedures

Training procedures in our occupational training program are also based on Marc Gold's (1976) approach. We plot the degree of power needed for each training trial to illustrate and monitor the learning that is taking place. To our knowledge we are the first program operationally and explicitly to apply the *Try Another Way* technology and philosophy to autistic people. We have found that in general the approach needs little modification to be successful with this group beyond our somewhat more explicit data system.

Perhaps equally important to its effectiveness in reaching instructional objectives, however, is the philosophical framework it provides for seeing all people, with or without the problem of autism, as capable of competence, with the ability to grow and live shoulder to shoulder with others as contributing members of a community.

Data Collection

In addition to assessment/reassessment trials, data are collected during all training sessions. Summary graphs are maintained and kept current to within 3 days for all data-based training sessions which are scheduled in accordance with the person's IPP. Figure 4 provides a typical training graph and portrays the degrees of power needed for one of the six clients as he learned the grounds maintenance task of raking over 77 trials. His initial assessment score was 98 degrees of power for the first trial. He demonstrated mastery during trials 67 through 71, needing less than 5 degrees of power, and maintained this level of performance across people and across settings (trial 72), and across time (trials 73–77) more than 60 days later. It is interesting to note the highly variable performance during training and, later, the stable performance after mastery.

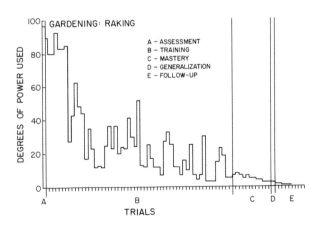

Figure 4. Sample data-based summary training graph.

Reliability of the Data

Reliability is calculated for the scores obtained during initial assessment, mastery, generalization, and follow-up phases. This is accomplished in the same manner described previously. Indices of reliability ranged from 0.96 to 1.00 for all the data collected during the four phases of assessment, mastery, generalization, and follow-up for the six clients.

Results and Discussion

Figure 5 shows the cumulative number of occupational skills mastered by the six residents of our first group home over their first 2½ years in the occupational training program. These skills cover a range of areas including grounds maintenance, industrial assembly, building maintenance, woodworking, and industrial machine work. Overall the clients mastered 239 skills in the 30 months from December 1978 to June 1981 (or an average of 40 skills per client), more than twice the number of skills mastered in the home program. Mastery was measured by a score of under 5 degrees of power needed for five trials in a row.

Figure 6 shows the average assessment, mastery, generalization, and follow-up scores for the six clients in the grounds maintenance course. During this course of study clients learned such things as watering, raking, transplanting, weeding, shoveling, planting, clipping, mowing, edging, hoeing, etc. During the initial trial on tasks such as these the clients

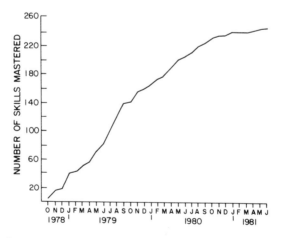

Figure 5. Cumulative number of skills mastered for six clients in the occupational training program.

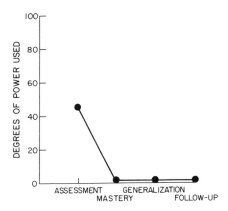

Figure 6. Average scores for six clients in the ground maintenance program during initial assessment, mastery, generalization, and follow-up.

obtained an average assessment score of 43 degrees of power. The average score at mastery was .5 degrees of power, and .3 and .2 during the generalization and follow-up phases, respectively. This is typical of the pattern of results we have seen for the other courses of study as well.

The results of the home program suggested the possibility of response generalization. The results in Figure 6 also suggest stimulus generalization and response maintenance over time since the skills assessed in novel settings with novel people and in later follow-up reflect scores at better than mastery levels. This raises the possibility that reported problems in generalization may be at least partially an artifact of the teaching techniques employed and not totally an inherent aspect of the problem of autism. That is, discrete trial procedures applied in artificial settings (e.g., Rincover & Koegel, 1975) may promote problems in generalization, while task-analysis procedures employing a fading hierarchy of power applied in natural (i.e., target) environments may promote stimulus and response generalization and maintenance over time.

The ultimate validation of any occupational training program can only come from the extent to which a person is productively earning enough money to pay for his or her own needs. For our population this not only means paying for room, board, and entertainment, but also for whatever support systems they may need to remain in the community. Only then will they be seen as "independent of the state" and no longer a drain on society. We are just now beginning to graph client earnings per month as a measure of social validation of our occupational training program. Their continuous growth on this dimension of independence is one of our goals.

Behavior Management

Because of state and federal mandates requiring deinstitutionalization, community programs face the challenge of serving those with the
problems typically associated with autism, including behavioral excesses
that are often extreme and very difficult to manage. To deal effectively
with these problems, a rich context of positive programming, nonaversive
behavior-management techniques, and when appropriate and necessary,
aversive techniques must be available. Both client and staff rights can
best be protected if certain preconditions are met before punishment is
used in applied settings. These include: (a) a context of constructive,
positive programming; (b) a behavior analysis that attempts to identify
the relevant variables maintaining the behavior targeted for reduction; (c)
written documentation of the alternatives to punishment that were fully
and properly implemented; (d) the availability of personnel qualified to
be experts in designing behavior-management programs; (e) informed,
written prior consent from the client's parents; (f) written guidelines for
the use of punishment and other behavior-management techniques; and
(g) an independent peer review committee to review the use of punishment
and other behavior-management programs (LaVigna, 1980).

The major thrust of the Jay Nolan Center program is the development
of increased competency on the part of the residents. Nevertheless many
behavior problems occur, as is expected with this population. It is also
expected that the staff will ordinarily be able to deal with most of these
problems through the use of nonaversive management procedures. For
those extreme problems that are not so easily brought under control, the
program staff includes a licensed clinical psychologist who specializes in
behavior therapy with autistic children, adolescents, and adults.

Although it is impossible to predict the exact interventions we will
eventually use in each case, it is possible to discuss major starting points.
Good treatment, however, goes where the data lead, and we anticipate
each assessment to dictate a specific approach. We have at this point
organized our thrust around 11 alternatives to the use of punishment which
we feel have promise in their application to the behavior problems typically associated with autism (LaVigna & Donnellan, Note 2):

1. *Differential reinforcement of competing behavior* is the reinforcement of those behaviors which are incompatible with the undesired response in intensity, duration, or topography.
2. *Differential reinforcement of low rates of responding (DRL)* is
   the reinforcement of the undesired response only if at least a
   specified period of time has elapsed since the last response or

only if fewer than a specified number of the undesired responses occurred during a preceding interval of time.

3. *Differential reinforcement of other behavior (DRO)* is reinforcement after a specified period of no undesired responding.

4. *Stimulus control* is establishing the discriminative control of an undesired behavior, either through differential reinforcement or fading.

5. *Stimulus change* is the noncontingent and sudden addition of a novel stimulus or an alternation of the incidental stimulus conditions.

6. *Instructional control* is the differential reinforcement of those responses which are in compliance with the verbal instruction presented.

7. *Shaping* is the gradual modification of some property of responses (usually, but not necessarily, topography) by the differential reinforcement of successive approximations to some criterion.

8. *Stimulus satiation* is the continued, noncontingent presentation or availability of a reinforcer that reduces the reinforcer's effectiveness.

9. *Additive procedures* are the combinations of two or more procedures in order to reduce or eliminate an undesired behavior.

10. *Programming* is an instructional sequence designed to help the subject reach certain behavioral objectives based on a behavior analysis and involving the systematic manipulation of stimulus conditions, consequences, instructional stimuli, and other variables that have a functional relationship with the behavior.

11. *Differential reinforcement of other behavior with progressive reinforcement (DROP)* is reinforcement after a specified period of no undesired responding with progressively larger amounts of reinforcement for successive intervals without undesired responding.

Nonaversive procedures were used exclusively to modify the behavior problems of the first six residential clients of the Jay Nolan Center. These behavior problems included aggression, self-injury, property destruction, screaming, stereotypic verbalizations, inappropriate conversations, severe noncompliance, and the like. The nonaversive procedures were applied in a series of *AB* and changing criterion designs. They included: instructional control, the differential reinforcement of competing behavior, the differential reinforcement of other behavior, and the differential reinforcement of low rates of responding. Once a target behavior is under control, the reinforcement schedule is gradually thinned until the procedures can be discontinued without causing a reversal of treatment gains. An acceptable level of control has accordingly been established and maintained without reverting to punishment techniques for any of the six original clients.

Since we opened we have only had two situations in our homes in which we thought an aversive procedure would be justified. In the first case we sought permission from the state to use such a procedure and were denied. Accordingly, the client had to be removed from the program because of the danger he presented to other clients and staff. In the second case permission was granted, and a time-out procedure has been effective in sharply reducing severe property destruction and aggression where nonaversive alternatives had previously proven ineffective. After almost 3 years and after serving 24 clients we feel confident in our original point of view that aversive procedures are only rarely necessary and most problems can be solved without resorting to the use of punishment.

CONCLUSION

Implications

There are a number of implications in these results for us to consider. We have created the beginnings of a model that appears to have contributed significantly to the general development of six young autistic adult men. Whether we have identified the crucial elements of that program will best be shown if we can continue to demonstrate development for our original six clients and replicate these results in our more recently opened homes. Demonstration that we have identified the basic program components will also come from the attempts of others to replicate these findings based on the Jay Nolan Center model.

We also believe that these results have implications for the concept of normalization and the movement toward community-based living arrangements. Four of the six clients described in this chapter had spent a considerable period of their lives in an institutional setting. Their transition to a community-based group home was remarkably without incident. We are unaware of any needs they have that could have been met better in a state hospital. The results obtained after 2½ years of operation support the major hypothesis that led to the establishment of the Jay Nolan Center—that institutional placement is primarily a function of the unavailability of appropriate community-based programs and not of training needs and behavior problems which can only be met in an institutional setting. Accordingly, these results provide empirical support for the concept of normalization and the movement toward community-based living arrangements.

It is sometimes argued that if we don't get autistic people into programs at the earliest age possible, all hopes for a good prognosis are lost. The implication is that adults with autism are less able to learn than they would have been as children. Nevertheless the results of our first 2½ years provide encouraging evidence that adults with autism can continue to develop, and in the case of those who have spent most of their years in a state hospital setting, perhaps begin to develop. If we place value on the process of *becoming* as a major source of human dignity, then the relative rate of development of children over adults becomes a moot point. All children become adults. Therefore the provision of programs for adults that establish a learning environment for continued development becomes the ultimate need for all those who are autistic.

Limitations

There are a number of weaknesses in what we have presented that require caution in attempts to replicate our findings with other autistic adults. Two and a half years is a short period when compared to a lifetime. Whether continued development can be sustained, given the present model, only follow-up studies will tell. Further, to the extent that our model has been effective we are not able to state with certainty what aspects of it are necessary and sufficient for successful replication. We have identified in the foregoing those aspects which we believe are the crucial ones. This remains, however, to be empirically verified through controlled studies. Controlled studies aimed at identifying the operational program variables and repeated replications will give further and needed substance to these encouraging but preliminary findings.

ACKNOWLEDGMENTS: The writing of this chapter resulted from the support of many individuals from inside as well as outside the Jay Nolan Center. The author wishes to thank Sue Anderson, Don Trout, Suzette Soviero, Jeri Dolan-Arnold, Mary McIlhany, and Jan Shapiro for their efforts at Cherry Street, the first home. Thanks are also due to Ruth Grigsby, Kathy Boyet, David Ellerd, and Diane Feheley for their efforts at the Occupational Training Center and to John Thvedt for his editorial assistance. Special thanks go to Carole French for her typing of the manuscript. The Jay Nolan Center for Autism acknowledges the continuing support of the Los Angeles Chapter of the National Society for Autistic Children. Additionally, we thank Dr. Tom Kelly and Ann Baerwald from the North Los Angeles County Regional Center, and Dr. David Loberg, director of the California Department of Developmental Services, for their support and encouragement of our efforts at local and state levels of government.

REFERENCES

Eisenberg, L. The autistic child in adolescence. *American Journal of Psychiatry*, 1956, *112*, 607–612.

Eisenberg, L. The course of childhood schizophrenia. *Archives of Neurological Psychiatry*, 1957, *78*, 69–83.

Gold, M. W. Task analysis of a complex assembly task by the retarded blind. *Exceptional Children*, 1976, *43*, 78–84.

Graziano, A. *Child without tomorrow*. Elmsford, N.Y.: Pergamon, 1975.

LaVigna, G. W. Reducing behavior problems in the classroom. *In Critical issues in educating autistic children and youth*. (B. Wilcox and A. Thompson, eds.), Washington, D.C.: U.S. Department of Education, Office of Special Education, 1980.

Liberman, R. P. Social and political challenges to the development of behavioral programs in organizations. *In Trends in behavior therapy*. (S. Bates, P. O. Sjoden, W. S. Dockens, K. G. Gotestam, eds.), New York: Academic Press, 1979.

Lovaas, O. I., Koegel, R. L., Simmons, J. Q., & Long, J. Some generalization and follow-up on autistic children in behavior therapy. *Journal of Applied Behavior Analysis*, 1973, *6*, 131–166.

Rincover, A., & Koegel, R. L. Setting generality and stimulus control in autistic children. *Journal of Applied Behavior Analysis*, 1975, *8*, 235–246.

Rutter, M., Greenfeld, D., & Lockyer, L. A five to fifteen year follow-up study of infantile psychosis. II. Social and behavioural outcome. *British Journal of Psychiatry*, 1967, *113*, 1183–1200.

Wolfensberger, W. (Ed.). *The principle of normalization in human services*. Toronto: National Institute on Mental Retardation, 1972.

REFERENCE NOTES

1. Lovaas, O. I. *Teaching homes: An alternative to institutionalization*. Paper presented at the annual meeting and conference of the National Society for Autistic Children, Orlando, Florida, June 1977.

2. LaVigna, G. W., & Donnellan, A. *Alternatives to the use of punishment in the control of undesired behavior*. Portions of this paper were presented at the Eighth Annual Southern California Conference on Behavior Modification, Los Angeles, October 1976, and the 10th Annual Meeting of the Association for the Advancement of Behavior Therapy, New York, December 1976.

19

Service Development for Adolescents and Adults in North Carolina's TEACCH Program

GARY B. MESIBOV, ERIC SCHOPLER,
and JERRY L. SLOAN

Childhood autism has only recently been recognized as a disorder which can best be treated and managed in the context of the child's own family and community. Such children have been provided with comprehensive, statewide services in North Carolina, a program for the Treatment and Education of Autistic and Communications handicapped CHildren (Division TEACCH). Beginning as a research project funded by the National Institute of Mental Health and the U.S. Office of Education in 1966, the TEACCH program has been serving autistic children and their families for the past 15 years. It became the first legally mandated statewide program for autistic children in 1972, and now includes a network of 5 regional centers, 34 public school classrooms, and 4 group homes located throughout the state of North Carolina. Over 1,000 children and their families have been evaluated and assisted since the program's inception.

TEACCH emphasizes the involvement of parents in a psychoeducational model using both developmental and behavioral theory for its implementation. As new knowledge has become available the program has changed and grown. One of the most important instances of this

GARY B. MESIBOV and ERIC SCHOPLER ● Division TEACCH, Department of Psychiatry, University of North Carolina School of Medicine, Chapel Hill, North Carolina 27514. JERRY L. SLOAN ● Southeastern TEACCH Center, Department of Psychiatry, University of North Carolina School of Medicine, Chapel Hill, North Carolina 27514.

evolution has been the recent recognition that even when autistic children improve in their adaptation, their handicapping condition usually continues in some form throughout their life cycle. In order to meet this range of needs the TEACCH legislative mandate has been extended to serve adolescents and adults with appropriate programs and services.

Because so little is known about the older age range, only a few model programs have been developed to date (See chapters 17 and 18). Accordingly, our own services for autistic adolescents and adults were developed from our extensive 15 years' experience with the younger children and their families. Our work with the younger age range has evolved five guiding principles useful with the older group. These can be summarized as follows:

1. *The concept of development* facilitates both understanding and treatment of autistic clients. Autism is now recognized as a developmental disorder rather than an emotional illness (Schopler, Rutter, & Chess, 1979). Moreover, the associated handicaps appear across a continuum of severity (Wing & Gould, 1978) requiring individualized and developmentally appropriate curriculum and services.
2. *Individualized diagnostic assessment* forms the basis for the identification of appropriate classification, educational curricula, and service programs. A distinction is made between diagnostic classification and individualized assessment.
3. *Parents of autistic children* as a group are similar to other parents with the noteable exception that they have a handicapped child. They are more the victims of their child's disorder than its cause (Schopler, 1971, 1976). They also continue to be the most effective allies for professionals developing appropriate services, even though their involvement changes as the autistic child reaches adulthood.
4. *Structured classrooms* in the public schools can provide an effective education, when implemented in small classes with an appropriate curriculum for each child (Schopler & Bristol, 1980).
5. *Specialized procedures and services* are required to meet the needs of autistic children. They differ sufficiently from their nonhandicapped peers that such special services frequently offer the most cost-effective treatment available.

The purpose of this chapter is to describe how the TEACCH program uses these five principles in developing comprehensive day and residential programs for autistic adolescents and adults in North Carolina. Specific examples will be given of how each principle is being applied in the context of more general programs and concerns. Although this chapter represents only a preliminary report, an outline of the needed and evolving services is presented for possible use by others developing community-based programs for this population.

THE CONCEPT OF DEVELOPMENT

This principle has played an important role in the TEACCH program at two different levels. The first pertains to the shift in definition of autism from a psychiatric disease to a developmental disability. The second level deals with the development of teaching programs. Because autistic children characteristically show quite uneven learning profiles it is necessary to individualize both behavior management and teaching programs according to the different developmental levels reflected in the same child. We will discuss each of these uses of the developmental concept below.

Autism as a Developmental Disability

Historically autism was considered a form of social withdrawal by vulnerable children from emotionally cold, rejecting, "refrigerator mothers" (Bettelheim, 1967; Kanner, 1943). This conception brought autistic children under the exclusive jurisdiction of mental health, with several important negative consequences for such children and their families. First, the children were frequently seen in inappropriate verbally oriented play therapy while their parents were seen in therapy aimed at correcting their "destructive attitudes." Second, the children were excluded from public schools. Educators did not recognize autism, and when they did they persisted in classifying it as an emotional disturbance.

More recently many investigators have recognized that this perspective is inconsistent with both their experiences and a growing body of empirical research (Rutter & Schopler, 1979). They recognized that autistic children frequently appear emotionally disturbed, but when they do it is in reaction to the frustration caused by their deficits rather than that the emotional difficulties cause their learning deficits.

In recent years autism is increasingly accepted as a developmental disability (Schopler, Rutter, & Chess, 1979). This conception has been incorporated in the definition of autism used by the National Society for Autistic Children (NSAC) (Schopler & Rutter, 1978). Autism is included under the Developmental Disabilities Act of 1975, and the U.S. Office of Education has also initiated reclassification (Martin, 1980) by removing autism from the emotionally disturbed category.

Programming Developmentally

The shift toward defining autism as a developmental disability has coincided with the emphasis on skill training and behavior management as opposed to psychotherapy. The TEACCH program has been of this position since its inception (Schopler & Reichler, 1971) as have several other nationally recognized programs for autistic people (see Chapters 17 and 18, and Fenichel, 1976). However, the concept of development has been important in the TEACCH program not just because it offers an explanation other than psychogenesis for the puzzling autistic behavior, but it also helped to define treatment procedures. Appropriate adult responses can often best be approximated from the normal response to a particular development level. For example, a 5-year-old autistic child may have age-appropriate motor coordination but the language level of a 2-year-old. While he could be taught to use a tricycle, this can best be done by the adult using simple speech appropriate to the 2-year-old level. Such consideration of the uneven development in autistic children has shaped our assessment procedures (described below) and contributed to the effectiveness of our individualized programming (Schopler, Mesibov, DeVellis, & Short, 1981).

Even though children, normal and otherwise, change with age more rapidly than do adults, developmental considerations continue to shape our teaching efforts with adolescents and adults. This developmental perspective can best be illustrated by our guidelines for sex education. Autistic people at different levels of development have different needs for sex education. Therefore it is not necessary, or even desirable, to provide each autistic person with the same kind of information. Autistic people in the severely retarded range of mental functioning need different information and training in sexuality than those functioning in the normal range intellectually, including good language abilities. In developing sex education as well as any other program for autistic people it is important to assess the amount of information needed, given an individual's level of functioning and expected life experiences.

In our program we have divided the sex education needs of autistic people into three separate groups. The first group includes our most severely handicapped clients, who have extremely limited expressive language and comprehension ability. For them the major sex education issue is their behavior concerning sexual matters, especially in public. The behaviors they must learn include going to the bathroom appropriately and privately, learning where and how to dress and undress themselves, and if they masturbate, learning to do this in the privacy of their own home. If they can learn these and other similar behaviors effectively, they will achieve an acceptable level for their abilities and probable life situations. Teaching them body parts or other words related to sexuality is probably not desirable. This group's communication skills are so limited that it is more appropriate to teach them words and concepts having more functional meaning in their day-to-day lives.

The second group includes less handicapped clients, who are still of limited ability to understand and communicate. This group should learn the appropriate behaviors described for the first group and will additionally need to develop a better understanding of their own anatomy and physical development. These clients are aware of their bodies and possible changes that are occurring, but will probably not be engaged in sexual activity with other people. For this group, some basic discussion of anatomy and self-help skills might be of greatest use. The program developed at Benhaven (Chapter 9) is ideally suited to the needs and skills of this group.

Finally, there is a third group of autistic people with average or near-average intelligence who are capable of and often concerned about heterosexual activities. This group must learn all the information designed for the already-designated groups, and in addition will need supplemental information about appropriate heterosexual functioning. Many curricula for mentally retarded people without autism are appropriate as a starting point for this population; however, certain modifications might be needed. For example, our discomfort with sexual issues often forces us to be somewhat more obscure and symbolic when discussing these matters. With autistic clients it is important to remain very concrete and specific, even though one might be a bit uncomfortable with the concepts or ambiguous notions. In our work with the younger population of autistic children we have found that such developmental differences must be considered in order to implement appropriate treatment programs. This is accomplished through individualized diagnostic evaluation and assessment.

DIAGNOSTIC EVALUATION AND ASSESSMENT

In the TEACCH program (Reichler & Schopler, 1976; Schopler & Olley, 1981) a distinction has always been made between diagnosis for the purpose of administrative or research grouping on the one hand and assessment for individualized education and management on the other. With the term "diagnosis" we refer to the identification of those features of the disorder which are shared by children designated as autistic, that is, the necessary components of the syndrome, while the term "assessment" is used for evaluating the host of unique characteristics and behaviors that are shared by some, but not necessarily by most autistic children. The evaluation of these more unique behavior clusters is essential to working out a developmentally appropriate treatment program for each individual.

Diagnosis

Our diagnosis of autism is based on the criteria developed by Creak (1964) and revised by Rutter and the NSAC (Schopler & Rutter, 1978). These represent primarily the following four cardinal features of the disorder: (1) the child is impaired in his interpersonal and social relationships; (2) speech and language are absent, delayed, or peculiar; (3) the child shows repetitive and ritualistic behaviors and becomes upset when these are interfered with; and (4) the onset of the disorder is early in life, before 3 years of age.

When autism was first introduced into the literature the diagnosis was only made by highly trained psychiatrists and professionals. Since then the accumulation of empirical research (Rutter & Schopler, 1979) has produced sufficient data about the condition to shift diagnosis into the public domain. Accordingly, we have developed a Childhood Autism Rating Scale (CARS) (Schopler, Reichler, DeVellis, & Daly, 1980) and use it for diagnosing children referred to the TEACCH program. It includes 15 scales based on the concept that autism is located on a continium of disabilities (Wing & Gould, 1978) from mild to severe, and that the nature of the disability meets the criteria cited above. We have rated about 1,000 children since the beginning of the program with an average age of 5 and a range from 2 to 33. They do not come from upper-middle-class parents as was once believed, but include the same family social class distribution found in the rest of the state. Most of them are mentally retarded as well as autistic, with over 50% in the moderate to severe range, 34% in the mild to moderate range, and only 15% in the near-normal range. All our autistic children share the autism features mentioned before, and all of them have problems and specific characteristics which will be discussed below.

The diagnoses of adolescents and adults share these features. That is, any adolescent or adult who met the criteria of autism as a child is also included in the diagnostic category as an adult. For this retrospective diagnosis the CARS can still be used with the older age range. However, a diagnosis based only on currently observable behavior will look somewhat different because of the developmental changes which occur in adolescence. These of course differ for the near-normal autistic adolescents from those with more severe degrees of retardation. To summarize a pilot study of Mesibov and Shea (Note 1), they found the following characteristics in a sample of higher level autistic adolescents: (1) they tend to talk too much, often with obsessive repetition; (2) they have trouble understanding what others are saying; (3) they are inattentive to details outside their special interest; (4) they have inappropriate responses to the feelings and thoughts of others; and (5) they show ritualistic behaviors. This study will be extended to a larger sample and cover a wider range of disability to confirm these behavioral features of autistic adolescents before they can be incorporated in an objective rating system.

Assessment

The assessment needed for individualized education and treatment of the younger children requires a wider range of information than is needed for diagnostic classification. In the TEACCH program we developed the Psychoeducational Profile (PEP) (Schopler & Reichler, 1978). It identifies the variations of developmental levels in 10 areas of educational functioning: imitation, perception, gross motor, fine motor, eye–hand integration, cognitive performance, expressive language, self-help skills, social skills, and behavior problems. The resulting profile is combined with assessment information from home and school in order to formulate appropriate teaching strategies (Schopler, Reichler, & Lansing, 1979), and specific teaching programs (Schopler, Lansing, & Waters, in press).

Our assessment procedure for the younger age group has been extended to the older population, but with adaptation to that older group's changed needs. As with the normal population developmental changes become less rapid as the child matures. Formal schooling terminates in adult life with an increased expectation to participate in work and in independent living, even when the young adult remains in the parents' home. The Psychoeducational Profile has been extended to assess these changing needs of adults and includes the following six function areas: (1) vocational behaviors, i.e., reactions to work interruption, ability to participate in work group projects, to manage snacks and the Coke machine; (2) work-related socialization, including relations with supervisors and co-workers; (3) vocational skills, the use of fine motor skills with tools necessary for completing vocational tasks; (4) self-help skills for personal care in dress, cleanliness, toileting, and eating behavior; (5) independent work skills or the ability to sustain work for designated periods after the necessary skills are mastered; and (6) leisure activities, including the capacity to use nonworking time in a socially acceptable and pleasurable activity.

The needed survival skills in each of these areas are evaluated in direct observation of the client. As with the PEP, the resulting profile distinguishes skills already mastered from those which are not or are still emerging. In addition these six function areas are also evaluated by parents or parent substitutes from observations in the actual living situation. An additional evaluation form is completed by the teacher or workshop supervisor to provide direct observation from the vocational segment of the client's life. The composite profile scores of these three assessment areas are used for determining an individualized plan of additional training and placement for each client. Parents continue to play a critical role in implementing these plans.

PARENT–PROFESSIONAL COLLABORATION

Since its beginning the TEACCH program has emphasized that parents are not the cause of their child's autism, but rather the most effective developmental agents and allies for professionals in developing ways of helping autistic people (Reichler & Schopler, 1976). With the younger age group we have found four different important roles that parents play in their interaction with our professional staff.

First is the parent as a trainee. In this role our staff have experience with many more children than do parents. Staff also usually have more experience with methods of teaching and management and with work of others in the same field. Parents assume the role of trainees in learning specific ways of teaching and shaping socially acceptable behavior for their child.

Second is the parent as trainer. In this role we recognize that parents have the most extensive experience with their own child and also the greatest motivation for achieving effective living and learning arrangements with their child. They instruct our staff with their own experiences, successes, and failures in understanding and managing their children, consistent with their own lifestyle requirements. In this area parents become the trainers and staff the trainees.

Third is parent–staff emotional support. This role is important for reducing burn-out and maintaining the primarily positive attitudes for the special struggles imposed by the child's developmental disability. The staff can provide this by recognizing the child's slow process of learning and frequent relapses into special behavior problems. This understanding will be reflected even when staff and parents are in disagreement about specific issues and procedures. Conversely, parents are expected to have a similar understanding of staff frustrations, especially those spending the most time with the child, including teachers or group home staff. Mutual support between parents and staff is a critical element in providing appropriate help for autistic children.

Fourth is the role of social advocate. This involves community education to the child's special needs, defining the needed cost-effective services, and soliciting community cooperation and help in making these available. In the TEACCH program this is provided through collaboration in parent groups formed around classrooms or centers and affiliated with state and national societies for autistic children. In this role the expertise of both staff and parents is combined in order to achieve even wider understanding and help.

Needless to say these four different roles overlap with each other, with one being more important at one phase of parent–staff relations than at another. For example, when first developing services for autistic adolescents and adults, the social action collaboration with parent groups was of primary importance in the TEACCH program. Parents called our attention to both their children's and their own changing needs as they grow older.

At home parents have struggled for more than a decade with the special needs of their child. They have made special accommodations, and arranged rooms, furniture, and supplies so as to be safe for their autistic child and at the same time available for and usable for the rest of the family. Some have built fenced-in yards to make a safe play area for the child without sense of boundaries. All have made special efforts to maintain communication and encourage the handicapped child's participation in family life. Some families' ties were strengthened along this special path while others experienced more hardship. Most have gone through at least some periods of special stress that families without handicapped children don't even know about. By the time their autistic child reaches adolescence the parents have grown older and tired, while the child grows stronger but not much more independent.

The upper age limit in school according to North Carolina state law is 18. For parents whose child approaches this age a new family crisis looms on the horizon. What are they to do with him or her after the termination of public schooling? Is further training available? Are there opportunities for the youngster to live away from home to be self-supporting, as is possible for parents with nonhandicapped adolescents? Or will the autistic adult need to remain at home for the rest of his or her parents' life? And if the young adult can remain at home, is any support or help available to the parents from relatives or from the community?

Members of the larger community are inevitably involved in the answers and the lack of answers to these questions. They can best be informed through the collaborative efforts of parents and concerned professionals.

In North Carolina the effectiveness of parent–staff collaboration was exemplified by the development of one of our most needed services, group homes for autistic adolescents and adults. These evolved from conflicting pressures first experienced by our parents. On the one hand many parents felt unable to continue providing the special care and supervision needed by their mature handicapped offspring without sacrificing their family stability and mental health. On the other hand they were told by increasing numbers of professionals that state institutions, the primary alternative to home care, were a living hell to which no decent human being would condemn a relative. The resolution of this conflict resulted in the first North Carolina group home (Triad Home) for autistic people. The Triad Group Home for Autistic Youth opened in Greensboro in early 1976. It was the product of a collaborative grant written by both the TEACCH program and the parents' group (North Carolina Society for Autistic Children) who identified a group home as their most important need when money became available for autistic children through the North Carolina Developmental Disabilities Council. Initially the parents assumed full responsibility for the home with their executive director serving concurrently as the group home director. Once the program was established, control was gradually shifted to a private, nonprofit board of directors who now hire their own independent group home director.

Even though the Triad Home and three subsequent group homes for autistic adolescents and adults are now directed by private, nonprofit boards of directors, an important parental role continues. Parents are heavily represented on these boards of directors and their influence is evident in many aspects of the programs, policies, and procedures (Boyd, Dossett, Marcus, Stager, & Woods, Note 2).

The Triad Group Home has served as a model for the others. Its guiding philosophy was forged by parent–staff collaboration. It reflects the family home environment in the overall design of the home as illustrated by the following excerpt from the Triad philosophy:

> It was agreed that the home environment is best for most, if not all, people. Therefore, the group home was the most logical alternative. It was the belief of the parents and professionals involved that autistic citizens have the same right as anyone else to live out their lives in a comfortable, supportive, growth-producing, home-like environment, in a place that feels like "home," where one can relax after a hard day's work or school. It was also the belief of these people that this home should be in a typical community with access to schools, parks, hospitals, grocery stores, movies, shopping centers, and all aspects of normal American culture. It was their belief that the residents of the group

home should participate in all aspects of the community. For these reasons, the philosophy of this particular group is to be home-like, a place where people live their daily lives. Secondary to that, it may be a school, or adaptive work, or a therapeutic environment, a treatment center, or even a respite care center for parents. While it is all those, it is first of all "Home" for the people who live there. (Boyd et al., Note 2, p. 2)

The management of the Triad Home includes strong parental involvement. The Personnel Committee has strong representation from parents who want to be sure that applicants have the potential for involvement and caring for the home's residents before they are hired.

The Admissions Committee consists of two professionals and four parents. Each applicant for residency in the home is interviewed by one parent and one professional, who try to determine the degree of stress that the autistic adolescent is causing and to formulate a recommendation for admission. A Human Rights Committee was designed to monitor the protection of the residents' rights, and at least a third of its members are parents.

Parent involvement is also evident in many of the procedures. When a child first moves into the home, a contract conference is held between the home's staff and the parents, explaining the privileges and responsibilities of each. Parents are encouraged to take their children home as frequently as possible and to make these visits as pleasant as possible. The home does not ask the parents to help with the active programming for their children, and in fact discourages this. Parents are encouraged to visit the home whenever they like, to be involved in their childrens' Individual Habilitation Plan and Individual Education Plan, and are sent copies of the bimonthly staffings notes for each child. Although each of the three group homes that has followed the Triad Home in North Carolina has its own unique flavor and philosophy, strong parental involvement and mutual respect between parent and professional epitomize these programs as well.

APPROPRIATE SMALL, STRUCTURED CLASSROOMS

The fourth guiding principle for adolescents derives from the recognized need for small, structured classrooms. In collaboration with the local educational authorities the TEACCH program has developed 28 such preadolescent classrooms located in public schools. TEACCH staff were involved in the hiring and training of teachers, evaluating and placing children in the classrooms, and providing ongoing consultation support. We soon learned that it was necessary to plan for special education in adolescence well before the child's 18th birthday. It is helpful already by age 13 to consider employment possibilities and to begin developing curricula for training vocational skills. Such early planning improves the child's ability to utilize classrooms designed for autistic adolescents.

In North Carolina there are six classrooms now serving autistic adolescents and developing appropriate learning opportunities for this group. One of the original classrooms is located in Wilmington, North Carolina, and is representative of our adolescent classroom programs. The overall goals of the Wilmington classroom are to provide training for those severely handicapped adolescents who had been previously excluded or inappropriately served in other public school classes, and to provide this training in an age-appropriate high school setting. More specifically, there are four major instructional goals reflected in the class curriculum and activities:

1. To provide training in the development of a functional alternative language system utilizing simultaneous communication (sometimes called "signing").
2. To provide training in realistic prevocational and vocational skills which may be applied either in competitive employment or in a sheltered workshop setting.
3. To stimulate improved self-help skills and to increase the student's ability to function without direct supervision at home and school.
4. To promote appropriate interaction and social skills among the students and their peers in the school setting.

Development of the Classroom

The classroom developed out of clinical experiences with the children when they were younger. Initially, work was begun with two adolescent students (ages 16 and 17), both diagnosed as severely communications-handicapped and severely retarded. Neither student had any expressive language, and both were estimated to have receptive language at about the 2- to 3-year-old level. Both students did, however, use some primitive gestural communication. They were prone to engage frequently in stereotypic and self-stimulatory behavior in unstructured settings, and one student had a severe bilateral sensorineural hearing loss. Both had been judged to be incapable of learning in the usual settings for the handicapped. Both students remained in their assigned classroom placements, but the local school system arranged to provide transportation to the center for two 90-minute training sessions each week. These sessions included two staff members, the children, and their parents, and consisted of training in attending skills and in the use of basic label signs, especially those involving food and basic needs. These sessions were continued over an entire school year and the following summer. Both students learned nearly 100 signs receptively, and although they acquired a smaller number expressively (about 25), each made some use of their signs for spontaneous expressive communication. At the same time additional home programs given to the families focused on self-help skills and some prevocational tasks such as sorting and simple two- or three-item assemblies.

As a result of these preliminary studies the local school system and TEACCH agreed to contract for the establishment of a class for these and other children. The contract provides for joint selection of teaching staff by TEACCH and the local schools, with diagnostic services, staff training, and ongoing consultant support provided by TEACCH. For the 1979–1980 school year six children were identified. Three students were female, and the six ranged from 13 to 18 years of age. All were moderately to severely retarded with mental ages on nonlanguage tests ranging from 4 to 7 years. The diagnoses varied, but include autism and autistic-like behavior, Down's syndrome, and even organic involvement such as meiplegia.

Classroom Organization and Curriculum

The class is located in a large (approximately 1,600 students) urban high school. It was the first class for such seriously handicapped students in this particular school. The overall arrangement of the classroom is somewhat different from traditional classes (see Figure 1) and was based on the Leicestershire open classroom system, with nine stations: language master, activities for daily living (bed and ironing), measurement, sorting, assembly, packaging, signing, snack, and cooking. Each of these stations has a number, although some areas of the room, such as the "free" or "recreational" area, are not marked. When the students arrive each day (most ride schoolbuses), each one "checks in" by placing a name card in an envelope marked "in." After routine class maintenance tasks are performed, each student picks up a clipboard which has a series of number tags which refer to the various work station numbers. On signal each student goes to the work station listed first on the clipboard, tears off the number, and places it in the receptacle provided. A task is given or the student removes the appropriate materials to perform a task (as in assembly procedures) and begins work. When the assigned task is completed, the student signals for a teacher to check the work performed. When the

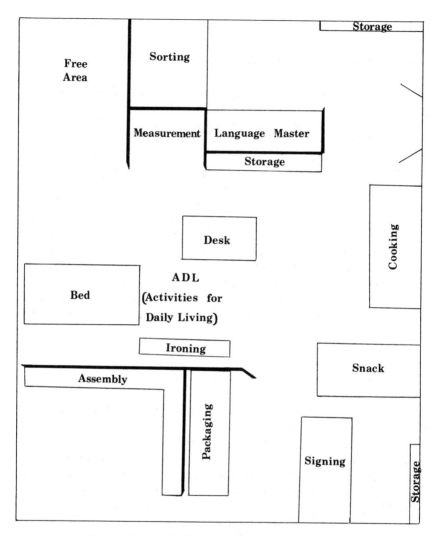

Figure 1. Floor plan of TEACCH classroom for adolescents.

students have completed their work or when a predetermined time has elapsed, students move on to the next station. Such activities encompass the majority of the day.

It is not sufficient, however, to involve students in individual tasks all day long. There is also an emphasis on cooperative work on complex tasks. Students in this class have an opportunity to work in groups on "assembly-line" tasks similar to those they might encounter in some competitive or sheltered workshop placements. They are also expected to cooperate in various classroom activities, such as preparing snacks. In a typical assembly-line task, one student might be required to sort out a group of small parts from a bin according to a pattern (or "jig") and place these in a small container. A second student would place these in an envelope and pass the envelope to a third student who seals it and places it with other envelopes in a shipping container. Such activities are of special value to students who have difficulties in relating, as is the case with autistic people, since working and relating with others are likely areas of difficulty in work settings.

We have frequently heard the complaint that it is difficult to replicate real working conditions in a classroom because of a lack of equipment or challenging tasks. We have not observed this to be the case. Virtually all of the equipment in this class is teacher-made, and some very common items provide opportunities for complex and challenging activities for the severely handicapped. For instance, three or four dozen inexpensive ball-point pens may be used for a 12-step assembly task. The task analysis for this task is as follows:

Step 1. Place bottom half of pen in hand
Step 2. Put one spring in bottom half
Step 3. Place ink cartridge in bottom half, point in first
Step 4. Place silver divider over ink cartridge
Step 5. Put assembled bottom half down
Step 6. Pick up top half of pen
Step 7. Place colored inner piece into top half of pen
Step 8. Place white plastic piece into top half of pen
Step 9. Pick up bottom half of pen
Step 10. Place top half over/into bottom half
Step 11. Push and screw on top to bottom
Step 12. Place completed pen in carton

In order to maintain vocational placement, the development of a viable communication system is also basic to independent functioning. In this class simultaneous communication is stressed as an alternative to verbal speech, and each student receives individual training in this area every day. Signing with whatever proficiency each student has is expected in all aspects of classroom work. Students sign to the staff and to each other in assembly-line work, in preparing snacks, and in the cafeteria, where even the kitchen staff has learned some basic food signs.

The staffing pattern and support network for the class are also important considerations in the success of the classroom. The teacher and assistant were both known to TEACCH previously, and were well experienced in teaching the severely handicapped. In addition regular (almost weekly) visits are made by the TEACCH Center–based consultant, who provides advice and feedback to the staff and acts as a liaison to the center. This person can also act as extra staff at times if there are special needs, and may assist in taking baseline data for behavior-management programs or videotaping.

Problems in Maintaining a Good Classroom

Any classroom which provides an active, challenging environment for severely handicapped students such as these will of necessity encounter problems in maintaining the critical balance of elements needed for successful teaching. At one level there are the staff problems presented by the demands of the type of teaching involved. Despite the small number of students served, a large amount of planning must be done in order to integrate the needs of the students and to continue to derive new tasks of a meaningful nature. The work requires more than the usual amount of space, and the staff spends much additional time preparing materials for the class. The nature of the instruction in this class also precludes enrolling a large number of children. One direct result of these demands is that the staff expends large amounts of energy and needs frequent support and feedback from the consultant.

Another problem has been the fact that the nature of the classroom and its curriculum does not seem suitable for all families and students, even among those who have severe handicaps. Some families feel that their children are better served in a more traditional class, arguing that those years represent the only opportunity their children will have to acquire academic skills. It also seems clear that those students who are able to read, have good language skills, and do mathematics are probably better placed in classes which stress these functions. As a consequence another class for older autistic and communication-handicapped children of higher ability has been established in a junior high school. This class also has something of a prevocational emphasis, but the potential for these students to obtain competitive employment is much better than for the students of the class described here.

A third problem, and a continuing source of frustration for parents and professionals alike, has been the lack of opportunities for the students of this class to use the skills they have learned, either in summer programs or in workshop or employment settings after formal education is completed. Knowing that such opportunities are quite scarce is somewhat demoralizing for all concerned, and makes it difficult for those involved to maintain their enthusiasm. This experience has demonstrated the importance of functional integration of teaching in the living context of the student (Brown, Branston, Hamre-Nietupski, Pumpion, Certo, & Gruenewald, 1979).

This issue of behavior management arises in the classroom as well. The program makes use of basic behavior-management principles and a token system is employed to systematically encourage the performance of certain behaviors such as attending, signing, signaling when a task is completed, and so on. Data on job performance are also taken in order to evaluate each student's progress. However, the staff tries to make use of rewards similar to those which occur in everyday life, such as praise, smiles, and handshakes, and these are dispensed on a variable-ratio schedule as soon as possible in order to simulate natural conditions. These provide the best potential for carry-over into other aspects of the child's life.

NEED FOR SPECIALIZED SERVICES

Our program has been influenced by the normalization principle (Mesibov, 1976; Wolfensberger, 1972) in trying to utilize existing community-based resources whenever possible. However, these efforts frequently encounter opposition. Autistic people are sufficiently different from their nonhandicapped peers that the same requirements and expectations do not reasonably apply to both groups. Most autistic people also suffer from mental retardation, hence their needs often overlap with those of non-autistic retarded people. However, because of their more obvious problems with social and communication skills, autistic people are frequently excluded from available services, including those for retarded citizens.

Our efforts to overcome this kind of discrimination has led to two trends. First, when the children were excluded from public schools, summer recreation programs, or summer camps, we developed these services especially for autistic children in collaboration with our parent groups. Once these services became established and working effectively, it was easier to obtain better acceptance for our children in services for non-autistic mentally retarded children. Some special staff training and understanding of the autistic handicap was needed. However, it soon became obvious that it was in the best interest of all handicapped children if placement were made by special need rather than by diagnostic label. Because of their additional cost and greater staff requirements, special services should only be developed when special needs cannot be met within existing programs. However, when the special community-based services needed by autistic people are not provided, the primary option is still placement in large, impersonal, institutional warehouses. Community-based programs designed to prevent unnecessary institutionalization are not only much less expensive than institutions, but they also provide more humane and cost-effective help.

The help needed for community functioning usually involves support for effective living arrangements and for successful vocational placement. Below is a brief description of services in each of these two areas being developed with our parent groups in the TEACCH program.

Living Arrangement Support

When we first became aware of the need for services for the older group in 1977, our parents' groups put as a first priority the establishment of group homes for autistic adolescents and adults. The most pressing need came from parents whose children developed disruptive behaviors that were threatening the families with disorganization. However, we soon learned that it was not sufficient to locate a group home in the community unless certain safeguards were built into the program. A group home can become as isolating and restricted as the most impersonal institution. Such safeguards include the following: Viable connecting links must be worked out between the group home residents and schools, workshops, medical care, shopping centers, and recreation areas. By requiring residents to be away from the home during the day, the possibility of overmedication and neglect are reduced. Additional safeguards against such neglect are provided by a private board of directors who, along with other members of the community, offer both support for staff and restraint against increase of potential isolation. In addition to community links, the Admissions Committee must consider how to balance the group into a viable living unit. One resident with severely self-injurious or aggressive behavior can be maintained in the group, sometimes even two, but not three or more. When group balance is ignored, staff burn-out is likely to increase. Balanced grouping is facilitated when cooperative or reciprocal admissions can be developed with group homes for mentally retarded residents. Some of our autistic adults have been admitted to such group homes. Unfortunately our existing group homes are insufficient for all our clients needing placement. Our parents' group is currently also considering the development of a vocational center in the country, including the potential for a summer camp, access to nearby urban work placement, farm work, and residential facilities. In spite of these developments many parents still prefer to keep their adolescent and older children in their own homes. This arrangement often is still the least restrictive environment. But even when good family adaptation has been achieved, periods of stress occur and parents may need respite from the stress of special care required to maintain their handicapped offspring at home.

Respite Care

This is a short-term service in which parents can be separated from their offspring for brief vacation periods. In North Carolina some 30 respite care programs are administered through mental health centers. These were not primarily designed for autistic people. However, as the potential for training staff regarding the special needs of autistic people increased, they were more readily included in existing respite care programs. This resource is generally delivered in two different ways.

A respite home, sometimes a reserved bed in a group home, is available for brief periods up to a month. The autistic person is placed there while the family regroups its energy and caring abilities. This kind of respite care does not work out in all cases. The adolescent or adult must adapt to brand-new people and living environments. For some this is more stressful than the second alternative—home-based respite care. For this service a trained housekeeper moves into the family's home while the parents are away. Although some special training is necessary, this has the advantage of being organized more readily and less expensively than a respite home, and it requires fewer new adjustments for the autistic person.

Neither parental homes nor group homes offer higher level functioning autistic persons the best opportunity to maintain the least restrictive living arrangements. These people can often maintain themselves in independent living units or apartments with minimum supervision or help in establishing satisfactory living arrangements. It is often especially difficult to find financial support for independent living units or supervision because these individuals are socially retarded but do not meet funding criteria for mental retardation.

Vocational Training and Placement Support

Autistic adults may be able to use special vocational placement from the entire range of placement services. At the higher end of the continuum this may include jobs like piano tuning, library work, electronic equipment assembly, dishwashing, and so on. Such placement can often be effected if a vocational advocate, someone trained in the problems of autistic adults, is available to work out initial adjustment. This includes not only training the client on the specific job requirements, but also orienting co-workers and supervisors to better understanding and support. This process is discussed in greater detail in Chapter 7.

Many autistic people could fit the supervised work opportunity offered by sheltered workshops. However, because of their social peculiarities or behavior problems they are too frequently denied access to sheltered workshops. Since the TEACCH program began its adolescent and adult services we have been able to obtain increasing acceptance of autistic clients in existing workshops. However, sufficient numbers are still excluded so that we are considering the possibilities for establishing some sheltered workshops especially to cope with the problems of autistic clients.

Even when the most appropriate living arrangement or vocational placement is obtained, autistic individuals are still likely to encounter special periods of stress. At those times their survival in the community is threatened. We have established the beginning of an intensive survival treatment program to help individuals cope with these periods. Each of our regional centers will be able to identify an intervention team to provide such intensive help when the need arises. At this time we do not have the resources for full-time intensive intervention across the entire state; however, part-time staff can be mobilized at critical times.

SUMMARY

In this chapter we have discussed how our 15 years' experience with young autistic and communication-handicapped children has evolved into programs for autistic adolescents and adults. The concept of development which had been demonstrated as most useful for the younger population is also essential for defining autism in adolescents and adults. It is useful for identifying emerging skills and formulating an appropriate educational program, as in the example of sex education. In order to identify appropriate levels of skill training, developmental assessment procedures were developed. These are used to identify autistic adults (CARS) and their individual needs (PEP). The involvement of parents continues to play an important part in our work with adolescents and adults, although this includes recognition of increasing independence between aging parents and children. Training toward this end is provided by small, structured classrooms, which begin prevocational skill training in early adolescence. These classrooms prepare adolescents for the utilization of special services including both living arrangements and vocational placements in the adult years.

REFERENCES

Bettelheim, B. *The empty fortress: Infantile autism and the birth of self.* London: Collier-Macmillan, 1967.

Brown, L., Branston, M., Hamre-Nietupski, S., Pumpion, I., Certo, N., & Gruenewald, L. A strategy for developing chronological age appropriate, functional curriculum for severely handicapped adolescents and adults. *Journal of Special Education,* 1979, *13,* 81–90.

Creak, M. Schizophrenic syndrome in childhood: Progress report of a working party. *Developmental Medicine and Child Neurology,* 1964, *6,* 530.

Fenichel, C. Socializing the severely disturbed child. In *Psychopathology and child development.* (E. Schopler & R. J. Reichler, eds.), New York: Plenum Press, 1976.

Kanner, L. *Childhood psychosis: Initial studies and new insights.* Washington, D.C.: Winston, 1974.

Martin, E. Implementing the right to education. *Proceedings, National Society for Children and Adults with Autism,* 1980, 95–114.

Mesibov, G. B. Implications of the normalization principle for psychotic children. *Journal of Autism and Childhood Schizophrenia,* 1976, *6,* 360–377.

Reichler, R. J., & Schopler, E. Developmental therapy: A program model for providing individual services in the community. In *Psychopathology and childhood development.* (E. Schopler & R. J. Reichler, eds.), New York: Plenum Press, 1976.

Rutter, M., & Schopler, E. *Autism: A reappraisal of concepts and treatment.* New York: Plenum Press, 1978.

Schopler, E. Parents of psychotic children as scapegoats. *Journal of Contemporary Psychotherapy,* 1971, *4,* 17–22.

Schopler, E. Towards reducing behavior problems in autistic children. In *Early childhood autism,* 2nd ed. (L. Wing, ed.), New York: Pergamon Press, 1976.

Schopler, E., & Bristol, M. Autistic children in public schools. *ERIC Exceptional Child Education Report.* 1980 ERIC Clearinghouse, Reston, Va.

Schopler, E., & Olley, J. G. Comprehensive educational services for autistic children: The TEACCH model. In *Handbook for school psychology.* (C. Reynolds & T. Guthins, eds.), New York: Wiley, 1981.

Schopler, E., & Reichler, R. J. Parents as cotherapists in the treatment of psychotic children. *Journal of Autism and Childhood Schizophrenia,* 1971, *1,* 87–102.

Schopler, E., & Reichler, R. J. *Psychoeducational profile: Individualized assessment for autistic and developmentally disabled children* (Vol. 1). Baltimore: University Park Press, 1979.

Schopler, E., & Rutter, M. Diagnosis and definition of childhood autism. *Journal of Autism and Developmental Disorders,* 1978, *8,* 137–169.

Schopler, E., Reichler, R. J., & Lansing, M. D. *Teaching strategies for parents and professionals,* Vol. 2, *Individualized assessment and treatment for autistic and developmentally disabled children.* Baltimore: University Park Press, 1980.

Schopler, E., Rutter, M., & Chess, S. Editorial: Change of journal scope and title. *Journal of Autism and Developmental Disorders,* 1979, *9,* 1–10.

Schopler, E., Reichler, R. J., DeVellis, R. F., & Daly, K. Toward objective classification of childhood autism: Childhood Autism Rating Scale (CARS). *Journal of Autism and Developmental Disorders,* 1980, *10,* 91–103.

Schopler, E., Mesibov, G. B., DeVellis, R. F., & Short, A. Treatment outcome for autistic children and their families. In *Frontiers of knowledge in mental retardation.* (M. Rutter, ed.), Baltimore: University Park Press, 1981.

Schopler, E., Lansing, M. D., & Waters, C. *Teaching activities for autistic children,* Vol. 3, *Individualized assessment and treatment for autistic and developmentally disabled children.* Baltimore: University Park Press, in press.

Wing, L., & Gould, J. Systematic recording of behaviors and skills of retarded and psychotic children. *Journal of Autism and Developmental Disorders,* 1978, *8,* 79–97.

Wolfensberger, W. *The principle of normalization in human services.* Toronto: National Institute of Mental Retardation, 1972.

REFERENCE NOTES

1. Mesibov, G. B., & Shea, V. *Social and interpersonal problems of autistic adolescents and adults.* Paper presented at the meeting of the Southeastern Psychological Association, Washington, D.C., March 1980.

2. Boyd, S., Dossett, B., Marcus, L., Stager, J., & Woods, A. *Group home model for autistic citizens—Triad Group Home.* Bylaws of the Triad Group Home, Greensboro, N.C., 1979.

Index